Breastfeeding A–Z

Terminology and Telephone Triage

Second Edition

Karin Cadwell, PhD, RN, FAAN, ANLC, IBCLC

The Healthy Children Project
The Center for Breastfeeding
East Sandwich, MA

Cindy Turner-Maffei, MA, ALC, IBCLC

The Healthy Children Project
The Center for Breastfeeding
East Sandwich, MA

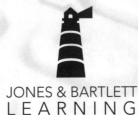

JONES & BARTLETT
LEARNING

World Headquarters
Jones & Bartlett Learning
5 Wall Street
Burlington, MA 01803
978-443-5000
info@jblearning.com
www.jblearning.com

Jones & Bartlett Learning books and products are available through most bookstores and online booksellers. To contact Jones & Bartlett Learning directly, call 800-832-0034, fax 978-443-8000, or visit our website, www.jblearning.com.

Substantial discounts on bulk quantities of Jones & Bartlett Learning publications are available to corporations, professional associations, and other qualified organizations. For details and specific discount information, contact the special sales department at Jones & Bartlett Learning via the above contact information or send an email to specialsales@jblearning.com.

Production Credits

Publisher: Kevin Sullivan
Acquisitions Editor: Amanda Harvey
Editorial Assistant: Rebecca Myrick
Production Editor: Cindie Bryan
Marketing Communications Manager: Katie Hennessy
V.P., Manufacturing and Inventory Control:
    Therese Connell
Composition: Paw Print Media
Cover Design: Kristin E. Parker
Cover Images:
    Top: © George Doyle/Stockbyte/Thinkstock;
    Bottom: © Hemera/Thinkstock
Printing and Binding: Edwards Brothers Malloy
Cover Printing: Edwards Brothers Malloy

Library of Congress Cataloging-in-Publication Data
Cadwell, Karin.
  Breastfeeding A-Z : terminology and telephone triage / Karin Cadwell, Cindy Turner-Maffei. -- 2nd ed.
    p. ; cm.
  Includes bibliographical references.
  ISBN 978-1-4496-8776-2 (pbk.) -- ISBN 1-4496-8776-8 (pbk.)
  I. Turner-Maffei, Cindy. II. Title.
  [DNLM: 1. Breast Feeding--Terminology--English. 2. Lactation--Terminology--English. WS 15]

  649'.33--dc23
                            2012025471

6048

Printed in the United States of America
17 16 15 14 13   10 9 8 7 6 5 4 3 2 1

Dedication

This book is dedicated to the volunteer and professional telephone helpers with whom we have worked over the past several decades, who have opened our eyes to the intricate skill of eliciting the mother's and baby's story.

Contents

Introduction

This book was developed to provide nurses, physicians, nutritionists, breastfeeding peer counselors, and lactation care providers with an evidence-based reference about common breastfeeding terms and issues that may present in telephone calls. The need for such a tool emerged as a result of our experiences answering calls on the Cape and Islands Breastfeeding Warmline, and counseling mothers in person at the Center for Breastfeeding, which serves Barnstable, Dukes, and Nantucket counties in Massachusetts, United States. In addition, this book is based on collected data related to our calls.[1] We have also spoken[2] and published[3,4] information about our experiences.

One of the questions we are often asked about our warmline is, "What is the difference between a helpline that is called a 'warmline' and one that is a 'hotline?'" For us, a warmline is a breastfeeding support telephone line answered in person during office hours, usually 5 days a week, with an opportunity for the caller to leave a voice mail message if the line is busy, after hours, and on weekends. The voice mail queries are answered the next business day. A hotline is answered in person 24 hours a day, 7 days a week.

Helping women with their breastfeeding concerns is a complex process. That complexity is amplified when the telephone answerer cannot see the mother or the baby, and the mother's description of the situation may be inadequate. The focus of the telephone interaction should be to decide the urgency and the best disposition of the case. In other words, the person answering the telephone must determine:

- Does the mother or baby need to be seen in person, or is this telephone interaction sufficient?
- If the mother or the baby needs to be seen in person, how urgently? Immediately? Later today? Tomorrow? Next week? Communities and health plans may have a variety of resources and options. The telephone answerer should be familiar with available community services. "Seek emergency care now" could mean a call to emergency services in one community or urgent care in another. "Seek medical care within 4 hours" means call the medical care provider now or, if the caller or baby does not have a provider, go to urgent care or an emergency care setting quickly. Agencies should give phone answerers explicit instructions regarding services in the communities they

serve. The form located in Appendix B provides a model for indicating which action triage workers should take.

- What is the best disposition of the case? Who should be the next person to see or talk to the mother?

This book will help breastfeeding support workers to triage problems and to appropriately answer breastfeeding questions on the telephone. Key words direct further questions and provide the support person with the information needed to clarify the situation and decide the appropriate urgency and disposition of the case.

Problems may be addressed under several headings to facilitate quick reference. For example, pain in the breast is addressed under "Breast pain" and "Painful breastfeeding."

Telephone evaluation requires asking simple questions in plain language. Therefore, this book contains simple keywords such as "breast pain" as well as medical terms such as "galactocele." The mother's tone of voice, sense of urgency, and concern, as well as the history of the mother and the baby must be considered. Referring to the mother or baby's chart or records is ideal, but not always possible.

It is important to always keep in mind the limitations of telephone support interactions. The telephone interaction cannot take the place of in-person assessment, evaluation, or teaching. However, for many mothers, especially those who are breastfeeding for the first time, the telephone can offer an opportunity to check out whether what they are experiencing is common, normal, or abnormal, and to ask questions as they arise.

Mothers may call the helpline when they have a specific question or problem. In some cases, the mother articulates her situation clearly, such as in the following examples:

"I called because my neighbor told me my 6-week-old baby is ready for solid foods."

"I think I have the flu. Can I still breastfeed?"

"I'm going back to work. Where can I get a breast pump?"

"I think that my baby has diarrhea. Did he get it from my milk?"

Other mothers' calls are less clear about their issues and require open-ended questions so that the telephone answerer can work with her to clarify her concerns. For example, the mother may say, "My baby isn't feeding right." We can never assume that our ideas of "feeding right" are the same as the mother's. We must work to try to gain a better understanding of what the mother means.

Breastfeeding supporters also need to be aware that mothers may construct a "door-opener" question or complaint that overlies a real concern that they are afraid is unworthy of attention. The mother may not have articulated her real concern to a point at which it can be easily communicated. For example, the mother may be worried about the quality of her milk but ask for help with her inverted nipple. Upon further discussion, the telephone answerer learns from the mother's own description that her nipples are indeed nicely everted. In this case, the mother does not need false reassurance, but a thoughtful exploration of other concerns or questions she may have.

Not all questions that come to a breastfeeding support telephone line are about breastfeeding. For example, a mother may be the victim of domestic abuse. She may want to know about government programs or housing. She may call the breastfeeding support line because it is a number she has handy or she has called before. How will these calls be handled? At our call center, we keep information about accessing community resources and refer mothers to specified nonbreastfeeding resources. Your agency will need to make its own policy regarding appropriate referrals.

This book constitutes a revision of our first attempt to provide a quick reference and triage tool. We welcome you to give us feedback and input to enrich future editions of this book. Please send us your suggestions, so that together we may build a rich reference for telephone helpers.

Karin Cadwell and Cindy Turner-Maffei
info@centerforbreastfeeding.org

References

[1] Philipp, B. (2001). Every call is an opportunity: Supporting breastfeeding mothers over the telephone. *Pediatric Clinics of North America, 48*(2), 525–532.

[2] Cadwell, K., & Turner-Maffei, C. (2002, July). *From concept to reality: Building a breastfeeding warmline.* Poster, Healthy Mothers Healthy Babies Coalition Biennial Conference, Tampa, FL.

Turner-Maffei, C., & Cadwell, K. (1999, April). *From reality to evaluation: Documenting and improving the work of a breastfeeding warmline.* Breastfeeding: The Odds-on Best; the 1999 National Conference on the Theory and Practice of Human Lactation and Breastfeeding Management, Las Vegas, NV.

Philipp, B., & Cadwell, K. (1998, November). *Calls to a breastfeeding warmline: Using the data to shape teaching curriculum.* Academy of Breastfeeding Medicine Third Annual Meeting; Kansas City, MO.

[3] Philipp, B. L., & Cadwell, K. (1999). Fielding questions about breastfeeding. *Contemporary Pediatrics, 16*(4).

[4] Cadwell, K., & Turner-Maffei, C. (2004). *Case studies in breastfeeding: Problem-solving skills & strategies.* Sudbury, MA: Jones and Bartlett.

How to Use This Book

This book is meant to be a quick reference for anyone who uses the phone to help support breastfeeding women. The following key features have been used throughout the text to draw attention to information that will be important to consider while on the phone. Please remember to watch for these items while you are using the book.

Terms

Common breastfeeding problems, concerns, and events are listed alphabetically. Note that many items (e.g., breast pain and painful breastfeeding) repeat for ease of quick reference during telephone calls. Remember that callers may report more than one concern.

DEFINITION/DESCRIPTION

If the caller gives a technical or medical name to her problem (e.g., engorgement), review the definition or description to ensure that the caller and the telephone helper agree on the nature of the problem and are using the appropriate definitions to describe the problem.

ASK ABOUT

Ask descriptive, simple questions in lay language about the items in this section to explore the severity of the mother's concern and possible contributing or complicating factors.

ASSESSMENT

This section presents questions designed to help the telephone answerer triage the need for referral to emergency, prompt, or routine care. Use the questions to determine the appropriate disposition of the case at hand.

SELF-CARE INFORMATION

Self-care information may be suggested for use until the mother receives a medical or lactation evaluation.

IMPORTANT CONDITIONS TO REPORT

Encourage the client to report any symptoms of concern, including those listed under this section.

NOTES

This section may contain information about the relevance of certain symptoms, as well as contact information for various support agencies and organizations.

See also is a section that suggests other related topics that may be appropriate to review with the caller.

General Recommendations for Telephone Triage

- Maintain a welcoming tone on the telephone. Many callers will be concerned about having silly questions or wasting your time. Tell callers that all questions are welcome and important.

- Make sure that you write down the caller's name and telephone number before beginning to discuss the presenting concern. This will allow you to call back if further information or discussion is needed, or if you lose connection with the caller.

- When possible, pull the caller's records or chart during the call. This may help provide important history or details to the case (e.g., this mother has already experienced mastitis, or this baby was born prematurely).

- Ask open-ended questions whenever possible. Callers will provide more information when asked questions that cannot be answered with a "Yes" or "No."

- Encourage callers to talk about the history of the problem or concern, when it was first noticed, and what they think caused the problem.

- If you do not know the answer to a question the caller asks, say so, and tell the caller you will find out the answer and call back. Do not forget to follow through on this promise.

- At the end of the call, review the triage plan. Make sure the caller has your name and telephone number in case she requires further assistance.

- Remember that callers may have more than one concern. Before ending the call, ask the caller what other concerns or problems she has.

- Document the call while you are speaking to the caller or immediately after the call. Develop a form that works for your needs and the needs of your program (see Appendix A of this book for a sample intake form).

About the Authors

Karin Cadwell, PhD, RN, FAAN, ANLC, IBCLC, is a nationally and internationally recognized speaker, researcher, and educator. She convened Baby-Friendly USA, implementing the WHO/UNICEF Baby-Friendly Hospital Initiative in the United States, is a delegate to the U.S. Breastfeeding Committee, was visiting professor and chair of the Health Communications master's degree program at Emerson College, and is a professor at the Union Institute and University. Dr. Cadwell served on the International Board of Lactation Consultant Examiners (IBLCE) panel of experts to develop the first lactation consultant certification exam. Her extensive clinical experience includes hospital and community practice, and she continues to counsel nursing mothers on Cape Cod in Massachusetts. Dr. Cadwell is the author of numerous publications, including *Maternal and Infant Assessment for Breastfeeding and Human Lactation: A Guide for the Practitioner, Case Studies in Breastfeeding, Pocket Guide for Lactation Management, Continuity of Care in Breastfeeding,* and *Reclaiming Breastfeeding for the U.S.: Protection, Promotion, and Support.* She was awarded the designation International Board Certified Lactation Consultant (IBCLC) in 1985 for significant contribution to the field and has since been recertified.

Cindy Turner-Maffei, MA, ALC, IBCLC, is a faculty member of the Healthy Children Project, Inc. She served as the national coordinator of Baby-Friendly USA, Inc., implementing the WHO/UNICEF Baby-Friendly Hospital Initiative in the United States, for 14 years. Ms. Turner-Maffei has extensive experience as a breastfeeding educator in the Special Supplemental Nutrition Program for Women, Infants, and Children (WIC) and other maternal child health programs and continues to counsel nursing mothers on Cape Cod in Massachusetts. A delegate to breastfeeding coalitions on the local, state, and national level, including the U.S. Breastfeeding Committee, she is also an affiliated faculty member of the Union Institute and University. She has coauthored numerous books with Dr. Cadwell, including those listed previously as well as *Ten Steps to Successful Breastfeeding: A 20-Hour Interdisciplinary Breastfeeding Management Course for the United States.*

Acknowledgments

We are eternally grateful to Kimberly G. Lee, MD, MS, IBCLC, who was Assistant Professor of Pediatrics, Harvard Medical School, and Assistant Director, Newborn Nursery, Beth Israel Deaconess Medical Center, Boston, Massachusetts, when she thoughtfully and insightfully reviewed the first edition of this book.

We thank our beloved colleagues, Sheri Garner, RN, BS, ANLC, IBCLC, for her careful review of the second edition of this book, Asia Roberge, CLC, for her grace and patience with the revision process, and Christine Rathbun Ernst for her meticulous and insightful edits.

We also gratefully acknowledge the support of our colleagues at the Center for Breastfeeding and our wonderful families.

The information contained in this book is intended for use in understanding and triaging clients' concerns in order to direct them to the most appropriate route of care. Information obtained from this publication is not intended as a substitute for professional care. If you have or suspect that you have a medical problem, please consult your healthcare provider immediately. Health care is an ever-changing science; as new research and clinical experience broaden our knowledge, changes in treatment are required.

The authors have checked with sources believed to be reliable in their efforts to provide information that is complete and generally in accord with the standards accepted at the time of publication.

➤ AA (ALSO KNOWN AS ARA)

See Arachidonic acid (AA, also ARA)

➤ AABC

See American Association of Birth Centers (AABC)

➤ AAFP

See American Academy of Family Physicians (AAFP)

➤ AAN

See American Academy of Nursing (AAN)

➤ AAP

See American Academy of Pediatrics (AAP)

➤ ABI

See American Breastfeeding Institute (ABI)

➤ ABM

See Academy of Breastfeeding Medicine (ABM)

➤ ABRUPT WEANING

DEFINITION   Sudden cessation of breastfeeding. May be initiated by either the mother or the baby.

ASK ABOUT

Onset.
Age of the baby.
Reason for abrupt weaning.
Whether initiated by the mother or the baby.

ASSESSMENT

EMERGENT CARE NEEDED?

Are any of the following present?

Extreme lethargy in the baby.
Extreme irritability in the baby.
Sudden change in the baby's muscle tone (extremely floppy or stiff).
Sudden disinterest in feeding.
Inability to wake the baby.
Inability to calm the baby, even with cuddles.

IF YES,   *Seek emergency care now.*

PROMPT MEDICAL CARE NEEDED?

Are any of the following present?

For mothers or for babies older than 3 months, fever higher than 101°F
   (38.5°C). In a baby under 3 months, fever higher than 100.4°F (38°C).
In mother, extreme breast discomfort or redness.
In mother, flu-like aching throughout body.

IF YES,   *Seek medical care within 4 hours.*

Are any of the following present?

Unexplained **breast refusal** by the baby.
Lack of appetite in baby lasting one day or more.

IF YES,   *Call pediatric care provider today.*

PROMPT LACTATION CARE NEEDED?

Are any of the following present?

Breast discomfort.

Difficulty relieving pressure in the breast.

Concern about effects of weaning on baby.

Sadness about weaning.

Nursing strike.

Mother has taken a drug which negatively affects milk supply

(e.g., pseudoephedrine).

IF YES, *Call lactation care provider today.*

ROUTINE CARE NEEDED?

Are any of the following present?

Mild breast swelling.

Mild breast discomfort.

Ongoing adjustment difficulty.

Give self-care information.

IF YES, *Report to lactation care provider if no improvement in 2 days.*

SELF-CARE INFORMATION

Consider supportive bra.

Nonprescription pain relief.

Expect some emotional response to abrupt weaning.

Talk out your feelings with a trusted friend, family member, or counselor.

The baby requires an appropriate substitute for breastfeeding (expressed breastmilk
or formula if younger than 12 months, other foods if older than 12 months).

Ensure that the baby receives emotional and physical comfort during adjustment
to weaning.

IMPORTANT CONDITIONS TO REPORT

Fever.

Signs of infection.

Ongoing discomfort.

Unresolved symptoms after 48 hours.

Weaning is best accomplished in a gradual manner. Slow weaning allows time for mother and baby to adjust physically and emotionally to this change. Rarely, **abrupt weaning** may be necessary for mothers to take one of the rare **contraindicated medications**, or experience separation from their babies for an extended period (e.g., women in the military who are deployed overseas).

Babies may abruptly refuse feeding. In this case, it is important to distinguish medical from developmental reasons for the infant's disinterest in breastfeeding. Rarely, babies can experience life-threatening infections or events that cause extreme lethargy and disinterest in feeding. They may be suddenly floppy or stiff. These symptoms indicate a medical emergency, as they may reflect botulism, meningitis, or other life-threatening infection.

More commonly, babies may refuse to nurse for developmental or other reasons. For babies 4–6 months old, this may be due to distractibility. Refusal to nurse is often considered a **nursing strike**, rather than weaning. Typically it is an indication that something is troubling the baby. Troubles can range from teething and ear infection to a negative reaction to mother–baby separation or family stress. When nursing strike persists, the baby should be examined to rule out ear infection or other contributing factors.

Strategies for overcoming nursing strike include not forcing nursing, offering lots of contact and holding, having the mom lie down beside a sleepy baby and offering the breast, having the mom and baby take a bath together, and applying peer pressure by bringing a baby in contact with other nursing babies.

The mother may need assistance with expressing milk to continue her milk supply during this phase. She may wish to discuss her reaction to the baby's refusal to feed.

While weaning abruptly, women usually need to remove some milk to relieve the pressure in their breasts. Women who are weaning permanently should remove as little milk as possible, as milk removal continues milk synthesis. Other women may be weaning temporarily due to short-term separation from the baby, or short-term use of a contraindicated medication. In this situation, mothers should be encouraged to hand express or pump milk as many times daily as their baby would nurse.

See also Nursing strike; Relactation; Weaning

➤ ABSCESS, BREAST

DEFINITION   A localized collection of pus resulting from the breakdown of breast tissue. Inflammation often occurs around the abscess. Breast abscess is often the outcome of unresolved breast infection or inflammation (mastitis).

Abscess may or may not be visible on the surface of the breast.

Abscesses are typically drained through aspiration or by surgical incision and drainage. Antibiotic treatment will be prescribed based on suspected or confirmed pathogen.

ASK ABOUT

Onset.
Prior breast infection.
Known drug allergies.

ASSESSMENT

EMERGENT CARE NEEDED?

Are any of the following present?

Visible or palpable breast abscess.

Maternal fever higher than 100°F (37.7°C).

Extreme breast discomfort.

Flu-like aching throughout body.

Chills.

Continuing fever after abscess drainage.

Reaction to antibiotic prescribed postdrainage.

Green or odorous change to fluid seeping from site after drainage.

IF YES, *Seek medical care within 4 hours.*

PROMPT CARE NEEDED?

Are any of the following present?

Continuation of pain, swelling, or redness after drainage.

Difficulty with breastfeeding following abscess drainage.

IF YES, *Seek medical care within 24 hours and call lactation care provider today.*

ROUTINE CARE NEEDED?

Are any of the following present?

Questions about resumption of breastfeeding on affected breast.

IF YES, *Call obstetric or surgical care provider today.*

SELF-CARE INFORMATION

Finish full course of antibiotics prescribed (unless told to stop by a physician).

Continue nonprescription pain relief as recommended.

Continue to monitor breasts for symptoms of recurring breast infection (redness, heat, fever, blockage, pain).

IMPORTANT CONDITIONS TO REPORT

Symptoms worsen or persist.

Signs of infection.

NOTES

Abscess indicates a need for urgent medical treatment. Symptoms include reddened areas of the breast, occasionally with a visible fluid-filled sac protruding through the surface of the breast, and overall body sensation of **malaise**, aching, fever, or fatigue. Abscess may follow **mastitis**. Typical treatment includes appropriate antibiotic administration and drainage by lancing or aspiration. Presence of one identified abscess may indicate presence of multiple other abscesses, some of which may be deep in the breast, visible only by imaging technology. When symptoms do not resolve after treatment, presence of additional abscesses must be considered.

Breastfeeding is not contraindicated on the noninvolved breast. Breastfeeding may continue on the affected breast if determined safe. Drainage may cause leaking of milk from severed ducts. Women may feel very ill and need practical and emotional support.

See also Acute infection; Breast infection

➤ **ABUSE**

DEFINITION   Improper treatment, misuse, or physical, emotional, or sexual maltreatment.

ASK ABOUT

Location.

Physical safety at this moment.

ASSESSMENT

EMERGENT CARE NEEDED?

Are any of the following present?

Physical safety of baby and caller in danger at this moment.

IF YES,   *Seek emergency protection now.*

PROMPT CARE NEEDED?

Are any of the following present?

The caller or the baby is endangered, but not at the current moment.

IF YES,   *Contact social services immediately.*

SELF-CARE INFORMATION

Contact local abuse resources.

Know local emergency assistance numbers.

Know the location of area police stations.

Physical and emotional abuse are disturbingly common. When individuals reach out for help with abuse, appropriate response is crucial.

Follow your office protocol for abuse referrals. Protocols should be based on existing state or territorial laws and resources. Know the rules regarding mandated reporting. Have the emergency social service numbers on hand for easy reference.

Careful response to the abuser is critical; otherwise the caller and her family may be further endangered. Refer abusive situations to the appropriate authorities.

➤ ACADEMY OF BREASTFEEDING MEDICINE (ABM)

DESCRIPTION   "The Academy of Breastfeeding Medicine is a worldwide organization of physicians dedicated to the promotion, protection and support of breastfeeding and human lactation. Its mission is to unite into one association members of the various medical specialties with this common purpose."[1(p1)]

The Academy of Breastfeeding Medicine
Email: ABM@bfmed.org
Web: www.bfmed.org
   ABM publishes clinical protocols on its website and in its journal, *Breastfeeding Medicine*.

Footnote

[1]The Academy of Breastfeeding Medicine. (2008). *About ABM*. Retrieved from http://www.bfmed.org/About/Default.aspx.

➤ ACADEMY OF LACTATION POLICY & PRACTICE (ALPP)

DESCRIPTION   "The Academy of Lactation Policy and Practice, Inc. is a non-profit organization that provides a national credentialing program in Breastfeeding and Human Lactation for nurses, physicians, dietitians, WIC personnel, peer counselors, independent lactation counselors, and others.

   Founded in 1999, ALPP is dedicated to improving the foundation of breast-feeding comprehension and understanding throughout the United States by providing certificates of added qualification in breastfeeding. The ALPP credentialed programs, including the CLC, ANLC, and ALC, are approved by the following: The American Nurses Credentialing Center (ANCC), the Commission on Dietetic Registration, the International Board of Lactation Consultant Examiners (IBLCE), The American College of Nurse Midwives, the Accreditation and Approval Review Committee (AARC) on Education in Human Lactation and Breastfeeding, and Lamaze International. The CLC, ANLC, and ALC are all accredited as nursing skills competency programs through the ANCC."[2(p1)]

The Academy of Lactation Policy and Practice
Email: info@talpp.org
Web: www.talpp.org

Footnote

[2]The Academy of Lactation Policy & Practice. (2011). *What Is ALPP?* Retrieved from http://talpp
.org/about-us.html

➤ ACADEMY OF NUTRITION AND DIETETICS (FORMERLY THE AMERICAN DIETETIC ASSOCIATION)

DESCRIPTION   "The Academy of Nutrition and Dietetics is the world's largest organization of food and nutrition professionals. The Academy is committed to improving the nation's health and advancing the profession of dietetics through research, education, and advocacy."[3(p1)]

Academy of Nutrition and Dietetics
Email: findnrd@eatright.org
Web: www.eatright.org
   The Academy of Nutrition and Dietetics publishes articles and policy statements about breastfeeding on its website and in its printed publications.

Footnote

[3]Academy of Nutrition and Dietetics. (2012). *About the Academy of Nutrition and Dietetics.* Retrieved from http://www.eatright.org/Media/content.aspx?id=6442467510

➤ ACCESSORY BREAST TISSUE

DEFINITION Extra breast and nipple tissue. Women may have extra accessory breast or nipple tissue anywhere on the ventral surface of their trunk, as well as in the axillary, groin, and upper thigh areas.

NOTES

Presence of accessory tissue does not contraindicate breastfeeding, though a small amount of milk may be produced. Refer questions and problems to the lactation care provider.

➤ ACNM

See American College of Nurse-Midwives (ACNM)

➤ ACOG

See American Congress of Obstetricians and Gynecologists (ACOG)

➤ ACOP

See American College of Osteopathic Pediatricians (ACOP)

➤ ACQUIRED IMMUNODEFICIENCY SYNDROME (AIDS)

DEFINITION A life-threatening disease of the immune system caused by the human immunodeficiency virus (HIV). People with AIDS have increased susceptibility to infections and rare cancers including Kaposi sarcoma. HIV is transmitted primarily by exposure to contaminated body fluids, especially blood and semen, and potentially by breastmilk.

ASK ABOUT

Onset of illness.
Age of the baby.

ASSESSMENT

EMERGENT CARE NEEDED?

Are any of the following present?

Breastfeeding mother with concern about possibility of recently contracting HIV.

Breastfeeding mother diagnosed with HIV.

IF YES,   *Seek medical care within 4 hours.*

PROMPT CARE NEEDED?

Are any of the following present?

Pregnant mother with concerns about possibility of recently contracting HIV.

Pregnant mother diagnosed with HIV.

IF YES,   *Call obstetric care provider today.*

ROUTINE CARE NEEDED?

Are any of the following present?

General questions about HIV.

IF YES,   *Call pediatric or obstetric care provider today.*

SELF-CARE INFORMATION

Know your HIV status.
Know your treatment options.
Know the HIV status of all sexual partners.
Practice safe sex.
Avoid intravenous drug use.

IMPORTANT CONDITIONS TO REPORT

Need for testing.

NOTES

In the United States, breastfeeding is contraindicated in women diagnosed as HIV positive or with AIDS. Women at high risk for **HIV** (e.g., women who are sex workers, women with an HIV-positive sexual partner, women using intravenous drugs, women whose sexual partners use intravenous drugs, and women who are raped or coerced to have sex) should receive testing and ongoing counseling regarding infant feeding.

See also Contraindicated conditions

➤ ACROCYANOSIS

DEFINITION   Blue color of the hands and feet. This condition is caused by constriction of the tiny arterioles (small arteries) and results in mottled blue or red discoloration of the wrists, hands, ankles, and toes.

➤ ACUTE INFECTION

DEFINITION   Invasion and reproduction of microorganisms in the cells or tissues of the body. Infectious microorganisms include bacteria, viruses, fungi, and others. Symptoms of infection may include fever and malaise. Lack of desire to feed can be an additional symptom of infection in the baby.

ASK ABOUT

Onset.
Age of the baby.
Medications taken.
Known drug allergies.

ASSESSMENT

EMERGENT CARE NEEDED?

Are any of the following present?

Extreme **lethargy** or **irritability** in baby.

Sudden change in baby's muscle tone (extremely floppy or stiff) or repetitive jerking movements (e.g., seizure activity).

Baby shows sudden disinterest in feeding.

Inability to wake baby.

IF YES,   *Call pediatrician now.*

PROMPT CARE NEEDED?

Are any of the following present?

About the mother:

Fever higher than 100°F (37.7°C).

Extreme breast discomfort.

Flu-like aching throughout body.

Extreme exhaustion.

Visible or palpable breast **abscess**.

About the baby:

Extreme discomfort.

Any fever in a baby younger than 3–4 months of age.

Fever higher than 100°F (37.7°C) in an older baby or child.

Vomiting and diarrhea that last for more than a few hours in a child of any age.

Rash, especially if there is also a fever.

Any cough or cold that does not improve within several days, or a cold that worsens and includes a fever.

Drainage from an ear.

Problems swallowing.

Sharp or persistent pains as described by older baby in the throat, ear, abdomen, or stomach.

Fever and vomiting at the same time.

Not eating for more than a day.

IF YES,   *Seek medical care within 4 hours.*

SELF-CARE INFORMATION

Feed the baby at least 10 times per 24 hours.

Soften breasts between feedings with gentle hand expression.

Finish full course of antibiotics prescribed (unless told to stop by a prescriber).

Continue nonprescription pain relief as recommended.

Continue to monitor for symptoms of recurring breast infection (redness, heat, fever, chills, pain).

IMPORTANT CONDITIONS TO REPORT

Symptoms worsen or persist.

Signs of infection.

NOTES

Rarely, babies experience life-threatening infections or events that cause extreme lethargy and disinterest in feeding. They may be suddenly floppy or stiff. These symptoms indicate a medical emergency, as they may reflect botulism, meningitis, or other life-threatening infection.

Many mothers experiencing **mastitis** may mistake symptoms of mastitis for flu. When a mother calls to ask for recommendations of safe flu medications, remember to ask her if she has any red, painful, hot spots on her breasts. See **Mastitis** and **Flu, maternal** for more information.

Few infections are incompatible with breastfeeding. Infections in the breastfeeding mother that are not compatible with breastfeeding include **HIV**; **HTLV-1**; brucellosis; active, untreated tuberculosis; and active **herpes** simplex lesion on the nipple or other area that will be in contact with the baby's mouth.[4]

Mothers with certain infections may breastfeed once a period of treatment is initiated. These infections include tuberculosis, hepatitis, and Lyme disease. The Centers for Disease Control & Prevention and health departments can provide further information.

See also Breast infection; Flu, maternal; Mastitis

Footnote

[4]AAP Section on Breastfeeding. (2012). Breastfeeding and the use of human milk. *Pediatrics*, *129*(3), e827–e841. doi:10.1542/peds.2011-3552

➤ ADOLESCENT BREASTFEEDING

DEFINITION   Adolescent mothers (ages 13–19) should be encouraged to breastfeed. Like all mothers, teens also need breastfeeding support.

ASK ABOUT

Age of the baby.

ASSESSMENT

PROMPT CARE NEEDED?

Are any of the following present?

Difficulty with breastfeeding.

Breast or nipple discomfort or trauma.

Misshapen nipple after feedings.

Visible fissures on nipples.

Concern about adequate milk production.

IF YES,   *Call lactation care provider today.*

ROUTINE CARE NEEDED?

Are any of the following present?

Mother has questions or concerns about breastfeeding.

IF YES,   *Call lactation care provider today.*

SELF-CARE INFORMATION

Practice skin-to-skin contact in the first hour after birth and frequently thereafter.

Feed the baby at the first sign of hunger cues (signs that say "feed me" include hand-to-face or hand-to-mouth movements, lip smacking, seeking with lips, rooting, and head bobbing).

Feed the baby at least 10 times per 24 hours.

Listen for signs of the baby swallowing.

Allow the baby to end feedings.

Expect at least three infant stools per 24 hours after the first 4 days of life.

Good positioning and attachment are crucial to prevent or reduce nipple pain.

If the baby is fed away from the breast, hand express or pump milk to maintain supply.

Eat well to preserve your energy.

IMPORTANT CONDITIONS TO REPORT

Discomfort with nursing.

Feeding or stooling expectations are not met.

NOTES

There is no reason to suspect that adolescent women will have difficulty making milk.

The Dietary Reference Intake for breastfeeding teens call for an additional 500 calories over the amount required to maintain prepregnant weight.[5] About 1,300 mg of **calcium** is recommended for pregnant and lactating teens younger than 18 in order to protect bone density.[6] Research indicates that breastfeeding is not detrimental to bone density in adolescent mothers, and it may be protective.[7] Eating more healthful foods is important to maintain mothers' energy levels and nutrient stores. Eating more or less healthfully will not change milk composition or affect infant growth.

See also Teenaged mothers

Footnotes

[5]Otten, J. J., Hellwig, J. P., Meyers, L. D., & National Academies Press (U.S.). (2006). *DRI, dietary reference intakes the essential guide to nutrient requirements.* Washington, DC: National Academies Press. Available at http://www.nap.edu/catalog.php?record_id=11537

[6]Institute of Medicine. (2010). *Dietary reference intakes for calcium and vitamin D.* Retrieved from http://www.iom.edu/~/media/Files/Report%20Files/2010/Dietary-Reference-Intakes-for-Calcium-and-Vitamin-D/Vitamin%20D%20and%20Calcium%202010%20Report%20Brief.pdf

[7]Chantry, C. J., Auinger, P., & Byrd, R. S. (2004). Lactation among adolescent mothers and subsequent bone mineral density. *Archives of Pediatric & Adolescent Medicine, 158*(7), 650–656.

➤ ADOPTION AND INDUCED LACTATION

DEFINITION Induced lactation is the process of establishing a milk supply in a woman who has not given birth.

ASK ABOUT

Age of the baby.

ASSESSMENT

ROUTINE CARE NEEDED?

Are any of the following present?

Mother wishes to induce lactation for an adopted infant.

IF YES,   *Call lactation care provider.*

SELF-CARE INFORMATION

Frequent stimulation may enable milk production.

Practice skin-to-skin contact in the first hour and frequently thereafter.

Feed the baby at the first sign of hunger cues. (Signs that say "feed me" include hand-to-face or hand-to-mouth mouth movements, lip smacking, seeking with lips, rooting, and head bobbing.)

Work with pediatric care provider to determine need for supplementation of the adopted baby.

Listen for signs of the baby swallowing.

Allow the baby to end feedings.

Expect at least three infant stools per 24 hours after the first 4 days of life.

Good positioning and attachment are crucial to prevent or reduce nipple pain.

If the baby is not yet with the mother or is fed away from the breast, hand express or pump milk to maintain supply.

IMPORTANT CONDITIONS TO REPORT

Arrival of baby.

First visible milk produced.

Lack of milk production after weeks of attempt.

NOTES

Feeding adopted babies at the breast can be a wonderful bonding experience for mothers and babies. Adoptive mothers can produce milk with frequent breast stimulation (from a baby, hand expression, or a pump). It may take weeks of stimulation for a partial supply to develop. There is a wide range of volume of milk produced. Women need much practical guidance and support during this time and should consult with a lactation care provider early and often while awaiting the arrival of their adopted child.

Adopted babies may take right to the breast or may take longer to learn to feed. Devices may be used to deliver supplements to the baby at the breast in the event that mother does not have a full milk supply.

See also At-breast supplementation; Increasing milk supply; Induced lactation; Relactation

➤ ADVANCED LACTATION CONSULTANT (ALC)

DEFINITION   A lactation credential awarded by the Academy of Lactation Policy & Practice and the American Nurses Credentialing Center.

See also Academy of Lactation Policy & Practice; American Nurses Credentialing Center

➤ ADVANCED NURSE LACTATION CONSULTANT (ANLC)

DEFINITION   A lactation credential awarded by the Academy of Lactation Policy & Practice and the American Nurses Credentialing Center.

See also Academy of Lactation Policy & Practice; American Nurses Credentialing Center

➤ AGA

DEFINITION   Appropriate for gestational age. Babies who are classified appropriate for gestational age are of weight, length, and development considered appropriate for their gestational age at birth.

➤ AHRQ

See DHHS/Agency for Healthcare Research and Quality (AHRQ)

➤ AIDS

DEFINITION   Acquired immunodeficiency syndrome. A life-threatening disease of the immune system caused by the human immunodeficiency virus (HIV). People with AIDS have increased susceptibility to infections and rare cancers including Kaposi sarcoma. HIV is transmitted primarily by exposure to contaminated body fluids, especially blood and semen and potentially breastmilk.

ASK ABOUT

Onset of illness.
Age of the baby.

ASSESSMENT

EMERGENT CARE NEEDED?
Are any of the following present?
Breastfeeding mother with concern about possibility of recently contracting HIV.
Breastfeeding mother diagnosed with HIV.

IF YES,   *Seek medical care now.*

PROMPT CARE NEEDED?

Are any of the following present?

Pregnant mother with concerns about possibility of recently contracting HIV.

Pregnant mother diagnosed with HIV.

IF YES, *Call obstetric care provider today.*

ROUTINE CARE NEEDED?

Are any of the following present?

General questions about HIV.

IF YES, *Call pediatric or obstetric care provider today.*

SELF-CARE INFORMATION

Know your HIV status.

Know your treatment options.

Know the HIV status of all sexual partners.

Practice safe sex.

Avoid dirty needles with intravenous drug use.

IMPORTANT CONDITIONS TO REPORT

Need for testing.

NOTES

In the United States, breastfeeding is contraindicated in women diagnosed as HIV positive or with AIDS. Women at high risk for **HIV** (e.g., women who are sex workers, women with an HIV-positive sexual partner, women using intravenous drugs, women whose sexual partners use intravenous drugs, and women who are raped or coerced to have sex) should receive testing and ongoing counseling regarding infant feeding.

See also Contraindicated conditions

➤ ALC

See Advanced Lactation Consultant

➤ ALCOHOL

DEFINITION   An intoxicating chemical component of fermented and distilled beverages.

ASK ABOUT

Age of the baby.
Status of alcohol consumption.

ASSESSMENT

EMERGENT CARE NEEDED?

Are any of the following present?

Symptoms of alcohol poisoning (confusion, vomiting, seizures, slow or irregular breathing, pale or blue-tinged skin, unconsciousness).

Symptoms of alcohol withdrawal (delirium tremens [confusion and hallucinations], fever, agitation, convulsions, blacking out).

IF YES,   *Seek emergency care now.*

PROMPT CARE NEEDED?

Are any of the following present?

Admission of chronic dependence on alcohol.

IF YES,   *Seek medical care within 4 hours.*

ROUTINE CARE NEEDED?

Are any of the following present?

Occasional social use of alcohol.

Plans to use alcohol occasionally.

IF YES,   *Call lactation care provider today.*

SELF-CARE INFORMATION

Avoid or limit alcohol consumption.

Avoid consuming alcohol with an empty stomach.

It takes about 2 hours for the body to metabolize the alcohol in one drink.

Alcohol is not trapped in breastmilk. When you have had an occasional drink of alcohol and you no longer feel the effects of alcohol, it is safe to breastfeed.

Do not give alcohol to a baby or child.

IMPORTANT CONDITIONS TO REPORT

Sleepiness in baby.

Difficulty waking baby.

NOTES

Alcohol passes quickly and easily into the mother's bloodstream and into her milk. As alcohol levels fall in her blood, alcohol is reabsorbed from her milk and metabolized by her body. Alcohol from a single drink (one drink is considered to be one 12-oz beer, one 4- to 5-oz glass of wine, or one shot of 80-proof alcohol) may be removed from her milk in approximately 2 hours. Mothers are best encouraged to avoid alcohol during the breastfeeding period. Citing the Institute of Medicine, the American Academy of Pediatrics Section on Breastfeeding (2012) states:

> ingestion of alcoholic beverages should be minimized and limited to an occasional intake but no more than 0.5 g alcohol per kg body weight, which for a 60 kg mother is approximately 2 oz liquor, 8 oz wine, or 2 beers.[8(p.e833)]

Other lines of inquiry and counseling surround the safety of the baby during the time mother is drinking. Who will care for the baby? Mother and other caregivers should be advised not to sleep in the same bed as the baby when caregivers are under the influence of alcohol and other medications that may alter awareness and sleep states.

Footnote

[8]AAP Section on Breastfeeding. (2012). Breastfeeding and the use of human milk. *Pediatrics*, *129*(3), e827–e841. doi:10.1542/peds.2011-3552

➤ ALLERGEN

DEFINITION   A protein perceived as foreign by the body, thus triggering an allergic response.

See also Allergy in the breastfed infant

➤ ALLERGY IN THE BREASTFED INFANT

DEFINITION   An abnormal immune reaction to substances consumed, breathed, touched, or injected in a baby consuming human milk.

ASK ABOUT

Onset.
Age of the baby.
Known allergies.

ASSESSMENT

EMERGENT CARE NEEDED?

Are any of the following present?

Difficulty breathing.
Difficulty swallowing.
Swelling of tongue.

IF YES,   *Seek emergency care now.*

PROMPT CARE NEEDED?

Are any of the following present?

Swelling of the face, hands, or feet.
Persistent rash, headache, or fever.
Persistent diarrhea, nausea, or vomiting.
Bloody stool.

IF YES,   *Seek medical care within 4 hours.*

ROUTINE CARE NEEDED?

Are any of the following present?

Suspected reaction to food or medication.

Occasional nausea, vomiting, or diarrhea.

Persistent runny nose.

Wheezing.

Mild rash.

Mild itching.

IF YES,   *Seek medical care today.*

SELF-CARE INFORMATION

Monitor symptoms.

Possibility of developing allergy to other proteins.

Comfort techniques for irritable baby (rocking, singing, skin-to-skin contact, bathing, seeking quiet, calm environment, etc.).

IMPORTANT CONDITIONS TO REPORT

Family history of allergy.

Symptoms worsen, persist, or reoccur.

NOTES

If breathing difficulty or other extreme symptoms are reported, refer the caller to emergency care immediately.

Babies born into allergic families are more likely to develop allergy, particularly those with two allergic parents or one allergic parent and an allergic sibling. Exclusive breastfeeding is the optimal feeding choice for these babies in particular. Should the baby develop allergy symptoms, the mother may be counseled to avoid consuming offending allergens such as cow's milk.

Mothers who have not chosen breastfeeding may **relactate** for their allergic infant. Babies whose mothers do not choose to relactate may be fed hypoallergenic formula.

In the event that the allergic response is to a solid food, that food should not be fed to the baby. The breastfeeding mother should avoid the food until directed by a medical care provider to reintroduce allergen.

Rarely, babies develop allergies to fragments of foreign proteins consumed by their breastfeeding mother. The most potent allergens in the diets of U.S. residents include cow's milk, fish, eggs, peanuts, and tree nuts. Infantile symptoms of an allergic reaction include hives, facial swelling, runny nose, wheezing, eczema, vomiting, irritability (colic), blood in the stool, and **anaphylaxis**. Treatment centers on identification and avoidance of the proteins that are triggering the allergic reaction.

If supplementation is required, babies with documented allergy should be fed protein hydrolysate formula identified by a medical care provider. There is no convincing evidence that soy-based formulas are hypoallergenic.[9]

Concern about infant allergy is much more predominant than actual allergy. The American Academy of Pediatrics reports that the prevalence of infant cow's milk allergy is 2–3%.[10] The overall prevalence of childhood food allergy is 4–6%.[11]

Counseling and education should include comfort techniques for the irritable baby and coping methods for parents.

See also Atopic eczema

Footnotes

[9]Greer, F. R., Sicherer, S. H., Burks, A. W., & the Committee on Nutrition and Section on Allergy and Immunology. (2008). Effects of early nutritional interventions on the development of atopic disease in infants and children: The role of maternal dietary restriction, breastfeeding, timing of introduction of complementary foods, and hydrolyzed formulas. *Pediatrics, 121*(1), 183–191. doi:10.1542/peds.2007-3022

[10]American Academy of Pediatrics Committee on Nutrition. (2000). Hypoallergenic infant formulas. *Pediatrics, 106*, 346.

[11]Ziegler, R. S. (2003). Food allergen avoidance in prevention of food allergy in infants and children. *Pediatrics, 111*, 1662–1671.

➤ **ALPP**

See Academy of Lactation Policy & Practice

➤ ALTERNATE BREAST MASSAGE

DEFINITION A technique used to encourage milk to flow from the breast. When the suckling baby pauses, the mother gently but firmly massages and compresses the breast to which the baby is attached, thereby increasing the flow of milk and starting the suckling again.

NOTES

This technique is used with sleepy or inefficient feeders, especially those who are premature or have low muscle tone.

➤ ALUMINUM IN BREASTMILK AND FORMULA

DEFINITION Aluminum is a toxic metal that is present in the environment. It affects the nervous system and other tissues.

NOTES

Aluminum levels are higher in formula than in human milk. Levels are highest in soy-based formulae.[12,13]

Infants born prematurely or with kidney disease are at greater risk for aluminum toxicity.

Footnotes

[12]American Academy of Pediatrics Committee on Nutrition. (1996). Aluminum toxicity in infants and children. *Pediatrics, 97*, 413–416.

[13]Dabeka, R., Fouquet, A., Belisle, S., & Turcotte, S. (2011). Lead, cadmium and aluminum in Canadian infant formulae, oral electrolytes and glucose solutions. *Food Additives & Contaminants. Part A, Chemistry, Analysis, Control, Exposure & Risk Assessment, 28*(6), 744–753. doi:10.1080/19393210.2011.571795

➤ ALVEOLI

DEFINITION   Tiny sacs containing milk producing cells within the breast.

NOTES

These cells produce droplets of milk in response to suckling and the resulting rise in maternal blood levels of the hormone prolactin. Milk produced passes through the cell membrane into the center (lumen) of the alveolar cluster, causing it to fill. The hormone oxytocin (which is released by nipple stretching, breast massage, and other stimuli) causes the myoepithelial bands around the alveoli to contract, squeezing the milk into the ducts, propelling it toward the nipple.

When the breast is very full, alveolar lobes and clusters may be palpable through the skin of the breast. Encouraging frequent feeding, good positioning, and using techniques such as **alternate breast massage** may assist mothers through this period.

If lumps or fullness do not resolve within a day or two, the mother should be seen by a physician to rule out other pathology in the breast.

➤ AMCHP

See Association of Maternal & Child Health Programs

➤ AMENORRHEA

DEFINITION   A period of cessation of menses (monthly flow of blood from the uterus).

ASK ABOUT

Age of the baby.

ASSESSMENT

ROUTINE CARE NEEDED?

Are any of the following present?

Concern about prolonged lack of menses.

Concern about contraceptive usage.

Desire to conceive again.

IF YES,   *Schedule routine obstetric visit.*

Are any of the following present?

Desire to extend amenorrhea.

IF YES,   *Call lactation care provider today.*

SELF-CARE INFORMATION

Characteristics of breastfeeding thought to increase the chances of amenorrhea include baby younger than 6 months, **exclusive breastfeeding**, unrestricted feeding (10–12 or more feeds per day), avoidance of pacifiers, and frequent feedings including at night.

Once any of these criteria no longer apply, secure another family planning method (unless pregnancy is desired at this time).

IMPORTANT CONDITIONS TO REPORT

Past fertility problems.

Resumption of menses.

NOTES

A woman who breastfeeds exclusively during the first 6 months of her baby's life is likely to experience amenorrhea (that is, no menstrual period). Many breastfeeding women experience amenorrhea of a year or more, as long as they continue to breastfeed frequently.

Lactational amenorrhea method (LAM) is a form of natural family planning that is 98% effective in the first 6 months of the baby's life, so long as the mother's menses have not returned, her baby is exclusively breastfed, and there are no long periods of time between feedings, day and night. Once the baby is older than 6 months, or any of the above criteria no longer apply, LAM is no longer effective, and mothers should utilize other forms of birth control or child spacing, if desired.

See also Bellagio Consensus; Lactational amenorrhea method (LAM); Menstrual cycle; Natural family planning

➤ AMERICAN ACADEMY OF FAMILY PHYSICIANS (AAFP)

DESCRIPTION   "The American Academy of Family Physicians is one of the largest national medical organizations, representing more than 100,300 family physicians, family medicine residents and medical students nationwide. Founded in 1947, its mission has been to preserve and promote the science and art of Family Medicine and to ensure high-quality, cost-effective health care for patients of all ages."[14(p1)]

NOTES

American Academy of Family Physicians
Email: contactcenter@aafp.org
Web: www.aafp.org
  The AAFP publishes articles regarding breastfeeding in its journals, *American Family Physician*, *Family Practice Management*, and *Annals of Family Medicine*. A breastfeeding position paper is available on its website.

Footnote

[14]American Academy of Family Physicians. (2012). About us. Retrieved from http://www.aafp.org/online/en/home/aboutus.html?navid=about+us

➤ AMERICAN ACADEMY OF NURSING (AAN)

DESCRIPTION   "The mission of the AAN is to serve the public and nursing profession by advancing health policy and practice through the generation, synthesis, and dissemination of nursing knowledge."[15(p1)]

NOTES

American Academy of Nursing
Web: www.aannet.org
   AAN convenes an expert panel on breastfeeding.

Footnote

[15]American Academy of Nursing. (n.d.). *Strategic plan 2011–2014*. Retrieved from http://www.aannet.org/assets/docs/strategic%20plan_2011-2014%201.4.12.pdf

➤ AMERICAN ACADEMY OF PEDIATRICS (AAP)

DESCRIPTION   "The mission of the American Academy of Pediatrics is to attain optimal physical, mental, and social health and well-being for all infants, children, adolescents, and young adults."[16(p1)]

NOTES

American Academy of Pediatrics
Web: www.aap.org
   The AAP publishes articles, policies, and protocols covering breastfeeding on its website and in its journals, *Pediatrics* and *Pediatrics in Review*.

Footnote

[16]American Academy of Pediatrics. (2011). *AAP agenda for children—strategic plan*. Retrieved from http://www.aap.org/en-us/about-the-aap/aap-facts/Pages/AAP-Agenda-for-Children-Strategic-Plan.aspx

➤ AMERICAN ASSOCIATION OF BIRTH CENTERS (AABC)

DESCRIPTION   The American Association of Birth Centers promotes and supports birth centers as means to uphold the rights of healthy women and their families, in all communities, to birth their children in an environment that is safe, sensitive, and cost effective with minimal interventions.[17]

NOTES

American Association of Birth Centers
Email: aabc@birthcenters.org
Web: http://www.birthcenters.org/

Footnote

[17]American Association of Birth Centers. (2010). *Mission*. Retrieved from http://www.birthcenters .org/about-aabc/mission

➤ AMERICAN BREASTFEEDING INSTITUTE (ABI)

DESCRIPTION   "The purpose of the American Breastfeeding Institute shall be to promote, protect and support breastfeeding in the United States through research and education."[18(p1)] The American Breastfeeding Institute includes the National Commission on Donor Milk Banking and M2M, which is coordinating the national infrastructure for mother-to-mother support.

NOTES

American Breastfeeding Institute
Web: http://www.facebook.com/pages/American-Breastfeeding-Institute /176421862426503
    The American Breastfeeding Institute was incorporated in 2000 as a nonprofit corporation.

Footnote

[18]Articles of Incorporation, American Breastfeeding Institute.

➤ AMERICAN COLLEGE OF NURSE-MIDWIVES (ACNM)

DESCRIPTION   "The American College of Nurse-Midwives (ACNM) is the professional association that represents certified nurse-midwives and certified midwives in the United States. With roots dating to 1929, ACNM is the oldest women's health care organization in the United States. ACNM provides research, administers and promotes continuing education programs, establishes clinical practice standards, and creates liaisons with state and federal agencies and members of Congress."[19(p1)]

NOTES

American College of Nurse-Midwives
Web: www.midwife.org
   The ACNM publishes policy papers on breastfeeding on its website and in the *Journal of Midwifery and Women's Health*.

Footnote

[19]American College of Nurse-Midwives. (2010). About ACNM. Retrieved from http://www.midwife.org/index.asp?sid=19

➤ AMERICAN COLLEGE OF OSTEOPATHIC PEDIATRICIANS (ACOP)

DESCRIPTION   "ACOP is the official pediatric organization of the American Osteopathic Association. Government agencies turn to ACOP when they want an official position on the practice of pediatrics. ACOP submits resolutions concerning the practice of pediatrics to the AOA House of Delegates, taking the lead on positions and standards concerning children."[20(p1)]

NOTES

American College of Osteopathic Pediatricians
Email: acop@acopeds.org
Web: http://www.acopeds.org/

Footnote

[20]American College of Osteopathic Pediatricians. (2011). What is the ACOP? Retrieved from http://www.acopeds.org/about.iphtml

➤ AMERICAN CONGRESS OF OBSTETRICIANS AND GYNECOLOGISTS (ACOG)

DESCRIPTION   "The Congress, as the premier organization for obstetricians and gynecologists and providers of women's health care, will provide the highest quality education worldwide, continuously improve health care for women through practice and research, lead advocacy for women's health care issues nationally and internationally, and provide excellent organizational support and services for our members."[21(p1)]

NOTES

The American Congress of Obstetricians and Gynecologists
Email: resources@acog.org
Web: www.acog.org
   ACOG publishes several documents addressing breastfeeding on its website and in its journal, *Obstetrics & Gynecology*.

Footnote

[21]American Congress of Obstetricians and Gynecologists. (2009). *Strategic plan*. Retrieved from http://www.acog.org/~/media/About%20ACOG/StrategicPlanCongress.pdf?dmc=1&ts=201205 02T1524047849

➤ AMERICAN NURSES ASSOCIATION (ANA)

DESCRIPTION "The American Nurses Association (ANA) is the only full-service professional organization representing the interests of the nation's 3.1 million registered nurses through its constituent and state nurses associations and its organizational affiliates. The ANA advances the nursing profession by fostering high standards of nursing practice, promoting the rights of nurses in the workplace, projecting a positive and realistic view of nursing, and by lobbying the Congress and regulatory agencies on health care issues affecting nurses and the public."[22(p1)]

NOTES

American Nurses Association
Email: info@ana.org
Web: http://nursingworld.org/
   The ANA publishes articles and policy statements about breastfeeding on its website and in its journals.

Footnote

[22]American Nurses Association. (2012). About ANA. Retrieved from http://nursingworld.org/FunctionalMenuCategories/AboutANA

➤ AMERICAN NURSES CREDENTIALING CENTER (ANCC)

DESCRIPTION "The American Nurses Credentialing Center (ANCC), a subsidiary of the American Nurses Association (ANA), provides individuals and organizations throughout the nursing profession with the resources they need to achieve practice excellence . . . ANCC is the world's largest and most prestigious nurse credentialing organization. ANCC certification exams validate nurses' skills, knowledge, and abilities. More than a quarter million nurses have been certified by ANCC since 1990. More than 80,000 advanced practice nurses are currently certified by ANCC."[23(p1)]

Footnote

[23]American Nurses Credentialing Center. (2012). About ANCC. Retrieved from http://www .nursecredentialing.org/FunctionalCategory/AboutANCC.aspx

➤ AMERICAN PUBLIC HEALTH ASSOCIATION (APHA)

DESCRIPTION "The American Public Health Association is the oldest and most diverse organization of public health professionals in the world and has been working to improve public health since 1872. The Association aims to protect all Americans, their families and their communities from preventable, serious health threats and strives to assure community-based health promotion and disease prevention activities and preventive health services are universally accessible in the United States."[24(p1)]

Footnote

[24]American Public Health Association. (2012). About us. Retrieved from http://www.apha.org /about/

➤ AMPHETAMINES

DEFINITION   A category of drugs that stimulate the central nervous system.

NOTES

Breastfeeding is not recommended when a woman uses amphetamines and methamphetamines.[25]

Street names for these drugs vary, but include speed, crank, crystal, crystal meth, ecstasy, and ice.

Women reporting use of these drugs should receive substance abuse counseling. Hale (2010)[26] recommends that breastfeeding mothers avoid using this drug, or pump and discard milk for at least 48 hours after usage.

See also Illegal drugs; Medications

Footnotes

[25]AAP Section on Breastfeeding. (2012). Breastfeeding and the use of human milk. *Pediatrics*, *129*(3), e827–e841. doi:10.1542/peds.2011-3552

[26]Hale, T. W. (2010). Medications and mothers milk (14th ed.). Amarillo, TX: Hale Publishing, p. 668.

➤ ANALGESIA

DEFINITION   A category of drugs used for pain relief.

SELF-CARE INFORMATION

When mothers receive pain medications during the birth process, extended skin-to-skin contact should be practiced immediately after birth and continued, uninterrupted, until the infant self-attaches for the first breastfeeding. When the mother has had pharmacological pain relief in labor, it may take 2 hours or longer for her baby to self-attach. Provide continuous, uninterrupted skin-to-skin contact during this time period.

Breastfeeding and skin-to-skin contact have been shown to decrease pain in babies undergoing painful procedures.[27,28]

IMPORTANT CONDITIONS TO REPORT
Feeding difficulties after labor pain medication.

NOTES

A wide range of drugs are used to relieve pain. Medical evaluation should determine what analgesic is appropriate for the mother's and baby's situation.

Aspirin should never be given to infants or children due to concern about Reye's syndrome.

An up-to-date drug reference should be consulted to determine the safety and possible side effects of individual drugs.

Breastfeeding and skin-to-skin contact have been demonstrated to be analgesic for infants and may be recommended for babies while undergoing painful procedures, e.g., immunization, blood draw, etc.[29]

Newborn and premature babies are at greater risk of side effects due to limited ability to clear drugs from their systems.[30]

See also Drugs, InfantRisk Center; Lactmed; Medication Resources (inside back cover)

Footnotes

[27]Gray, L., Miller, L. W., Philipp, B. L., & Blass, E. M. (2002). Breastfeeding is analgesic in healthy newborns. *Pediatrics, 109*(4), 590–593.

[28]Phillips, R. M., Chantry, C. J., & Gallagher, M. P. (2005). Analgesic effects of breast-feeding or pacifier use with maternal holding in term infants. *Ambulatory Pediatrics: The Official Journal of the Ambulatory Pediatric Association, 5*(6), 359–364. doi:10.1367/A04-189R.1

[29]Gray, L., Watt, L., & Blass, E. M. (2000). Skin-to-skin contact is analgesic in healthy newborns. *Pediatrics, 105*(1), e14.

[30]Carbajal, R., Veerapen, S., Couderc, S., Jugie, M., & Ville, Y. (2003). Analgesic effect of breast feeding in term neonates: Randomised controlled trial. *The British Medical Journal, 326*(7379), 13.

➤ ANAPHYLAXIS

DEFINITION   A potentially life threatening, full body response to an allergen consumed, touched, inhaled, or injected.

Anaphylactic reactions are serious medical conditions. Symptoms may involve the skin and respiratory, digestive, circulatory, and nervous systems. Common symptoms include swelling, itching, and burning of the face (especially the lips, tongue, and inside of the mouth), flushing, nausea, vomiting, abdominal pain, diarrhea, difficulty breathing, coughing, constriction of the throat, wheezing, itching of the skin, hives, swelling of the eyelids, hands, and feet, rapid or irregular heartbeat, dizziness, low blood pressure (leading to loss of consciousness), confusion, and panic. Skin and respiratory reactions are the most common symptoms in children with anaphylaxis.[31]

The Canadian Paediatric Society recommends that when anaphylaxis has been diagnosed in a child, "On discharge, all patients should be prescribed epinephrine autoinjectors, and referred to an allergist or immunologist for further evaluation and education."[32(p35)]

Anaphylaxis in the mother has also been associated with breastfeeding. Researchers have referred to this as a "rare but potentially life-threatening event."[33(p415)] Shank and colleagues (2009) suggest avoidance of nonsteroidal anti-inflammatories in these cases, and recommend treatment with corticosteroids and antihistamines, which may offer the best protection. The etiology of breastfeeding-related anaphylaxis is not currently understood but is thought to be related to hormonal changes of the postpartum period. Many of the cases in the literature involve treatment of the woman with aspirin or other nonsteroidal anti-inflammatory medications as potential triggers for the reaction.[34]

See also Allergy in the breastfed infant

Footnotes

[31]Cheng, A., & Canadian Paediatric Society. (2011). Emergency treatment of anaphylaxis in infants and children. *Paediatrics & Child Health, 16*(1), 35–40.

[32]Cheng & Canadian Paediatric Society. (2011).

[33]Shank, J. J., Olney, S. C., Lin, F. L., & McNamara, M. F. (2009). Recurrent postpartum anaphylaxis with breast-feeding. *Obstetrics and Gynecology, 114*(2 Pt 2), 415–416. doi:10.1097/AOG.0b013e3181a20721

[34]McKinney, K. K., & Scranton, S. E. (2011). A case report of breastfeeding anaphylaxis: Successful prophylaxis with oral antihistamines. *Allergy, 66*(3), 435–436. doi:10.1111/j.1398-9995.2010.02486.x

➤ ANCC

See American Nurses Credentialing Center (ANCC)

➤ ANEMIA

DEFINITION   A deficiency in the oxygen-carrying capacity of blood cells, typically caused by iron deficiency (although other nutrient deficiencies and medical conditions can cause anemia).

NOTES

Iron deficiency anemia is a common problem in childbearing women. In a nonpregnant woman older than 18 years, hemoglobin levels below 12.0 g/dL and hematocrit levels lower than 35.7% are considered anemia. In children between 6 months and 2 years of age, hemoglobin levels of less than 11.0 g/dL and hematocrit of less than 32.9% are considered anemia.[35]

Currently, the need for iron supplementation in healthy term breastfed infants is a matter of controversy. The AAP's Section on Breastfeeding recommends "Supplementation of oral iron drops before 6 months may be needed to support iron stores,"[36(p.e835)] while AAP's Committee on Nutrition states:

> For partially breastfed infants, the proportion of human milk versus formula is uncertain; therefore, beginning at 4 months of age, partially breastfed infants (more than half of their daily feedings as human milk) who are not receiving iron-containing complementary foods should also receive 1 mg/kg per day of supplemental iron.[37(p1047)]

Preterm infants are at risk for anemia due to decreased transfer of iron prenatally. The American Academy of Pediatrics[38,39] recommends supplementation of 2 mg/kg/day in exclusively breastfeeding premature infants for the first year of life.

More commonly, anemia may influence energy levels and coping behaviors. Anemic women may not initiate an adequate number of feedings daily and may be more likely to use formula or pacifiers due to their exhaustion.

Rarely, women who have experienced a severe blood loss during childbirth may be at risk for **Sheehan's syndrome**, a failure of the pituitary gland caused by altered blood flow to the brain. Symptoms of this syndrome include sudden onset of hypothyroidism, diabetes insipidus, and hair loss along with menstrual irregularities.[40] Medical evaluation should include measurement of prolactin levels before and after suckling. The extent to which women recover from Sheehan's syndrome is variable with the degree of infarct.

Anemic children should be evaluated for developmental delays, behavioral disturbances, and lead poisoning.

Several other conditions and nutrient deficiencies can contribute to anemia.

Anemia should be treated and monitored in an ongoing manner.

See also Iron; Retained placental fragments; Sheehan's syndrome

Footnotes

[35]Centers for Disease Control and Prevention. (1998). Recommendations to prevent and control iron deficiency in the United States. *Morbidity and Mortality Weekly Report, 47*(RR-3).

[36]American Academy of Pediatrics. (2012). AAP Section on Breastfeeding. Breastfeeding and the Use of Human Milk. *Pediatrics, 129*(3), e827–e841. doi:10.1542/peds.2011-3552, p. e835.

[37]Baker, R. D., Greer, F. R. & the Committee on Nutrition. (2010). Diagnosis and Prevention of Iron Deficiency and Iron-Deficiency Anemia in Infants and Young Children (0-3 Years of Age). *Pediatrics, 126*(5), 1040–1050. doi:10.1542/peds.2010-2576, p. 1047.

[38]American Academy of Pediatrics. (2010).

[39]American Academy of Pediatrics. (2012).

[40]Lawrence, R. A., & Lawrence, R. M. (2011). Breastfeeding: A guide for the medical profession (7th ed., pp. 562–563). St. Louis, MO: Elsevier/Mosby.

➤ ANESTHESIA

DEFINITION Administration of drugs used to cause total or partial loss of sensation for surgical or other medical purposes.

SELF-CARE INFORMATION

When mothers receive pain medications during the birth process, extended skin-to-skin contact should be practiced immediately after birth and continued, uninterrupted, until the infant self-attaches for the first breastfeeding.

IMPORTANT CONDITIONS TO REPORT
Feeding difficulties after anesthesia.

NOTES

A wide range of drugs are used as anesthesia during surgical procedures. An up-to-date drug reference should be consulted to determine the safety and possible side effects of individual drugs.

Newborn and premature babies are at greater risk of side effects due to limited ability to clear drugs from their systems.

See also Medication Resources (inside back cover)

➤ ANIMAL MILKS

DEFINITION   Referring to the nutritive mammary secretions of mammals.

NOTES

Parents occasionally read that goat or other milks are preferable for their infant. Human milk and infant formula are the only safe milks for children younger than the age of 1.

Other mammalian milks are inadequate nutritionally for human babies. Children old enough (older than 1 year) to consume some cow's milk in their diet should drink whole milk. Low-fat and skim milk should not be offered until children are older than 2.

➤ ANKYLOGLOSSIA

DEFINITION   A tight lingual frenulum (the membrane attaching the tongue to the bottom of the mouth). This condition is also referred to as **tongue-tie.**

When the frenulum is tight, it can restrict the movement of the tongue, resulting in breastfeeding problems for some mothers and babies.

ASK ABOUT

Age of the baby.
Appearance of tongue.

ASSESSMENT

PROMPT MEDICAL CARE NEEDED?
Are any of the following present?
> Inadequate urine or stool output.
> Baby not back to birthweight by 2 weeks of age.
> Poor growth of breastfed infant.

IF YES, *Seek medical care within 4 hours.*

Are any of the following present?
> Presence of tight lingual frenulum in baby in conjunction with feeding or breast/nipple problems in breastfeeding mother.

IF YES, *Call pediatric care provider today.*

PROMPT LACTATION CARE NEEDED?
Are any of the following present?
> Tight lingual frenulum in baby.
> Nipple or breast pain.
> History of recurrent breast infection.
> Milk supply problems.

IF YES, *Call lactation care provider today.*

SELF-CARE INFORMATION
Practice skin-to-skin contact in the first hour and frequently thereafter.
Watch for hunger cues (signs that say "feed me" include hand-to-face or hand-to-mouth movements, lip smacking, seeking with lips, rooting, and head bobbing).
Feed the baby at the first sign of hunger cues.
Practice good attachment:
> Offer the breast as soon as it is seen.
> Wait for the baby to open his or her mouth wide (greater than a 140° angle).

Pull the baby in so that the chin touches the breast first, and the nipple enters the open space in the top part of the mouth; this should result in a wide-open mouth on the breast.

The baby may need to be in a semi-upright position to assist in attaining the widest mouth angle.

The baby's lips should be flanged outward.

The baby's lips should look off center when compared with the areola; the bottom lip should be farther away from the nipple than the top lip.

IMPORTANT CONDITIONS TO REPORT

Unresolved symptoms.

Ongoing concerns.

NOTES

Babies with ankyloglossia may have difficulty performing the tongue motions required to feed from a breast or sometimes even a bottle of milk. On visual assessment, the tongue may appear to be heart-shaped at the tip. The infant may be unable to extend the tongue beyond the lower gum ridge. The tongue may be held tightly in the posterior part of the mouth as well.

Breastfeeding mothers of babies with tongue-tie may experience sore nipples, mastitis, and milk supply problems.

Babies with ankyloglossia should be evaluated for their tongue mobility, and possibly for frenotomy or frenectomy.[41,42,43] Mothers should receive lactation assistance to improve positioning and milk removal. Occupational therapists and/or speech language pathologists have specialized skills for assisting babies with ankyloglossia.

See also Nipple pain

Footnotes

[41]Buryk, M., Bloom, D., & Shope, T. (2011). Efficacy of neonatal release of ankyloglossia: A randomized trial. *Pediatrics, 128*(2), 280–288. doi:10.1542/peds.2011-0077

[42]Geddes, D. T., Langton, D. B., Gollow, I., Jacobs, L. A., Hartmann, P. E., & Simmer, K. (2008). Frenulotomy for breastfeeding infants with ankyloglossia: Effect on milk removal and sucking mechanism as imaged by ultrasound. *Pediatrics, 122*(1), e188–194. doi:10.1542/peds.2007-2553

[43]Manfro, A. R. G., Manfro, R., & Bortoluzzi, M. C. (2010). Surgical treatment of ankyloglossia in babies—case report. *International Journal of Oral and Maxillofacial Surgery, 39*(11), 1130–1132. doi:10.1016/j.ijom.2010.06.007

➤ ANLC

See Advanced nurse lactation consultant

➤ ANTIBACTERIAL AGENTS IN BREASTMILK

DEFINITION   Referring to immunologically active components found in human milk.

NOTES

Human milk is a rich source of active immune factors. Breastfeeding children receive several different types of immunoglobulins as well as live immune cells and factors from their mother's milk.

With very few exceptions (see the section on Contraindicated conditions), mothers may continue to breastfeed their babies through illness.[44]

See also Antibodies; Contraindicated conditions

Footnote

[44]AAP Section on Breastfeeding. (2012). Breastfeeding and the use of human milk. *Pediatrics*, *129*(3), e827–e841. doi:10.1542/peds.2011-3552

➤ ANTIBIOTICS

DEFINITION   A group of drugs that fight infection.

NOTES

A wide range of drugs are used as antibiotics. An up-to-date drug reference should be consulted to determine the safety and possible side effects of individual drugs.

Newborn and premature babies are at greater risk of side effects due to limited ability to clear drugs from their systems.

See also Antibacterial agents in breastmilk; Medication Resources (inside back cover)

➤ ANTIBODIES

DEFINITION   Referring to specific proteins on the surface of immune cells that are secreted in response to the presence of a specific antigen (bacteria, viruses, or other invader) in the body. An antibody attacks and neutralizes the specific antigen to which it is sensitized.

NOTES

Human milk is a rich source of active immune factors, including antibodies.

Breastfeeding children receive several different types of immunoglobulins as well as live immune cells and factors from their mother's milk.

With very few exceptions (see the section on Contraindicated conditions), mothers should continue to breastfeed their babies through illness.[45] Mothers are usually exposed to the same illnesses as their babies and are producing specific antibodies that help the baby to mount an immune response.

See also Acute infection; Antigen; Contraindicated conditions; Immunoglobulin; Secretory IgA

Footnote

[45]AAP Section on Breastfeeding. (2012). Breastfeeding and the use of human milk. *Pediatrics*, *129*(3), e827–e841. doi:10.1542/peds.2011-3552

➤ ANTIDEPRESSANTS

DEFINITION   A category of drugs used to treat clinical depression. Depression is a state of extreme sadness, feelings of hopelessness, difficulty concentrating, difficulty sleeping, and often decreased appetite.

ASK ABOUT

Onset.
Age of the baby.
History of depression.

ASSESSMENT

EMERGENT CARE NEEDED?

Are any of the following present?

Suicidal thoughts.

Thoughts of harming the baby.

IF YES,   *Seek emergency medical and protective care now.*

PROMPT CARE NEEDED?

Are any of the following present?

Persistent sadness.

Inability to function.

IF YES,   *Seek medical care within 4 hours and seek psychological counseling today.*

SELF-CARE INFORMATION

Mood swings are normal in the postpartum period but may become more severe. Report symptoms and any worsening of symptoms to health care provider immediately.

Seek support.

IMPORTANT CONDITIONS TO REPORT

Worsening of depression.

Failure of treatment in alleviating symptoms.

Reoccurrence of depression.

History of depression, mood disorders, premenstrual syndrome, or thyroid disorders.

NOTES

Postpartum mood disorders affect most new mothers. Mood disorders cover a broad spectrum from baby blues to postpartum psychosis. While mood disorders are common, they are not to be ignored. Avoid giving false reassurance. Depression can be life-threatening for the mother and the baby.

Women who experienced depression during pregnancy and those with a history of depression, mood disorders, or premenstrual syndrome are at greater risk for postpartum depression.

Hypothyroidism, anemia, and other physical disorders share many symptoms with postpartum depression.

Consider using the Edinburgh Postnatal Depression scale to evaluate the need for referral for diagnosis and treatment.[46]

A wide range of drugs are used as antidepressants. An up-to-date drug reference should be consulted to determine the safety and possible side effects of individual drugs. Many antidepressants are compatible with breastfeeding. The Academy of Breastfeeding Medicine protocol on use of antidepressant medications (#18) is a valuable, evidence-based resource.[47]

Newborn and premature babies are at greater risk of side effects due to limited ability to clear drugs from their systems.

See also Baby blues; Medication Resources (inside back cover); Postpartum depression

Footnotes

[46]Cox, J. L., Holden, J. M., & Sagovsky, R. (1987). Detection of postnatal depression. Development of the 10-item Edinburgh Postnatal Depression Scale. *The British Journal of Psychiatry: The Journal of Mental Science, 150,* 782–786. Tool accessible on the Web: http://www.fresno.ucsf.edu /pediatrics/downloads/edinburghscale.pdf

[47]ABM Protocol Committee. (2008). ABM clinical protocol #18: Use of antidepressants in nursing mothers. *Breastfeeding Medicine: The Official Journal of the Academy of Breastfeeding Medicine, 3*(1), 44–52. doi:10.1089/bfm.2007.9978

➤ ANTIFUNGAL MEDICATIONS

DEFINITION A category of drugs used to treat clinically significant overgrowth of fungus, a condition that may cause pain for the mother and/or her breastfeeding baby.

NOTES

A number of drugs are used as antifungal agents. An up-to-date drug reference should be consulted to determine the safety and possible side effects of individual drugs.

Newborn and premature babies are at greater risk of drug side effects due to limited ability to clear drugs from their systems.

Antifungal agents intended for use in the vulvar or other areas may not be appropriate for use on the breast of a lactating woman, unless they are safe for consumption by her infant.

See also Candidiasis; Medication Resources (inside back cover); Thrush; Yeast infection

➤ ANTIGEN

DEFINITION A foreign substance that stimulates the production of an antibody when introduced into the body.

➤ ANTIHISTAMINES

DEFINITION A category of drugs that reduce the histamine response in allergic reactions and upper respiratory infections. Histamine response includes vasodilation, constriction of the bronchial muscles, and increased gastric secretion.

NOTES

A wide range of drugs are used as antihistamines. An up-to-date drug reference should be consulted to determine the safety and possible side effects of individual drugs.

Some antihistamines have been noted to suppress lactation.

Newborn and premature babies are at greater risk of drug side effects due to limited ability to clear drugs from their systems.

See also Allergen; Allergy in the breastfed infant; Medication Resources (inside back cover)

➤ ANTI-INFECTIVE AGENTS IN BREASTMILK

DEFINITION   Referring to immunologically active components found in human milk. These include antimicrobial, antiviral, antibacterial, and anti-inflammatory properties.

NOTES

Human milk is a rich source of active immune factors. Breastfeeding children receive several different types of immunoglobulins as well as live immune cells and factors from their mother's milk.

   With very few exceptions (see the section on Contraindicated conditions), mothers may continue to breastfeed their babies through illness. [48]

See also Antibodies; Anti-inflammatory agents in breastmilk

Footnote

[48]AAP Section on Breastfeeding. (2012). Breastfeeding and the use of human milk. *Pediatrics*, *129*(3), e827–e841. doi:10.1542/peds.2011-3552

➤ ANTI-INFLAMMATORY AGENTS IN BREASTMILK

DEFINITION   Substances that reduce the body's inflammatory response (a reaction of the immune system to injury or infection that results in pain, redness, swelling, and sometimes impaired function of the affected area).

NOTES

Human milk is a rich source of anti-inflammatory agents, including oligosaccharides and cytokines. These agents assist in maintaining health and fighting disease.

See also Allergy in the breastfed infant; Bioactive components of breastmilk

➤ ANTIRETROVIRAL MEDICATIONS

DEFINITION A category of drugs used to treat infection with retroviruses, especially the human immunodeficiency virus (HIV).

NOTES

A number of drugs are used as antiretroviral agents. An up-to-date drug reference should be consulted to determine the safety and possible side effects of individual drugs.

In the United States, breastfeeding is not recommended when the woman is HIV positive.[49]

Newborn and premature babies are at greater risk of drug side effects due to limited ability to clear drugs from their systems.

See also Contraindicated conditions; HIV; Medication Resources (inside back cover)

Footnote

[49]AAP Section on Breastfeeding. (2012). Breastfeeding and the Use of Human Milk. *Pediatrics*, *129*(3), e827–e841. doi:10.1542/peds.2011-3552

➤ APHA

See American Public Health Association (APHA)

➤ APPROPRIATE FOR GESTATIONAL AGE (AGA)

DEFINITION Babies who are classified appropriate for gestational age are of weight, length, and development considered appropriate for their gestational age at birth.

➤ ARA

See Arachidonic acid (AA, also ARA)

➤ ARACHIDONIC ACID (AA, ALSO ARA)

DEFINITION   A long-chain polyunsaturated fatty acid (LCPUFA) found naturally in human milk. These fatty acids assist in the development of nerve and brain tissue and may account for some of the differences between formula-fed and breastfed children in terms of IQ, test scores, and visual acuity.

NOTES

While LCPUFAs have been added to formula in recent years, there is no clear evidence of beneficial outcomes in children who have consumed them.[50,51] Supplements are also being marketed for mothers to consume during pregnancy and lactation, also with little evidence of efficacy.[52]

See also Docosahexaenoic acid; Fat in breastmilk; LCPUFAs

Footnotes

[50]Schulzke, S. M., Patole, S. K., & Simmer, K. (2011). Longchain polyunsaturated fatty acid supplementation in preterm infants. *Cochrane Database of Systematic Reviews (Online)*, (2), CD000375. doi:10.1002/14651858.CD000375.pub4

[51]Simmer, K., Patole, S. K., & Rao, S. C. (2011). Longchain polyunsaturated fatty acid supplementation in infants born at term. *Cochrane Database of Systematic Reviews (Online)*, (12), CD000376. doi:10.1002/14651858.CD000376.pub3

[52]Dziechciarz, P., Horvath, A., & Szajewska, H. (2010). Effects of n-3 long-chain polyunsaturated fatty acid supplementation during pregnancy and/or lactation on neurodevelopment and visual function in children: A systematic review of randomized controlled trials. *Journal of the American College of Nutrition*, *29*(5), 443–454.

➤ AREOLA

DEFINITION   The area of darkened pigmentation around the nipple. The size and color of the areola varies among women.

NOTES

It is normal for the areola to become much darker during pregnancy and lactation. **Montgomery's glands** or tubercles are mixed sebaceous and milk glands that look like goose bumps on the surface of the areola. These glands become more prominent during pregnancy and lactation.

It is normal for the areolar area to be slightly enlarged and darkened. Any reddening or lumpiness in this area should be examined by a medical care provider to rule out anomalies.

➤ ASSOCIATION OF MATERNAL AND CHILD HEALTH PROGRAMS (AMCHP)

DESCRIPTION   "The Association of Maternal & Child Health Programs is a national resource, partner, and advocate for state public health leaders and others working to improve the health of women, children, youth, and families, including those with special healthcare needs.

AMCHP's members come from the highest levels of state government and include directors of maternal and child health programs, directors of programs for children with special healthcare needs, and other public health leaders who work with and support state maternal and child health programs. The members directly serve all women and children nationwide and strive to improve the health of all women, infants, children, and adolescents, including those with special healthcare needs, by administering critical public health education and screening services, and coordinating preventive, primary and specialty care."[53] (p1)

NOTES

Association of Maternal & Child Health Programs
Email: info@amchp.org
Web: www.amchp.org

Footnote

[53]Association of Maternal & Child Health Programs. (n.d.). About AMCHP. Retrieved May 3, 2012 from http://www.amchp.org/AboutAMCHP/Pages/default.aspx

➤ ASSOCIATION OF MILITARY SURGEONS OF THE UNITED STATES

DESCRIPTION   "AMSUS was organized in 1891 and chartered by Congress in 1903 to advance the knowledge of healthcare within the federal agencies and to increase the effectiveness of its members. It is dedicated to all aspects of federal medicine—professional, scientific, educational and administrative. Presently our nearly 8,000 members represent all healthcare disciplines and serve in the Active and Reserve Components of all of the uniformed services as well as the Department of Defense and the Department of Veterans Affairs."[54(p1)]

NOTES

Association of Military Surgeons of the United States
Email: amsus@amsus.org
Web: www.amsus.org/
    AMSUS cosponsors the Breastfeeding Coalition of the Uniformed Services, a group of breastfeeding experts from different branches of the service, who endeavor to support breastfeeding servicewomen and their families.

Footnote

[54]Association of Military Surgeons of the United States. (2011). About AMSUS. Retrieved from http://www.amsus.org/index.php/about-amsus

➤ ASSOCIATION OF STATE & TERRITORIAL PUBLIC HEALTH NUTRITION DIRECTORS (ASTPHND)

DESCRIPTION "The Association of State & Territorial Public Health Nutrition Directors develops leaders in public health nutrition who strengthen policy, programs and environments making it possible for everyone to make healthy food choices and achieve healthy, active lifestyles."[55(p1)]

NOTES

Association of State & Territorial Public Health Nutrition Directors
Web: http://www.astphnd.org/

Footnote

[55]Association of State & Territorial Public Health Nutrition Directors. (2011). About ASTPHND. Retrieved from http://www.astphnd.org/newsletter.php?sid=544125&issue_id=11

➤ ASSOCIATION OF TEACHERS OF MATERNAL AND CHILD HEALTH (ATMCH)

DESCRIPTION "The Association of Teachers of Maternal and Child Health (ATMCH) aims to provide leadership in education, research, and service in the field of maternal and child health. ATMCH offers an interdisciplinary forum through which MCH faculty from schools of public health and other institutions of higher learning can share the knowledge, ideas, and skills essential to educating students, advancing MCH research, and applying research results to MCH policies, programs, and services."[56(p1)]

NOTES

Association of Teachers of Maternal and Child Health
Email: jpetrush@asph.org
Web: www.atmch.org/

Footnotes

[56]Association of Teachers of Maternal and Child Health. (n.d.) ATMCH. Retrieved May 3, 2012 from http://atmch.org/

➤ ASSOCIATION OF WOMEN'S HEALTH, OBSTETRIC, AND NEONATAL NURSES (AWHONN)

DESCRIPTION   "The Association of Women's Health, Obstetric and Neonatal Nurses (AWHONN) is a 501(c)3 nonprofit membership organization that promotes the health of women and newborns. Our mission is to improve and promote the health of women and newborns and to strengthen the nursing profession through the delivery of superior advocacy, research, education and other professional and clinical resources to nurses and other health care professionals."[57(p1)]

NOTES

Association of Women's Health, Obstetric, and Neonatal Nurses
Email: customerservice@awhonn.org
Web: www.awhonn.org
    Articles and policy statements about breastfeeding can be found in the *Journal of Obstetric, Gynecologic, and Neonatal Nursing*, and on the AWHONN's website.

Footnotes

[57]Association of Women's Health, Obstetric and Neonatal Nurses. (2012). About us. Retrieved from http://www.awhonn.org/awhonn/content.do;jsessionid=8B469FC2E537DBC08DAE5A861676F195?name=10_AboutUs/10_AboutUs_landing.htm

➤ ASTHMA AND LACTATION

DEFINITION   Asthma is a chronic respiratory disease characterized by difficulty breathing, constriction of the airways, and coughing attacks often triggered by allergens.

NOTES

Research has indicated that breastfeeding may reduce the risk and severity of asthma in susceptible children.

Mothers with asthma may breastfeed their babies. Any medications used by a mother with asthma should be reviewed. Consult an up-to-date drug reference to determine the safety and possible side effects of individual drugs.

Asthmatic women who take theophylline may need to be monitored for cumulative effects of this drug in combination with any dietary caffeine.

Newborn and premature babies are at greater risk of side effects due to limited ability to clear drugs from their systems.

See also Medication Resources (inside back cover)

➤ ASTPHND

See Association of State & Territorial Public Health Nutrition Directors (ASTPHND)

➤ ASYMMETRIC BREASTS

DEFINITION   Lack of similarity of appearance, size, or other characteristic of one breast as compared with the other.

ASK ABOUT

Onset.
Age of the baby.

ASSESSMENT

PROMPT CARE NEEDED?

Are any of the following present?

Reported breast asymmetry coupled with concern about milk supply or infant's weight gain.

IF YES,   *Call pediatric care provider and lactation care provider today.*

ROUTINE CARE NEEDED?

Are any of the following present?

Reported asymmetry with no concerns about milk supply or infant's growth.

| IF YES, | *Call lactation care provider today.* |

SELF-CARE INFORMATION

Practice skin-to-skin contact in the first hour and frequently thereafter.

Feed the baby at the first sign of hunger cues (signs that say "feed me" include hand-to-face or hand-to-mouth movements, lip smacking, seeking with lips, rooting, and head bobbing).

Feed the baby at least 10 times per 24 hours.

Listen for signs of the baby swallowing.

Allow the baby to end feedings.

Expect at least three infant stools per 24 hours after the first 4 days of life.

Good positioning and attachment are crucial to prevent or reduce nipple pain.

If the baby is fed away from the breast, hand express or pump milk to maintain supply.

IMPORTANT CONDITIONS TO REPORT

Feeding or stooling expectations are not met.

NOTES

Most women have some discrepancy between their breasts in terms of size, shape, position, etc. The hormones of pregnancy may alter the discrepancy, either exacerbating or lessening it. Minor asymmetry is common and normal.

When a lactating woman's breasts are markedly different, particularly with one or both breasts appearing underdeveloped, insufficient glandular tissue may exist in one or both breasts.

Marked asymmetry indicates the need for careful medical and lactation evaluation and monitoring. The baby's weight gain should be closely followed to ensure that adequate milk is being made and transferred.

See also Breast, insufficient glandular tissue; Insufficient milk supply; Milk transfer, estimating

➤ ASYMMETRIC LATCH

DEFINITION An ideal way for baby to remove maximal milk from the breast, referring to the position of the mother's nipple in the baby's mouth.

NOTES

In order to allow the baby to get as much breast tissue into the mouth as possible, an asymmetric latch position is recommended. In this position, baby's mouth is open to a 140° or larger angle, and the baby grasps more of the underside of the breast than the tissue above the nipple. The baby's lips will appear to be off-center on the nipple, with the upper lips closer to the nipple than the lower.

Because nipple and breast pain is a major reason for discontinuing breastfeeding, any woman reporting such pain should be seen within 24 hours by a skilled breastfeeding helper. The baby's growth should also be evaluated, as painful breastfeeding is associated with poor growth.

See also Latch-on; Taking the baby off the breast

➤ AT-BREAST SUPPLEMENTATION

DEFINITION Administration of extra fluids (expressed breastmilk or formula) to the baby through a tube device attached to the breast.

NOTES

At-breast supplementation is useful when a baby is not receiving an adequate amount of milk from the breast. This may be due to a temporary or permanent problem with milk supply on the part of the mother. It may also result from weak or inefficient suckling on the part of the baby, due to temporary or permanent conditions (e.g., prematurity, undernourishment, Down syndrome, cardiac problems).

See also Adoption and induced lactation

➤ ATOPIC ECZEMA

DEFINITION   An allergic inflammation of the skin characterized by itching, redness, and scaling.

ASK ABOUT

Onset.
Age of the baby.
Medications used.

ASSESSMENT

PROMPT CARE NEEDED?

Are any of the following present?

Eczema on the breast.
Eczema in the baby.
Concerns about medications to treat eczema.

IF YES,   *Seek medical care today.*

SELF-CARE INFORMATION

Follow instructions from the healthcare provider and report problems as directed.

IMPORTANT CONDITIONS TO REPORT

Allergy and eczema in parents and siblings.
Infant symptoms of blood in stool, wheezing, hives, facial swelling, runny nose, vomiting, or irritability.

NOTES

Research has identified that exclusive breastfeeding reduces the risk of atopic eczema in susceptible children.

In adults, atopic eczema is typically treated with topical steroid creams. The specific cream indicated should be examined in an up-to-date drug reference to ensure that it is safe for use by the breastfeeding mother.

Steroid cream use is of greater concern when the affected area is on the breast where the baby's mouth will be placed, as the baby could then absorb the steroid both through direct contact and through the milk.

In the breastfed baby, atopic eczema may be a symptom of food allergy or related to an allergen in food that the mother or baby is consuming. The mother and the baby should avoid consuming offending allergens such as cow's milk, fish, eggs, peanuts, and tree nuts.

Infantile symptoms of an allergic reaction include hives, facial swelling, runny nose, wheezing, eczema, vomiting, irritability (colic), blood in the stool, and **anaphylaxis**. Treatment centers on identification and avoidance of the proteins that are triggering the allergic reaction.

Babies born into allergic families are more likely to develop allergy, particularly those with two allergic parents or one allergic parent and an allergic sibling. Exclusive breastfeeding is the optimal feeding choice for these babies in particular.

If babies with documented allergy are supplemented, a protein hydrolysate formula should be considered.

See also Allergy in the breastfed infant; Medication Resources (inside back cover)

➤ ATMCH

See Association of Teachers of Maternal and Child Health (ATMCH)

➤ ATTACHMENT

DEFINITION Refers to the way in which the nursing baby latches on to the breast.

NOTES

Correct attachment of the baby to the breast is crucial to comfortable breastfeeding, to adequate milk manufacture and transfer, and ultimately to infant growth. When a baby is attached well, the mother should feel no pain or discomfort and should hear sounds of swallowing on the part of the baby.

Since concerns about pain and inadequate milk are major reasons mothers stop breastfeeding, mothers should be seen for a feeding evaluation within 48 hours of expressing breastfeeding concerns.

See also Asymmetric latch

➤ ATTACHMENT PARENTING

DEFINITION   A phrase used to describe a parenting style that includes continuous, nurturing contact between a baby and its parents. The goal of attachment parenting is to develop a secure emotional bond between the baby and its primary caregivers.

NOTES

Attachment parenting typically includes carrying babies in a sling, breastfeeding exclusively, cosleeping, and avoiding prolonged parent–baby separation.

See also Cosleeping

➤ AUGMENTATION SURGERY

DEFINITION   Saline or silicone filled medical prosthesis surgically inserted into the breast to increase its size. Implants can affect milk-making ability to some extent by reducing storage capacity in the breast.

ASK ABOUT

Date of surgery.
Age of the baby.
Location of surgical incision.

ASSESSMENT

PROMPT CARE NEEDED?
Are any of the following present?

History of augmentation surgery.
Concerns about milk supply.
Poor stool output in breastfed baby.
Poor weight gain in breastfed baby.

IF YES,   *Call pediatric care provider and lactation care provider today.*

SELF-CARE INFORMATION

Practice skin-to-skin contact in the first hour and frequently thereafter.

Feed the baby at the first sign of hunger cues (signs that say "feed me" include hand-to-face or hand-to-mouth movements, lip smacking, seeking with lips, rooting, and head bobbing).

Feed the baby at least 10 times per 24 hours.

Listen for signs of the baby swallowing.

Allow the baby to end feedings.

Expect at least three infant stools per 24 hours after the first 4 days of life.

Good positioning and attachment are crucial to prevent or reduce nipple pain.

If the baby is fed away from the breast, hand express or pump milk, or both, to reduce fullness or engorgement and maintain supply.

IMPORTANT CONDITIONS TO REPORT

Fewer than four bowel movements daily beginning on the fourth day after birth.

Ongoing problems with the baby's weight gain.

Ongoing concerns or problems with milk supply.

Ongoing concerns or problems with full breasts or engorgement.

NOTES

The location and extent of the incision may impact the sensation of the nerves in the nipple area. Loss of or decreased sensation may decrease milk-making potential. Trauma to the nerves may hinder the stimulation of the brain to release prolactin (the milk-making hormone) in response to suckling. Periareolar incisions suggest more potential nerve and duct injury than do incisions underneath the breast.

Babies of women who have had breast augmentation surgery should be followed closely even after the first 2 weeks to ensure milk transfer and growth.

If the mother reports that she had an implant in one breast only, inquire about the reason for this surgery. If augmentation corrected breast asymmetry, there may be increased concern regarding the mother's ability to make a full milk supply. Marked asymmetry may indicate insufficient glandular tissue in both breasts. The baby and the mother should be closely followed. (Breasts are rarely identical in shape and size. Minor asymmetry is common and normal.)

See also Asymmetric breasts; Breast surgery; Breast augmentation; Engorgement; Weight gain, baby—low

➤ AUSTRALIAN POSTURE

DEFINITION   A breastfeeding position where the baby is above the mother (or the mother is "down under" the baby—the reason for the name of the posture).

NOTES

This posture is suggested to deal with fast milk flow, which may cause the baby to pull away from the breast gasping.

Some mothers are successful managing the flow by nursing while lying on their back with the baby positioned flat on top. The baby has more head control in this position.

See also **Reclining posture**

➤ AUTOIMMUNE DISEASES

DEFINITION   Chronic illnesses caused by a person's immune cells acting on the body's own cells and tissues. Crohn's disease, lupus, and type 1 diabetes are examples of autoimmune diseases.

NOTES

A reduction in development of autoimmune diseases such as diabetes, some thyroid diseases, and multiple sclerosis has been documented in people who were breastfed as infants.

Autoimmune diseases are more common in women. A wide range of drugs are used to treat autoimmune disorders. An up-to-date drug reference should be consulted to determine the safety and possible side effects of individual drugs if they should be prescribed to the breastfeeding mother.

Newborn and premature babies are at greater risk of drug side effects due to limited ability to clear drugs from their systems.

See also **Diabetes; Thyroid disease**

➤ AUTOMATIC ELECTRIC BREAST PUMPS

DEFINITION   These fully automated devices are designed to remove milk from the lactating breast with minimal work on the part of the woman.

SELF-CARE INFORMATION

A breast pump cannot tell you how much milk you are making.

If you have concerns about milk supply, please call or see a lactation care provider.

Automatic electric breast pumps are ideally suited for women who are pumping for a baby from whom they are separated many hours daily. This includes women pumping for babies who are hospitalized in special care, as well as women who are separated from their babies due to work or school.

Automatic electric pumps can be rented or purchased from representatives of various companies.

There is no one pump that works best for all women. Please note that it is never appropriate to recommend mixing one manufacturer's pump kits with another manufacturer's pump.

Women will sometimes request a breast pump when they have doubts about their milk supply. Pumps should not be used to quantify a woman's milk supply. Refer women to a lactation care provider regarding this concern.

Hand expression may increase milk yield for women using breast pumps.

See also Breast pump

➤ AWHONN

See Association of Women's Health, Obstetric, and Neonatal Nurses (AWHONN)

➤ BABY

DEFINITION   A child younger than 12 months of age.

➤ BABY BLUES

DEFINITION   Transient mood swings experienced by more than 50% of women during the early days postpartum. Women may feel alternately giddy, sad, tearful, and anxious.

ASK ABOUT

Onset.
Age of the baby.
History of depression.

ASSESSMENT

EMERGENT CARE NEEDED?
Are any of the following present?
> Suicidal thoughts.
> Thoughts of harming baby.

IF YES,   *Seek emergency care and protective services now.*

PROMPT CARE NEEDED?
Are any of the following present?
> Persistent sadness.
> Inability to function.

IF YES,   *Seek medical care within 4 hours and seek psychological counseling today.*

SELF-CARE INFORMATION
Mood swings are normal in the postpartum period, but may become more severe.
Seek support from friends and family members.
Practice skin-to-skin contact in the first hour and frequently thereafter.
Feed the baby at least 10 times per 24 hours.

IMPORTANT CONDITIONS TO REPORT
Continuation of baby blues.
Worsening of symptoms.
History of depression, mood disorders, premenstrual syndrome, or thyroid disorders.

NOTES

While the baby blues are a common postpartum experience, women can progress to postpartum depression among other postpartum mood disorders. It is important to encourage mothers to report any worsening of symptoms.

Women who experienced depression during pregnancy and those with a prior history of depression, mood disorders, or premenstrual syndrome are at greater risk for postpartum depression.

Hypothyroidism, anemia, and other physical disorders share many symptoms with postpartum depression.

The Edinburgh Postnatal Depression Scale identifies women at risk for postpartum depression.[58]

See also Antidepressants; Edinburgh Postnatal Depression Scale; Medication Resources (inside back cover); Postpartum depression

Footnote

[58]Cox, J. L., Holden, J. M., & Sagovsky, R. (1987). Detection of postnatal depression. Development of the 10-item Edinburgh Postnatal Depression Scale. *The British Journal of Psychiatry: The Journal of Mental Science, 150,* 782–786.

Tool accessible on the Web: http://www.fresno.ucsf.edu/pediatrics/downloads/edinburghscale.pdf

➤ BABY FOOD

DEFINITION   Refers to ground, mashed, or blended foods intended for use by babies between the ages of 6 and 12 months. Baby foods may be made at home or purchased.

ASK ABOUT

Age of the baby.
Foods already introduced.

ASSESSMENT

EMERGENT CARE NEEDED?

Are any of the following present in the baby?

Difficulty breathing or swallowing.

Swelling of tongue.

IF YES, *Seek emergency care now.*

PROMPT CARE NEEDED?

Are any of the following present in the baby?

Swelling of the face, hands, or feet.

Persistent rash, headache, or fever.

Persistent diarrhea, nausea, or vomiting.

Bloody stool.

Wheezing.

IF YES, *Seek medical care within 4 hours.*

ROUTINE CARE NEEDED?

Are any of the following present in the baby?

Suspected reaction to food or medication.

Occasional nausea, vomiting, or diarrhea.

Persistent runny nose.

Rash and itching.

IF YES, *Schedule a pediatric appointment.*

SELF-CARE INFORMATION

Monitor the baby's symptoms.

Be aware of the possibility of developing allergy to other proteins.

IMPORTANT CONDITIONS TO REPORT

Family history of allergy.

Symptoms occur, worsen, persist, or reoccur.

NOTES

Exclusive breastfeeding is the ideal food for infants younger than 6 months. Around 6 months of age, babies may be introduced to solid foods as advised by their pediatric care provider. Around 12 months of age, whole cow's milk and other dairy foods may be introduced. There is limited need for commercial baby foods—family foods are often fresher and tastier.

In children of allergic families, potent allergenic foods such as cow's milk, egg whites, peanuts, and other tree nuts should be introduced per medical advice.

Care should be taken to avoid introducing foods that present choking hazards to babies and young children, including peanut butter, popcorn, hot dogs, and other sticky, hard, and rigid foods that can become lodged in the throat.

Mothers should be encouraged to continue breastfeeding as they wish throughout and beyond the first year of life.

See also Allergy in the breastfed infant; Baby-led weaning; Mixed feeds; Solid foods for breastfed babies

➤ BABY-FRIENDLY HOSPITAL INITIATIVE (BFHI)

DESCRIPTION   The Baby-Friendly Hospital Initiative (BFHI) is an international project of the United Nations Children's Fund (UNICEF) and the World Health Organization (WHO). The BFHI seeks to encourage hospitals and birth centers to implement the Ten Steps to Successful Breastfeeding, a set of best practices to ensure positive breastfeeding outcomes.

NOTES

For more information about this international program, see UNICEF: http://www.unicef.org/programme/breastfeeding/baby.htm

World Health Organization: http://www.who.int/nutrition/topics/bfhi/en/

➤ BABY-FRIENDLY USA, INC. (BFUSA)

DESCRIPTION   Baby-Friendly USA, Inc. is the national organization responsible for the implementation of the United Nations Children's Fund (UNICEF) and World Health Organization (WHO) Baby-Friendly Hospital Initiative (BFHI) in the United States. BFUSA is the accrediting body for the Baby-Friendly Hospital Initiative in the United States.

NOTES

Baby-Friendly USA
Email: info@babyfriendlyusa.org
Web: www.babyfriendlyusa.org

➤ BABY-LED WEANING

DEFINITION   A term referring to offering family foods to babies at and after the age of 6 months, rather than pureed baby foods.[59] This method has been associated with decreased obesity risk in children.[60]

Footnotes

[59]Rapley, G., & Murkett, T. (2010). *Baby-led weaning: The essential guide to introducing solid foods and helping your baby to grow up a happy and confident eater.* New York: The Experiment.

[60]Townsend, E., & Pitchford, N. J. (2012). Baby knows best? The impact of weaning style on food preferences and body mass index in early childhood in a case-controlled sample. *BMJ Open, 2*(1), e000298. doi:10.1136/bmjopen-2011-000298

➤ BACTERIA IN MOTHER'S MILK

DEFINITION   Bacteria are single celled microorganisms. Of concern in this context are those bacteria that are pathogenic.

Bacteria are a special concern in milk expressed for a premature or ill baby, or in milk collected for a donor milk bank. To avoid bacterial contamination of expressed milk for well babies, it is also important to employ careful hand-washing techniques and careful cleaning of any equipment used to collect, store, and feed milk. Breast pumps are more likely to introduce bacteria than manual expression.[61]

In the event of infant infection, it may be necessary to test mother's milk to identify if the pathogen originates with the mother or a contaminant in the expression, collection, or feeding process.

See also Antibacterial agents in breastmilk

Footnote

[61]Lawrence, R.A., & Lawrence, R. M. (2011). *Breastfeeding: A guide for the medical profession* (7th ed.). St. Louis, MO: Elsevier/Mosby.

➤ **BALT**

DEFINITION Bronchus-associated lymphoid tissue. Immunologically active tissue found within the lungs.

NOTES

The breast is thought to act as an extension of bronchus-associated lymphoid tissue (BALT). When a pathogen is breathed into the lung, BALT tissue responds by triggering the production of an immunoglobulin to attach the pathogen. The breast may also respond to the BALT trigger by manufacturing and releasing appropriate immunoglobulins to fight the organism through the milk.

See also Bioactive components of breastmilk

➤ BATTERY-OPERATED BREAST PUMP

DEFINITION   A motorized device designed to remove milk from the lactating breast using battery power.

SELF-CARE INFORMATION

A breast pump cannot tell you how much milk you are making.

If you have concerns about milk supply, please call or see a lactation care provider.

NOTES

Battery operated pumps may be suitable for women who need to pump occasionally. They can be purchased from representatives of various companies or from retailers.

There is no one pump that works best for all mothers. It is never appropriate to recommend mixing one manufacturer's pump kits with another manufacturer's pump unless the manufacturer states in writing that this is okay. Pumps in this category are not intended to be used by more than one woman. It is possible for the interior part of the pump motor to be contaminated.

Women will sometimes request a breast pump when they have doubts about their milk supply. Pumps should not be used to quantify a woman's milk supply. Hand expression may increase milk yield for women using breast pumps.

See also **Automatic electric breast pumps; Breast pump**

➤ BELLAGIO CONSENSUS

DEFINITION   A statement made in 1998 by a group of experts about the efficacy of the lactational amenorrhea method of family planning.

NOTES

In 1998, a group of specialists met in Bellagio, Italy to review what was known about the cessation of menses, or lactational amenorrhea, experienced by exclusively breast-feeding women. This group produced the Bellagio Consensus, which set forth what has been named the lactational amenorrhea method (LAM) of family planning.

Research suggests that LAM is 98% effective in the first 6 months following the birth of a baby, so long as the mother's menses have not returned (**amenorrhea**), her baby is exclusively breastfed, receiving no other foods or drinks, nursing at least eight times daily, and there are no long periods of time (6 hours or greater) between feedings, day and night. Once the baby is older than 6 months, or any of the other criteria above is no longer true, LAM is no longer effective, and women should utilize other family planning methods.

See also Amenorrhea; Lactational amenorrhea method (LAM)

➤ BENEFITS OF BREASTFEEDING

DEFINITION   Advantages of human milk over artificial replacement foods.

NOTES

Breastfeeding has innumerable positive effects for children, mothers, and society in general.
   Benefits include (but are not limited to):

Child: Optimal growth and development as well as protection against chronic and acute diseases.

Mother: Respite to recover physically from childbirth as well as protection against some chronic diseases.

Society: Less healthcare expenditure on acute and chronic illness for mothers and children; less environmental waste; far-reaching advantages from optimally healthy and bonded families.

When clients have questions about advantages of breastfeeding, refer them to a lactation care provider or medical care provider. Fathers may be particularly receptive to messages about the benefits of breastfeeding.

➤ BEST FOR BABES FOUNDATION

DESCRIPTION   "The mission of Best for Babes is to change the cultural perception of breastfeeding and Beat the Breastfeeding Booby Traps®–the cultural, institutional and legal barriers that prevent parents from making informed feeding decisions and that prevent moms from achieving their personal breastfeeding goals (whether that's 2 days, 2 months or 2 years) without judgment, pressure or guilt."[62(p1)]

Best for Babes Foundation, Inc.
P.O. Box 454
Little Silver, NJ 07739
(917) 612-8182
Email: info@bestforbabes.org
Web: www.bestforbabes.org/
   Best for Babes works to change the perception of breastfeeding through its social media presence, celebrity spokespersons, and with advertising campaigns.

Footnote

[62]Best for Babes. (2011). About us. Retrieved from http://www.bestforbabes.org/mission

➤ BETA-AGONISTS

DEFINITION   A category of drugs that mimic the effects of adrenaline on the body's beta receptors. These drugs are often used to relax the muscles of the airway, making breathing easier and reducing bronchial spasms.

NOTES

There are several different beta-agonists in use. An up-to-date drug reference should be consulted to determine the safety and possible side effects of individual drugs.
   Newborn and premature babies are at greater risk of side effects due to limited ability to clear drugs from their systems.

See also Medication Resources (inside back cover)

➤ BETA-BLOCKERS

DEFINITION   A category of drugs that block the effects of adrenaline on the body's beta receptors. These drugs are often used to reduce high blood pressure.

NOTES

There are several different beta-blockers in use. An up-to-date drug reference should be consulted to determine the safety and possible side effects of individual drugs.

Newborn and premature babies are at greater risk of side effects due to limited ability to clear drugs from their systems.

See also Medications; Medication Resources (inside back cover)

➤ BFHI

See Baby-Friendly Hospital Initiative (BFHI)

➤ BICYCLE-HORN BREAST PUMP

DEFINITION   A manually operated device designed to remove milk from the lactating breast. This particular manual pump employs a rubber bulb syringe which is compressed to generate pressure.

SELF-CARE INFORMATION

A breast pump cannot tell you how much milk you are making.

If you have concerns about milk supply, please call or see a lactation care provider.

NOTES

These inexpensive hand pumps are named for a rubber bulb syringe that the mother compresses to withdraw milk. These pumps are not recommended, due to two problems: (1) compression of the bulb can generate very high pressure, possibly injuring the breast and nipple, and (2) milk can flow backward into the bulb of most pumps of this type, creating a potential contamination problem (as the interior of the bulb cannot be cleaned thoroughly).

There is no one pump that works best for all mothers. It is never appropriate to recommend mixing one manufacturer's pump kits with another manufacturer's pump.

Pumps in this category are not intended to be used by more than one woman. It is possible for the interior of the pump to be contaminated with pathogens.

Women will sometimes request a breast pump when they have doubts about their milk supply. Pumps should not be used to quantify a woman's milk supply. Refer women to a lactation specialist regarding this concern. Hand expression may increase milk yield for women using breast pumps.

See also Breast pump

➤ BIFIDUS FACTOR

DEFINITION A group of components of human milk that stimulate the growth of *Lactobacillus bifidus*, a "friendly" bacterium, in the gut of the breastfed baby.

> **NOTES**

Lactobacillus bifidus is the predominant bacterium present in the gut of the breastfed baby. This friendly microbe helps to protect the baby's gut from infection.
  Infant formula does not contain bifidus factor.

➤ BILATERAL

DEFINITION Meaning two sides. In this context, the term refers to something occurring in or on both breasts or nipples.

➤ BILATERAL MASTITIS

DEFINITION The presence of mastitis (breast inflammation) in both breasts at the same time. Mastitis can be infective or noninfective.

> **ASK ABOUT**

Onset.
Prior breast inflammation.
Sore nipples.
Known drug allergies.

ASSESSMENT

EMERGENT CARE NEEDED?

Are any of the following present?

Visible red areas on the breast(s).

Maternal fever higher than 101°F (38.5° C).

Extreme breast discomfort.

Flu-like aching throughout body.

Continuing fever after treatment.

Reaction to antibiotic prescribed.

IF YES, *Seek emergency care now.*

PROMPT CARE NEEDED?

Are any of the following present?

Continuing symptoms after treatment.

Difficulty breastfeeding.

IF YES, *Call obstetric care provider today and call lactation care provider today.*

ROUTINE CARE NEEDED?

Are any of the following present?

Questions about treatment.

Questions about breastfeeding.

IF YES, *Call obstetric care provider today and call lactation care provider today.*

SELF-CARE INFORMATION

Breastfeed on both breasts, keeping them as soft as possible.

Take care of yourself as though you have the flu (rest in bed, drink plenty of fluids, and request help for other children and household chores).

Take medications as they have been prescribed, even after you feel better.

Call your health care provider or lactation care provider if you have questions.

IMPORTANT CONDITIONS TO REPORT

Symptoms that worsen or do not resolve.

NOTES

Bilateral presentation may indicate infection with *Streptococcus*. Lawrence and Lawrence state "bilateral mastitis should always be treated as Streptococcus unless . . . cultures disprove it. The infant needs to be treated as well."[63(p560)]

See also Breast infection; Breast inflammation

Footnote

[63]Lawrence, R. A., & Lawrence, R. M. (2011). *Breastfeeding: A guide for the medical profession* (7th ed.). St. Louis, MO: Elsevier/Mosby.

➤ BILIRUBIN

DEFINITION   A breakdown product of red blood cells. When bilirubin accumulates in the blood stream, a yellow discoloration of the skin and the whites of the eyes called **jaundice** can occur.

NOTES

Jaundice is the most common condition requiring medical treatment in the newborn period.
     Although the condition of jaundice may be benign, it can be a symptom of other serious conditions, including **kernicterus**.

See also Jaundice; Late onset jaundice

➤ BIOACTIVE COMPONENTS OF BREASTMILK

DEFINITION   Referring to living cells and other active components in human milk that stimulate growth, build the baby's immune response, and promote health.

Human milk is a rich source of bioactive factors, including antibodies, antiviral factors, white blood cells, enzymes, immune-active proteins, fats, sugars, and numerous growth and immune factors.

See also Antibacterial agents in breastmilk; Antibodies; Anti-infective agents in breastmilk; Anti-inflammatory agents in breastmilk; Bifidus factor; Bronchus-associated lymphoid tissue (BALT); Cytokine; Epidermal growth factor; Enzymes in breastmilk; Fat-soluble vitamins in breastmilk; Gut-associated lymphoid tissue (GALT); Hormones; IgA; IgE; IGF-I; Immunoglobulin; Lactoferrin; Lymphocytes; Macrophages; Mucosa-associated lymphoid tissue (MALT); Oligosaccharides in breastmilk; Secretory IgA

➤ BIOPSY, BREAST

DEFINITION   A surgical procedure performed to remove a sample of breast tissue for diagnostic purposes.

ASK ABOUT

Reason for the biopsy.
Date of biopsy.
Age of the baby.

ASSESSMENT

PROMPT CARE NEEDED?

Are any of the following present?

Biopsy scheduled in a lactating woman.
Breast or feeding problems post biopsy.

IF YES,   *Call lactation care provider today.*

ROUTINE CARE NEEDED?

Are any of the following present?

Concern about effect of past biopsy on breastfeeding.

IF YES,   *Call lactation care provider.*

SELF-CARE INFORMATION

Follow instructions about caring for biopsy site.

IMPORTANT CONDITIONS TO REPORT

Excessive leakage from biopsy site.
Increased pain.
Fever.

NOTES

Breast biopsy may be performed during lactation due to concern about masses in the breast. While many masses in the lactating breast are often associated with plugged milk ducts, galactocele growths—including cancerous ones—are possible.

Women can continue to breastfeed after biopsy, assuming they are not taking contraindicated medications. Women often need support and assistance in breastfeeding during the healing process.

Women who have had past biopsy surgery may experience decreased milk production in the segments of the breast surgically involved.

See also Abrupt weaning; Breast surgery

➤ BIRTH, CESAREAN

DEFINITION   Delivery of baby through surgical incision made through the abdomen and uterus.

ASK ABOUT

Date of cesarean section.
Age of the baby.
Feeding status.

ASSESSMENT

EMERGENT CARE NEEDED?

Are any of the following present?

The baby refuses to feed for more than 6 hours.

Exclusively breastfed baby stools less than one time daily after the first day of the newborn period.

Extreme **lethargy** or **irritability** in the baby.

Sudden change in the baby's muscle tone (extremely floppy or stiff) or repetitive jerking movements (e.g., seizure activity).

Baby shows sudden disinterest in feeding.

Inability to wake the baby.

The baby does not calm, even with cuddles.

IF YES,   *Call pediatric care provider now.*

PROMPT MEDICAL CARE NEEDED?

Are any of the following present?

Maternal temperature higher than 100.4°F.

Foul-smelling drainage or fluid from the incision.

Increased tenderness or soreness at the incision.

Incision edges are no longer together.

Redness or swelling at the incision site.

Exclusively breastfed baby stools fewer than three times daily in the newborn period (after 4th day).

IF YES,   *Call medical care provider today.*

PROMPT LACTATION CARE NEEDED?

Are any of the following present?

Breast engorgement.

Difficulty latching baby onto breast.

Difficulty finding comfortable feeding positions postsurgery.

Concerns about adequacy of milk supply.

Concerns about adequacy of infant growth.

IF YES,   *Call lactation care provider today.*

SELF-CARE INFORMATION

Practice skin-to-skin contact in the first hour and frequently thereafter.

Feed the baby at the first sign of hunger cues (signs that say "feed me" include hand-to-face or hand-to-mouth movements, lip smacking, seeking with lips, rooting, and head bobbing).

Feed the baby at least 10 times per 24 hours.

Listen for signs of the baby swallowing.

Allow the baby to end feedings.

Expect at least three infant stools per 24 hours after the first 4 days of life.

Good positioning and attachment are crucial to prevent or reduce nipple pain.

If the baby is being fed away from the breast, hand express or pump milk to maintain supply.

IMPORTANT CONDITIONS TO REPORT

Maternal fever.

Ongoing discomfort at incision site.

Ongoing difficulty with breastfeeding.

Ongoing concerns about infant growth.

Lethargy or irritability in baby.

NOTES

Mothers and babies who experience cesarean birth have greater risk of mother–baby separation, delayed breastfeeding initiation, delayed development of mature milk, and early supplementation. Mothers should be monitored to ensure that they are healing well after surgery and receiving appropriate postoperative pain relief.

A wide range of drugs are used to relieve pain. An up-to-date drug reference should be consulted to determine the safety and possible side effects of individual drugs.

Newborn and premature babies are at greater risk of side effects due to limited ability to clear drugs from their systems.

Face-to-face lactation counseling can assist mothers in finding comfortable breastfeeding positions and learning their baby's feeding cues.

See also Analgesia; Anesthesia; Childbirth; Medication Resources (inside back cover)

➤ BIRTH CONTROL

DEFINITION   Devices and drugs used to reduce fertility.

NOTES

Many contraceptive methods are compatible with breastfeeding, including all barrier methods (condoms, foam, diaphragms, and cervical caps), intrauterine devices (IUDs), and progestin-only hormonal methods.[64] Combined estrogen/progestin methods are generally not recommended as they may reduce milk supply and affect infant growth.

   The **lactational amenorrhea method (LAM)** is a form of natural family planning that is 98% effective in the first 6 months following the birth of a baby, so long as the mother's menses have not returned, her baby is exclusively breastfed, and there are no long periods of time between feedings, day and night. Once the baby is older than 6 months, or any of the above criteria is no longer true, LAM is no longer effective and mothers should utilize other forms of family planning.

See also Amenorrhea; Birth interval; Lactational Amenorrhea Method (LAM); Medications; Progestin-only contraceptives

Footnote

[64]Progestin-only injectable hormones are intended for use in breastfeeding women only after 6 weeks postdelivery, or when full milk supply is developed. Use prior to that time may decrease milk supply due to high circulating progestin levels, simulating a state of pregnancy.

➤ BIRTH INJURY

DEFINITION   Damage to the infant's body sustained during delivery.

ASK ABOUT

Type, degree, and effects of injury.

ASSESSMENT

EMERGENT CARE NEEDED?

Are any of the following present?

The baby refuses to feed for more than 6 hours.

Extreme **lethargy** or **irritability** in the baby.

Sudden change in the baby's muscle tone (extremely floppy or stiff) or repetitive jerking movements (e.g., seizure activity).

The baby shows sudden disinterest in feeding.

Unable to wake the baby.

The baby does not calm, even with cuddles.

IF YES,   *Seek emergency care now.*

PROMPT MEDICAL CARE NEEDED?

Are any of the following present?

Inadequate urine/stool output.

Infant discomfort during feeding.

IF YES,   *Seek medical care within 4 hours.*

PROMPT LACTATION CARE NEEDED?

Are any of the following present?

The baby has difficulty latching on to the breast.

The baby has difficulty sustaining feeding.

Difficulty finding comfortable feeding positioning on one breast or both.

Milk leaking from the baby's mouth during feeding.

IF YES,   *Call lactation care provider today.*

SELF-CARE INFORMATION

Practice skin-to-skin contact in the first hour and frequently thereafter.

Feed the baby at the first sign of hunger cues (signs that say "feed me" include hand-to-face or hand-to-mouth movements, lip smacking, seeking with lips, rooting, and head bobbing).

Feed the baby at least 10 times per 24 hours.

Listen for signs of the baby swallowing.

Allow the baby to end feedings.

Expect at least three infant stools per 24 hours after the first 4 days of life.

Good positioning and attachment are crucial to prevent or reduce nipple pain.

If the baby is fed away from the breast, hand express or pump milk to maintain supply.

IMPORTANT CONDITIONS TO REPORT

Persistent unresolved symptoms.

NOTES

Birth injuries are sometimes identified because of feeding problems. Birth injuries (e.g., fractured clavicle) may affect the baby's ability to feed well temporarily or permanently. Babies with birth injuries should be closely monitored for healing, development, and growth. Feeding positions may need adjustment to accommodate the baby's comfort.

Mothers may also experience injuries to soft tissue and coccyx that affect their comfort level.

A wide range of drugs are used to relieve pain. An up-to-date drug reference should be consulted to determine the safety and possible side effects of individual drugs.

Newborn and premature babies are at greater risk of side effects due to limited ability to clear drugs from their systems.

See also Breast refusal; Medication Resources (inside back cover)

➤ BIRTH INTERVAL

DEFINITION   Birth interval refers to the length of time from one birth date to the next birth date.

NOTES

Women who are exclusively breastfeeding a young baby are likely to experience a lack of menses (**amenorrhea**). Women may be amenorrheic for more than 1 year while breastfeeding.

Birth intervals of 2 years or more (international health agencies recommend 3 years or more[65]) are recommended to allow time for the mother's body to recover and replenish nutrient stores.

Women who wish to become pregnant again may consider breastfeeding less intensively to trigger resumption of their menses. Nutritionally appropriate foods should be offered to the baby when the mother begins to **wean**.

See also Amenorrhea; Lactational Amenorrhea Method (LAM); Birth control; Natural family planning

Footnote

[65]WHO. (2006). *Report of a WHO technical consultation on birth spacing.* Geneva, Switzerland: WHO. Retrieved from http://www.who.int/maternal_child_adolescent/documents/birth_spacing.pdf

➤ BIRTHWEIGHT

DEFINITION   The weight of the baby at the time of birth. Full-term babies are expected to weigh more than 5 lb, 8 oz (2,500 g). The average full-term baby born in the United States weighs more than 7 lb at birth.

Low birthweight babies weigh less than 2,500 g (5 lb, 8 oz) at birth. **Very low birthweight** babies weigh between 1,000 and 1,500 g (2 lb, 3 oz to 3 lb, 5 oz) at birth. Many low birthweight babies are born prematurely. Others are full-term babies who have experienced slow growth in the uterus—these babies are also considered small for gestational age (**SGA**).

Babies born above the 90th percentile for gestational age are considered large for gestational age (**LGA**).

NOTES

Low birthweight babies may be more challenging to feed, as they are usually premature and thus may be sleepier and more lethargic. Even if they are not premature, their smaller size and lower muscle mass may make it more difficult for them to latch well. Ongoing lactation support and attention to stool output, feeding frequency, and weight is indicated.

Babies of diabetic mothers are at increased risk of hypoglycemia and concomitant LGA status. Due to screening procedures and possibly treatment, these babies may experience more separation from their mother and a more difficult start to breastfeeding than appropriate gestational age (**AGA**) babies. Ongoing lactation support can assist in overcoming early difficulties.

➤ BITING

DEFINITION   This action occurs when the baby closes its teeth or jaw on the nipple and breast.

ASK ABOUT

Age of the baby.

ASSESSMENT

ROUTINE CARE NEEDED?

Are any of the following present?

Runny or stuffy nose in baby.

Difficulty nursing.

IF YES,   *Call pediatric care provider today and call lactation care provider today.*

Are any of the following present?

New onset of sore nipples.

Biting at the breast.

Questions about soothing the teething baby.

IF YES,   *Call lactation care provider today.*

SELF-CARE INFORMATION

Teething is a temporary (but reoccurring) stage. Teething can be difficult for some babies and families. Allowing the baby to bite down on a cool, textured teething toy prior to feeding may make feeding more comfortable.

IMPORTANT CONDITIONS TO REPORT

Difficulty breathing.

Wheezing.

Fever.

Babies do not need to be weaned because they are teething or because they have teeth, although mothers may be told this by friends or family.

Because their gums are uncomfortable, teething babies may try chewing at the breast.

Mothers may have sore nipples when the baby is teething.

Babies often have stuffy noses at the teething ages.

See also Clenching or clamping onto the nipple/areola; Sore nipples; Teething

➤ BLEB

DEFINITION   A tiny white, milky blockage of a single duct opening on the surface of the nipple. Mothers often describe excruciating, pinpoint pain at the site of the blockage, radiating back to their spine. Blebs may need to be lanced by a medical care provider.

ASK ABOUT

Onset.

Age of the baby.

History of herpes lesions or other skin conditions on breast or nipple.

ASSESSMENT

EMERGENT CARE NEEDED?

Are any of the following present?

History of herpes lesions on the nipple.

History of herpes lesions elsewhere on the mother's or partner's body with current bleb or lesion on the nipple or breast.

IF YES,   *Seek medical care now.*

PROMPT CARE NEEDED?

Are any of the following present?

Painful, protuberant bleb on nipple.

> **IF YES,**   *Seek medical care today and call lactation care provider today.*

SELF-CARE INFORMATION

If lanced, follow directions for postlancing care.

Breastfeeding can usually resume right away.

Some mothers find manual massage of the area helps the bleb to dislodge and move out of the breast. Others prefer warmth, such as a warm, wet towel.

IMPORTANT CONDITIONS TO REPORT

Symptoms of infection (fever, aching, chills, redness at site).

NOTES

Blisters may appear on the nipple and breast for several reasons, including poor latch, trauma, damage from nipple shields, abscess, and blebs.

Emergency differential diagnosis is crucial in women with history of herpes lesions on the nipple or elsewhere on the mother's or partner's body. As herpes can be fatal to the newborn, breastfeeding should be discontinued on the affected nipple until differential diagnosis is obtained. *Active herpes or chicken pox lesions on the nipple and breast are potentially life threatening to the baby.* Herpes lesions elsewhere on the body do not contraindicate breastfeeding. However, parents should practice very careful hand-washing techniques to avoid touching lesions and then touching the baby.

Other conditions to consider include poison ivy, allergic response to surface antigens (contact dermatitis), and eczema.

A bleb is a tiny white, milky blockage of a single duct opening on the surface of the nipple. Mothers often describe excruciating, pinpoint pain at the site of the blockage. Counseling and visual inspection may be required to assure correct diagnosis. A bleb "may be 'cured' or disappear when the health professional opens it with a sterile needle or lances it. It may reappear and have to be opened again."[66(p267)]

See also Blisters on nipple or breast; Nipple pain

Footnote

[66]Lawrence, R. A., & Lawrence, R. M. (2011). *Breastfeeding: A guide for the medical profession* (7th ed.). St. Louis, MO: Elsevier/Mosby.

➤ BLEEDING, BREAST

DEFINITION   Visible evidence of blood flow from the breast.

ASK ABOUT

Onset.
Age of the baby.
History of trauma or surgery to the breast.

ASSESSMENT

EMERGENT CARE NEEDED?

Are any of the following present?

Persistent bleeding from the breast between feedings.

Symptoms of infection (redness or pus at the site of bleeding, fever, chills, achiness, malaise).

Mass or lump in the breast that does not move in response to suckling or expression for 24–40 hours.

IF YES,   *Seek medical care within 4 hours.*

PROMPT CARE NEEDED?

Are any of the following present?

Bleeding during feedings.

Pain on latch.

IF YES,   *Seek lactation care within 4 hours.*

SELF-CARE INFORMATION

Practice skin-to-skin contact in the first hour and frequently thereafter.

Feed the baby at the first sign of hunger cues (signs that say "feed me" include hand-to-face or hand-to-mouth movements, lip smacking, seeking with lips, rooting, and head bobbing).

Wait for the baby to open mouth wide (greater than a 140° angle)

Pull the baby in so that his or her chin touches the breast first, and the nipple enters the mouth along the top of the tongue; this should result in a wide open mouth full of breast tissue.

The baby's lips should be flanged outward.

The baby's lips should look off-center when compared with the areola; the bottom lip should be farther away from the nipple than the top lip.

Feed the baby at least 10 times per 24 hours.

Observe for signs of the baby swallowing (sounds, pauses, etc.).

Allow the baby to end feedings.

Expect at least three infant stools per 24 hours after the first 4 days of life during the newborn period.

Good positioning and attachment are crucial to prevent or reduce nipple pain.

If the baby is fed away from the breast, hand express or pump milk to maintain supply.

IMPORTANT CONDITIONS TO REPORT

Any substance or item being used to decrease pain.

Worsening symptoms.

Persistent symptoms.

NOTES

Due to its highly vascular nature, the lactating breast may be more prone to bleeding. Blood may be seen in pumped milk. It may also appear on injured nipples. The nursing baby may spit up blood-tinged milk. Blood in the milk or coming from the breast indicates need for medical evaluation. Breast trauma, **intraductal papilloma**, and other findings are possible.

Mothers may be concerned about the safety of nursing the baby when they are bleeding. There is no reason for concern about the infant consuming small amounts of blood.

See also Bleeding, nipple; Papilloma, intraductal

➤ BLEEDING, NIPPLE

DEFINITION   Visible evidence of blood flow from the nipple.

ASK ABOUT

Onset.

Age of the baby.

History of trauma or surgery to the breast.

ASSESSMENT

EMERGENT CARE NEEDED?

Are any of the following present?

Persistent bleeding from nipple between feedings.

Symptoms of infection (redness or pus at the site of bleeding, fever, chills, achiness, malaise).

Mass or lump in the breast that does not move in response to suckling or expression for 24–40 hours.

IF YES, *Seek medical care within 4 hours.*

PROMPT CARE NEEDED?

Are any of the following present?

Bleeding during feedings.

Pain on latch.

IF YES, *Seek lactation care within 4 hours.*

SELF-CARE INFORMATION

Practice good attachment:

Watch for feeding cues and offer the breast as soon as cues are seen.

Wait for the baby to open his or her mouth wide (greater than a 140° angle).

Pull the baby in so that his or her chin touches the breast first, and the nipple enters the mouth along the top of the tongue; this should result in a wide-open mouth full of breast tissue.

Lips should be flanged outward.

The baby's lips should look off center when compared with the areola; the bottom lip should be farther away from the nipple than the top lip.

IMPORTANT CONDITIONS TO REPORT

Any substance or item being used to decrease pain.

Worsening symptoms.

Persistent symptoms.

> **NOTES**

Bleeding nipples are most often due to nipple trauma from poor breastfeeding positioning and attachment. The degree of pain women express varies widely.

Nipple pain is one of the main reasons women stop breastfeeding before they intended to do so. Nipple pain indicates need for a consultation with the lactation care provider.

Mothers may be concerned about the safety of nursing the baby when they are bleeding. There is no reason for concern about the infant consuming small amounts of blood.

See also Bleeding, breast; Nipple pain

➤ BLEEDING, POSTPARTUM HEMORRHAGE

DEFINITION   An abnormally high amount (generally more than 500 ml) of blood loss during or after delivery.

> **NOTES**

Postpartum hemorrhage is of concern related to breastfeeding because extreme blood loss can cause **Sheehan's syndrome**, an insult to the **pituitary gland**, where the hormones of lactation (**prolactin** and **oxytocin**) are manufactured. Women affected by Sheehan's syndrome may be unable to make an adequate amount of milk.

Other symptoms of this syndrome include sudden onset of hypothyroidism, diabetes insipidus, and hair loss along with menstrual irregularities. Medical evaluation should include measurement of prolactin levels before and after suckling. The extent to which women recover from Sheehan's is variable with the degree of infarct.[67]

Babies of mothers who suffered postpartum hemorrhage should be closely monitored for signs of adequate milk intake (e.g., swallowing, milk transfer, stool output) and growth.

See also Sheehan's syndrome

Footnote

[67]Lawrence, R. A., & Lawrence, R. M. (2011). *Breastfeeding: A guide for the medical profession* (7th ed.). St. Louis, MO: Elsevier/Mosby, p. 562.

➤ BLEEDING, POSTPARTUM VAGINAL

DEFINITION   Vaginal blood flow is expected after delivery. This is also called "lochia." Three types of lochia are recognized, including lochia rubra (red), lochia serosa (pink), and lochia alba (white).

Lochia rubra, a red discharge, begins after delivery and continues for 2–3 days.

Lochia serosa, a paler, pinkish discharge continues for the next week or so.

Lochia alba, a whitish discharge, starts around the 10th day postpartum and should be resolved within a month.[68]

ASK ABOUT

Onset.
Date of delivery.

ASSESSMENT

EMERGENT CARE NEEDED?

Are any of the following present?

Soaking more than one pad per hour.

Offensive odor to lochia.

Green color to lochia.

PROMPT CARE NEEDED?

Are any of the following present?

Sudden resumption of lochia rubra (bright red blood flow).

Lack of cessation of lochia rubra after 4 days postpartum.

Lack of cessation of lochia serosa.

Signs of infection (fever, chills, pain, malaise, overall aching).

Milk supply problems coupled with ongoing lochia rubra or serosa.

IF YES,   *Seek medical care within 4 hours.*

SELF-CARE INFORMATION

Monitor blood flow.

IMPORTANT CONDITIONS TO REPORT
Continuation of symptoms.
Sudden gushing of blood.
Multiple blood clots passed.
Concerns about milk supply.

NOTES

As time progresses, the volume of lochia should also decrease. Sudden return of bright red bleeding is of concern and should be evaluated medically. Retained placental fragments can be indicated by ongoing lochia rubra. In this event, mature milk production may not occur until placental fragments are expelled or removed.

See also Lochia; Retained placental fragments

Footnote
[68]Varney, H., Kriebs, J. M., Gegor, C. L. (Eds.). (2004). *Varney's midwifery* (4th ed., p. 1043). Sudbury, MA: Jones and Bartlett Publishers.

➤ BLISTERS ON NIPPLE OR BREAST

DEFINITION   A local swelling of the skin of the nipple or breast that contains fluid. May be caused by pressure of the baby's mouth or device, or by infectious or inflammatory process.

Because of the serious nature of some infectious conditions, including Herpes, women reporting rashes or lesions on the breast or nipple should be seen immediately by medical personnel to rule out contraindicated infections.

ASK ABOUT

Onset.
Age of the baby.
Known history of herpes lesions or other skin conditions.

ASSESSMENT

PROMPT MEDICAL CARE NEEDED?

Are any of the following present?

History of herpes lesions on the nipple or breast.

Blisters plus fever, aching, and systemic symptoms in the mother or baby.

History of herpes lesions elsewhere on the mother or partner's body with current bleb or lesion on the nipple or breast.

IF YES,   *Seek medical care within 4 hours.*

PROMPT LACTATION CARE NEEDED?

Are any of the following present?

Pain during breast pumping or feeding.

Trauma to the nipple or breast from pumping or feeding.

Concerns about adequacy of supply.

IF YES,   *Call lactation care provider today.*

SELF-CARE INFORMATION

Practice good attachment:

Watch the baby for hunger cues, and offer the breast as soon as cues are seen.

Place the baby so that his or her nose is opposite the nipple.

Wait for the baby to open his or her mouth wide (greater than a 140° angle).

Pull the baby in so that his or her chin touches the breast first, and the nipple enters the mouth along the top of the tongue; this should result in a wide-open mouth full of breast tissue.

The baby's lips should be flanged outward.

The baby's lips should look off center when compared with the areola; the bottom lip should be farther away from the nipple than the top lip.

IMPORTANT CONDITIONS TO REPORT

History of other skin conditions.

Known skin reaction.

Blisters may appear on the nipple and breast for several reasons, including poor latch, trauma, damage from **nipple shields**, **abscess**, and **blebs**.

Emergency differential diagnosis is crucial in women with history of herpes lesions on the nipple or elsewhere on mother's or partner's body. As herpes can be fatal to the newborn, breastfeeding should be discontinued on the affected nipple until differential diagnosis is obtained. *Active herpes or chicken pox lesions on the nipple and breast are potentially life threatening to the baby.* Herpes lesions elsewhere on the body do not contraindicate breastfeeding. However, parents should practice very careful handwashing techniques to avoid touching lesions and then touching the baby.

Other conditions to consider include poison ivy, allergic response to surface antigens (contact dermatitis), and eczema.

A **bleb** is a tiny white, milky blockage of a single duct opening on the surface of the nipple. Mothers often describe excruciating, pinpoint pain at the site of the blockage. Counseling and visual inspection may be required to assure correct diagnosis. A bleb "may be 'cured' or disappear when the health professional opens it with a sterile needle. It may reappear and have to be opened again."[69(p267)]

See also Bleb; Nipple pain; Milk blister, bleb

Footnote

[69]Lawrence, R. A., & Lawrence, R. M. (2011). *Breastfeeding: A guide for the medical profession* (7th ed.). St. Louis, MO: Elsevier/Mosby.

➤ BLOCK NURSING

DEFINITION   Nursing on the same breast for two or more feedings without nursing or otherwise releasing milk from the other breast. This strategy is often used to decrease an overly abundant milk supply.

While using this strategy to decrease milk production, mothers should be encouraged to examine their breasts frequently for any signs of inflammation or mastitis.

See also Engorgement; Mastitis; Oversupply; Plugged ducts

➤ BLOOD IN MILK

DEFINITION   Visible blood in expressed or dripped milk.

ASK ABOUT

Onset.
Age of the baby.
Trauma or injury to the breast.

ASSESSMENT

EMERGENT CARE NEEDED?

Are any of the following present?

Persistent bleeding from breast between feedings.

Symptoms of infection (redness or pus at the site of bleeding, fever, chills, achiness, malaise).

Breast lump or mass that does not move in response to suckling or expression for 24–40 hours.

IF YES,   *Seek medical care within 4 hours.*

PROMPT CARE NEEDED?

Are any of the following present?

Bleeding during feedings.

Pain on latch.

IF YES,   *Call lactation care provider today.*

ROUTINE CARE NEEDED?

Are any of the following present?

Bloody tinge to pumped milk with no other symptoms.

IF YES,   *Call lactation care provider.*

SELF-CARE INFORMATION

Practice good attachment:

Watch for feeding cues and offer the breast as soon as cues are seen.

Hold the baby so that his or her nose is opposite the nipple.

Wait for the baby to open his or her mouth wide (greater than a 140° angle).

Pull the baby in so that his or her chin touches the breast first, and the nipple enters the mouth along the top of the tongue; this should result in a wide open mouth full of breast tissue.

The baby's lips should be flanged outward.

The baby's lips should look off center when compared with the areola; the bottom lip should be farther away from the nipple than the top lip.

IMPORTANT CONDITIONS TO REPORT

Worsening symptoms.

Persistent symptoms.

NOTES

Due to its highly vascular nature, the lactating breast may be more prone to bleeding. Blood may be seen in pumped milk. It may also appear on injured nipples. The nursing baby may spit up blood-tinged milk. Blood in the milk or coming from the breast indicates need for medical evaluation. Breast trauma, intraductal **papilloma**, and other findings are possible.

Mothers may be concerned about the safety of nursing the baby when there is blood in their milk. There is no reason for concern about the infant consuming small amounts of blood.

See also Bleeding, breast; Bleeding, nipple; Rusty-pipe syndrome

➤ BLOOD IN STOOL

DEFINITION   Visible evidence of blood in the infant's stool. This finding needs immediate medical evaluation.

Blood in stool may indicate infection, reaction to protein in formula, physiologic disorder, or, in the breastfed infant, a reaction to protein in the mother's diet. If the infant is reacting to a protein in its mother's diet, the problem may be improved by an allergen avoidance diet. In this case, the mother may benefit from consultation with a dietitian or nutritionist.

See also Proctocolitis

➤ BMD

See also Bone mineral density (BMD)

➤ BONDING

DEFINITION   The complex process of parent–baby attachment, which develops over a period of weeks and months.

Mothers may feel guilty if they do not feel immediately bonded to their infant.

Several experiences can interfere with bonding, including childbirth trauma and pain, real or perceived problems for the baby, separation from the baby due to prematurity or illness, postpartum mood disorders, and familial or life stress.

Skin-to-skin contact, breastfeeding, learning soothing techniques for the baby, and receiving emotional and practical support enhance bonding.

Blanket reassurance does not help mothers with perceived bonding problems—genuine listening does. Refer mothers with concerns about bonding to a lactation care provider or parent educator.

➤ BONE LOSS

DEFINITION   Referring to the liberation of calcium from bone(s) during lactation.

NOTES

Bone mineral density (BMD) generally peaks in young adulthood. Some BMD is lost during extended breastfeeding, as calcium is liberated to be used in milk manufacture. After weaning, BMD is regained and often increased from prenatal BMD.

While eating calcium-rich foods is a healthful choice, it will not prevent bone loss from occurring during extended breastfeeding.

Women who entered pregnancy with osteoporosis or other bone density problems need ongoing medical and dietary counseling during this time.

See also Osteoporosis

➤ BONE MINERAL DENSITY (BMD)

DEFINITION   A measure of the abundance of calcium phosphate, the major mineral composing bone.

NOTES

Bone mineral density (BMD) generally peaks in young adulthood. Some BMD is lost during extended breastfeeding, as calcium is liberated to be used in milk manufacture. During and after weaning, BMD is regained and often increased from prenatal BMD.

While eating calcium-rich foods is a healthful choice, it will not prevent bone loss from occurring during extended breastfeeding.

Women who entered pregnancy with **osteoporosis** or other bone density problems need special medical and dietary counseling during this time.

See also Osteoporosis

➤ BOTTLE FEEDING

DEFINITION   Giving a baby expressed breastmilk or formula with a feeding bottle.

ASK ABOUT

Age of the baby.

Reason for bottle feeding.

PROMPT CARE NEEDED?

Are any of the following present?

The baby refuses to breastfeed after having a bottle.

The baby refuses to accept the bottle.

Questions about weaning.

IF YES,   *Call lactation care provider today.*

ROUTINE CARE NEEDED?

Are any of the following present?

Questions about bottle feeding methods or equipment.

IF YES,   *Call lactation care provider.*

SELF-CARE INFORMATION

Offer the baby comfort during change (cuddling, rocking, walking, etc.).

IMPORTANT CONDITIONS TO REPORT

Persistent feeding refusal.

NOTES

Mothers may have heard that offering a bottle to their newborn babies will cause **nipple confusion** or other problems. While there is no scientific evidence of nipple confusion, some babies seem to have more difficulty sensing the mother's softer, more pliable nipple in their mouth after being bottle fed. This may be particularly true of preterm babies and those with low muscle tone and/or neurological issues.

There are many different bottle and nipple shapes with a variety of flow rates available on the market. However, few have been studied scientifically to support any claims that they are most like the breast.

There are many alternative ways to supplement breastfed babies, including spoons, cups, **paladai**, droppers, and other feeding devices. The cup is one of the easiest feeding devices to clean. A nurse or lactation care provider should teach parents the safe method for cup feeding infants.

If a mother does not wish to or is unable to express her milk as a supplement, then the baby younger than 1 year of age should receive properly prepared infant formula in the bottle.

See also Feeding methods, alternate; Formula, infant; Paladai

➤ BOTULISM, INFANTILE

DEFINITION   An illness caused by a nerve toxin produced by *Clostridium botulinum*, resulting in symptoms of constipation, lethargy, and lack of muscle control (e.g., sudden inability to hold up one's head). These findings indicate the need for emergency care.

ASK ABOUT

Onset.
Age of the baby.

ASSESSMENT

EMERGENT CARE NEEDED?
Are any of the following present?
Extreme **lethargy** in the baby.
Sudden change in baby's muscle tone (extremely floppy or hypertense).
Sudden disinterest in feeding.

IF YES,   *Seek emergency care.*

IMPORTANT CONDITIONS TO REPORT
Administration of honey to the baby.

Botulism is uncommon in exclusively breastfed infants, whose guts are less hospitable to the *C. botulinum* spores that create this illness.

Feeding honey to a baby younger than 12 months (including putting honey on the breast or bottle nipples) is not recommended, as honey may contain botulism spores. Botulism spores are also found in the environment, particularly in soil.

See also Acute infection; Constipation; Lethargy

➤ BOVINE MILK

DEFINITION   The fluid produced by the lactating cow. Cow's milk is not recommended for children younger than 1 year of age.

Human milk and infant formula are the only appropriate milks for babies younger than 1 year of age. While cow's milk-based formula is a substitute for breastmilk, unaltered cow's milk is not, as it may lead to mineral and nutrient imbalance and bleeding in the gut. Similarly, soy and rice "milks" are not appropriate replacements for human milk or infant formula.[70]

For children between 1 and 2 years of age, whole cow's milk may be offered. Low-fat milk should not be offered until children are older than 2 years.

Concern about infant allergy is much more common than actual allergy. The American Academy of Pediatrics reports that the prevalence of infant cow's milk allergy is 2–3%.[71] The overall prevalence of childhood food allergy is 4–6%.[72]

Counseling and education should include comfort techniques for the irritable baby and coping methods for parents.

See also Allergy in the breastfed infant; Colic, infantile

Footnotes

[70]Greer, F. R., Sicherer, S. H., Burks, A. W., & and the Committee on Nutrition and Section on Allergy and Immunology. (2008). Effects of early nutritional interventions on the development of atopic disease in infants and children: The role of maternal dietary restriction, breastfeeding, timing of introduction of complementary foods, and hydrolyzed formulas. *Pediatrics, 121*(1), 183–191. doi:10.1542/peds.2007-3022

[71]American Academy of Pediatrics Committee on Nutrition. (2000). Hypoallergenic infant formulas. *Pediatrics, 106*, 346–349.

[72]Ziegler, R. S. (2003). Food allergen avoidance in prevention of food allergy in infants and children. *Pediatrics, 111*, 1662–1671.

➤ BOWEL MOVEMENTS, INFANT

DEFINITION   Fecal matter produced by the infant. In this context, stools passed daily are a good indicator of the adequacy of feeding. Exclusively breastfed newborn babies should pass at least three stools daily (fewer stools may be produced during the first 4 days of life). Four stools are expected daily beginning on day 4 with a change to yellow color. Fewer stools daily may be normal in the older breastfed baby.

ASK ABOUT

Age of the baby.
Stooling pattern.
Supplements given.

ASSESSMENT

EMERGENT CARE NEEDED?

Are any of the following present?

Exclusively breastfed newborn baby with less than one stool per day.
Meconium bowel movements after day 5 of life.
Constipation (hard stool) in a breastfed baby.
Blood in stool.
Persistent mucus in stool.
Pain with stooling.

IF YES,   *Call pediatric care provider now.*

PROMPT CARE NEEDED?

Are any of the following present?

Concern about inadequate feeding.

Concern about inadequate stooling.

Fewer than three stools daily in the exclusively breastfed baby over 4 days old.

IF YES,   *Call pediatric and lactation care provider today.*

SELF-CARE INFORMATION

Practice skin-to-skin contact in the first hour and frequently thereafter.

Feed the baby at the first sign of hunger cues (signs that say "feed me" include hand-to-face or hand-to-mouth movements, lip smacking, seeking with lips, rooting, and head bobbing).

Feed the baby at least 10 times per 24 hours.

Observe for signs of the baby swallowing (sounds, pauses, etc.).

Allow the baby to end feedings.

Expect at least three infant stools per 24 hours after the first 4 days of life during the newborn period.

Good positioning and attachment are crucial to prevent or reduce nipple pain.

If the baby is fed away from the breast, hand express or pump milk to maintain supply.

IMPORTANT CONDITIONS TO REPORT

Worsening of symptoms.

Persistent problems with bowel movements.

NOTES

Stool appearance:
All babies pass thick, black-green, tarry stool called **meconium** in the first days after birth. In the breastfed baby, meconium gives way to transitional stool, which is brownish and very soft. After 5 days of life, exclusively breastfed babies pass stool that is mustard-like in color and consistency.

Until they are started on solid foods or formula, breastfed babies have very soft, liquid stools with flecks of curd. Once other foods are introduced, the color of the stool may change back to a brownish color and be harder and more formed in shape.

Stool frequency:

Breastfed newborns pass small amounts of stool frequently during the day. They may stool during or after every feeding. *It is not normal for a breastfed newborn to go days without a bowel movement.* More than four stools daily are expected in the newborn period.

Infrequent stooling in the breastfed newborn may indicate inadequate feeding frequency (fewer than 10 feeds per 24 hours) or poor feeding dynamics. Consultation with a lactation care provider is indicated.

Rarely, constipation may be a symptom of **infantile botulism**.

See also Botulism, infantile; Constipation

➤ BRAS

DEFINITION   Clothing worn to support the breasts. Special bras that allow ease of feeding are made for breastfeeding mothers.

NOTES

Finding a comfortable nursing bra often takes some work. It is helpful to have referral information to a shop or service that will determine the appropriate size bra, as breast size changes during pregnancy and lactation. If a breastfeeding woman chooses to wear a bra, one specifically designed for breastfeeding is indicated. Pulling a regular or sports bra up over a woman's breasts or squeezing the breasts out over the top of the bra cup to feed can be the start of breast problems.

Bras that are too tight or constricting can also cause breast problems including reduced milk supply, plugged ducts, and mastitis. Some women have been told to wear a bra day and night. This is unnecessary and may cause problems. Many nursing mothers are more comfortable wearing natural fiber camisoles, sleeveless T-shirts, or tank tops with shelf bras.

There is no need for nursing mothers to wear bras around the clock. Bras are even more likely to cause breast problems when worn continuously.

See also Mastitis

➤ BREAST ABSCESS

DEFINITION   A localized collection of pus resulting from the breakdown of breast tissue. Inflammation often occurs around the abscess. Breast abscess is often the outcome of unresolved mastitis. Abscesses are typically drained through needle aspiration or by surgical incision and drainage. Antibiotic treatment will be prescribed based on suspected or cultured pathogen.

ASK ABOUT

Onset.
Prior breast infection.
Known drug allergies.

ASSESSMENT

EMERGENT CARE NEEDED?

Are any of the following present?

> Visible or palpable breast abscess.
> Fever higher than 100°F (37.7°C).
> Extreme breast discomfort.
> Flu-like aching throughout body.
> Chills.
> Continuing fever after abscess drainage.
> Reaction to antibiotic prescribed postdrainage.
> Green or odorous fluid seeping from the site after drainage.

IF YES,   *Seek medical care within 4 hours.*

PROMPT CARE NEEDED?

Are any of the following present?

> Continuation of symptoms after drainage.
> Difficulty with breastfeeding following abscess drainage.

IF YES,   *Seek medical care today and call lactation care provider today.*

ROUTINE CARE NEEDED?

Are any of the following present?

Questions about resumption of breastfeeding on the affected breast.

| IF YES, | *Call obstetric care provider today.* |

SELF-CARE INFORMATION

Finish the full course of antibiotics prescribed (unless told to stop by a prescriber).

Continue nonprescription pain relief as recommended.

Continue to monitor breasts for symptoms of recurring breast infection (redness, heat, fever, blockage, pain).

IMPORTANT CONDITIONS TO REPORT

Symptoms worsen or persist.

Signs of infection.

NOTES

Abscess indicates a need for urgent medical treatment. Symptoms include reddened areas of the breast, occasionally with a visible fluid filled sac protruding through the surface of the breast, and overall body sensation of **malaise**, aching, fever, and fatigue. Abscess may follow **mastitis**. Typical treatment includes appropriate antibiotic administration and drainage by lancing or aspiration. Presence of one identified abscess may indicate presence of multiple other abscesses, some of which may be deep in the breast, visible only by imaging technology. When symptoms do not resolve after treatment, the presence of additional abscesses must be considered.

Breastfeeding is not contraindicated on the noninvolved breast. Breastfeeding may continue on the affected breast if it is determined safe. Drainage may cause leaking of milk from severed ducts. Women may feel very ill and need practical and emotional support.

See also Acute infection; Breast infection

➤ BREAST AUGMENTATION

DEFINITION   A procedure that increases the size of the breast, typically by inserting a saline or silicone implant in the breast.

Date of the surgery.

Age of the baby.

Location of the surgical incision.

ASSESSMENT

PROMPT CARE NEEDED?

Are any of the following present?

Concerns about milk supply.

Failure of the breastfed baby to grow adequately.

IF YES,   *Seek medical care today and call lactation care provider today.*

SELF-CARE INFORMATION

Practice skin-to-skin contact in the first hour and frequently thereafter.

Feed the baby at the first sign of hunger cues (signs that say "feed me" include hand-to-face or hand-to-mouth movements, lip smacking, seeking with lips, rooting, and head bobbing).

Feed the baby at least 10 times per 24 hours.

Listen for signs of the baby swallowing.

Allow the baby to end feedings.

Expect at least three infant stools per 24 hours after the first 4 days of life.

Good positioning and attachment are crucial to prevent or reduce nipple pain.

If the baby is fed away from the breast, hand express or pump milk to maintain supply.

IMPORTANT CONDITIONS TO REPORT

Fewer than four bowel movements daily in the first month of life, after the fourth day.

Ongoing concerns or problems with milk supply.

NOTES

The location and extent of the incision may impact the sensation of the nerves in the nipple area. Loss of or decreased sensation may decrease milk-making potential. Trauma to the nerves may hinder the stimulation of the brain to release prolactin (the milk-making hormone) in response to suckling. Periareolar incisions suggest more potential injury than do incisions underneath the breast.

Babies of women who have had breast augmentation surgery should be followed closely to ensure proper milk transfer and growth even after the early weeks.

If the mother reports that she had an implant in one breast only, inquire about the reason for this surgery. If augmentation corrected breast asymmetry, there may be increased concern regarding the mother's ability to make a full milk supply. Marked asymmetry may indicate insufficient glandular tissue in both breasts.

The baby and the mother should be closely followed.

See also Breast surgery

➤ BREAST, BLEEDING FROM

DEFINITION   Visible evidence of blood flow from the breast.

ASK ABOUT

Onset.

Age of the baby.

History of trauma or surgery to the breast.

ASSESSMENT

EMERGENT CARE NEEDED?

Are any of the following present?

Persistent or significant amounts of bleeding from the breast between feedings.

Symptoms of infection (redness or pus at the site of bleeding, fever, chills, achiness, malaise).

IF YES,   *Seek medical care now.*

PROMPT CARE NEEDED?

Are any of the following present?

Small amount of bleeding after or before feedings.

Pain on latch.

IF YES,   *Call lactation care provider today.*

SELF-CARE INFORMATION

Practice good attachment:

Watch for feeding cues and offer the breast as soon as cues are seen.

Wait for the baby to open his or her mouth wide (greater than a 140° angle).

Pull the baby in so that his or her chin touches the breast first, and the nipple enters the mouth along the top of the tongue; this should result in a wide open mouth full of breast tissue.

The baby's lips should be flanged outward.

The baby's lips should look off center when compared with the areola; the bottom lip should be farther away from the nipple than the top lip.

The angle of the corner of the baby's mouth should be 140°–160°.

IMPORTANT CONDITIONS TO REPORT

Any substance or item being used to decrease pain or promote healing.

Worsening symptoms.

Persistent symptoms.

NOTES

Due to its highly vascular nature, the lactating breast may be more prone to bleeding. Blood may be seen in pumped milk. It may also appear on injured nipples. The nursing baby may spit up blood-tinged milk. Blood in the milk or coming from the breast indicates need for medical evaluation. Breast trauma, intraductal **papilloma**, and other findings are possible.

Mothers may be concerned about the safety of nursing the baby when they are bleeding. There is no reason for concern about the infant consuming small amounts of blood.

See also Bleeding, nipple; Papilloma, intraductal; Rusty-pipe syndrome (rusty-pipe milk)

➤ BREAST CANCER

DEFINITION Malignant growth within the tissues of the breast. Unexplained and unusual lumps in the lactating breast must be examined by a qualified healthcare provider.

NOTES

While many masses in the lactating breast are often associated with plugged milk ducts, other types of growths, including cancerous ones, are possible. When lumps in the breast do not resolve within 48 hours or are accompanied by other symptoms such as bleeding, fever, chills, etc., a complete breast evaluation should be performed.

Women who have previously been diagnosed and treated for breast cancer can breastfeed. Those who have had past breast surgery may experience decreased milk production in the segments of the breast surgically involved.

When cancer is identified in the lactating breast, weaning is generally indicated because of the nature of the drugs and other therapies used to treat cancer.

Breastfeeding reduces the risk of developing breast cancer in the mother and possibly the child.

See also Abrupt weaning; Biopsy, breast; Breast lumps; Breast refusal; Breast surgery; Goldsmith's sign

➤ BREAST ENGORGEMENT

DEFINITION Swelling in the breast associated with increase in the flow of blood and lymph to the breast, as well as the manufacture of milk. More common in the first days postpartum, engorgement may also occur whenever feedings are infrequent.

ASK ABOUT

Onset.
Age of the baby.
Feeding pattern.

ASSESSMENT

EMERGENT CARE NEEDED?

Are any of the following present?

Symptoms of infection (fever, aching, chills, malaise).

Red streaks on the breast.

IF YES, *Seek medical care within 4 hours.*

PROMPT CARE NEEDED?

Are any of the following present?

The baby is unable to latch on to the breast.

Engorgement is not resolving after latch-on.

IF YES,   *Call lactation care provider now.*

SELF-CARE INFORMATION

Consider soaking breasts in warm water before feeding

Gently hand express to soften breasts especially the area of the areola before feedings.

Nonprescription anti-inflammatory agents may also be helpful.

IMPORTANT CONDITIONS TO REPORT

Lack of resolution of engorgement in 24–48 hours.

Symptoms of infection (fever, chills, aching, redness, malaise).

NOTES

Engorgement is best resolved by softening the breast so that the baby can latch on to the breast. Nursing the baby offers more relief than does pumping or hand expression.

See also Breast infection; Hand expression of breastmilk

➤ BREASTFEEDING

DEFINITION   Feeding a baby milk produced by the breast.

See also Exclusive breastfeeding; Full breastfeeding

➤ BREASTFEEDING ASSESSMENT TOOLS

DEFINITION   Refers to documents or rubrics used to evaluate the adequacy of feeding. Documents include the IBFAT,[73] LAT,[74] LATCH,[75] MBA,[76] and SAIB[77] tools.

Footnotes

[73]Matthews, M. K. (1993). Assessment and suggested interventions to assist newborn breastfeeding behavior. *Journal of Human Lactation, 9*(4), 243–248.

[74]Blair, A., Cadwell, K., Turner-Maffei, C., & Brimdyr, K. (2003). The relationship between positioning, the breastfeeding dynamic, the latching process and pain in breastfeeding mothers with sore nipples. *Breastfeeding Review, 11*(2), 5–10.

[75]Jensen, D., Wallace, S., & Kelsay, P. (1994). LATCH: A breastfeeding charting system and documentation tool. *Journal of Obstetrics, Gynecology and Neonatal Nursing, 23*(1), 27–32.

[76]Mulford, C. (1992). The mother-baby assessment (MBA): An "APGAR" score for breastfeeding. *Journal of Human Lactation, 8,* 79–82.

[77]Shrago, L., & Bocar, D. (1990). The infant's contribution to breastfeeding. *Journal of Obstetrics, Gynecology and Neonatal Nursing, 19*(3), 209–215.

➤ BREASTFEEDING DURING PREGNANCY

DEFINITION If a mother becomes pregnant while she is breastfeeding a baby from a prior pregnancy, she may experience extremely sore nipples, a decrease in her milk supply, and production of colostrum. It is possible to continue breastfeeding through the pregnancy and then continue nursing the two babies together. This is called "tandem nursing."

SELF-CARE INFORMATION

Nursing during pregnancy and tandem nursing are individual choices that the mother makes for herself and her family. Although there are no reported problems with nursing during pregnancy and increased risk of premature labor, mothers with a prior history of premature birth or threatened premature labor should consider the risk as they make their decision.

Mothers should seek help for sore nipples and other discomforts of breastfeeding during pregnancy.

See also Tandem nursing

➤ BREAST, FIBROCYSTIC

DEFINITION A common breast condition in women that includes variable lumpiness, tenderness, and palpable cysts (pockets of fluid). Symptoms may change during the menstrual period. This benign condition is compatible with breastfeeding.

NOTES

Plugged ducts respond to improving breast milk drainage by moving in 24–48 hours. Lumps that do not resolve should be examined by the woman's healthcare provider to rule out plugged ducts and other problems.

   Women who have experienced fibrocystic breasts may misdiagnose plugged ducts and other breastfeeding problems as fibrocystic changes.

See also Breast lumps

➤ BREAST INFECTION

DEFINITION Invasion of the breast tissue by *Staphylococcus aureus* or other common pathogens, resulting in symptoms of red, hot, painful, swollen wedges of tissue of the breast, malaise, and overall aching. This condition is usually unilateral. Bilateral presentation may indicate infection with *Streptococcus*. Breast infection is a type of mastitis.

ASK ABOUT

Onset.
Breast involvement.

ASSESSMENT

EMERGENT CARE NEEDED?

   Are any of the following present?

      Sudden bilateral red streaks with fever, aching, chills, etc.

   IF YES,   *Seek emergency care now.*

PROMPT CARE NEEDED?

Are any of the following present?

Unilateral red streaks.

Symptoms of infection (fever, aching, chills).

IF YES,   *Call obstetric care provider now.*

SELF-CARE INFORMATION

Feed the baby at least 10 times per 24 hours.

Soften breasts between feedings with gentle hand expression.

Finish full course of antibiotics prescribed (unless told to stop by a healthcare provider).

Continue nonprescription pain relief as recommended.

Continue to monitor for symptoms of recurring breast infection (redness, heat, fever, chills, pain).

IMPORTANT CONDITIONS TO REPORT

Worsening of symptoms.

Persistence of symptoms.

Recurrence of symptoms.

NOTES

The Academy of Breastfeeding Medicine states that preferred antibiotics are "are usually penicillinase-resistant penicillins, such as dicloxacillin or flucloxacillin, 500 mg four times a day."[78(p178)]

Mothers should continue to breastfeed through the infection. There is no reason to cease breastfeeding due to concern about infecting the infant.

Occasionally breast infection does not respond to antibiotic treatment. In this case, clean-catch culture of the breastmilk may be taken to determine presence of infective organisms.

The symptoms listed previously may also indicate noninfectious inflammation due to a local reaction to overfull breast tissue. Mastitis can have both inflammatory and infectious causes.

See also Acute infection; Bilateral mastitis; Breast inflammation; Mastitis

Footnote

[78]Academy of Breastfeeding Medicine Protocol Committee. (2008). ABM clinical protocol #4: Mastitis. Revision, May 2008. *Breastfeeding Medicine: The Official Journal of the Academy of Breastfeeding Medicine*, 3(3), 177–180. doi:10.1089/bfm.2008.9993.

➤ BREAST INFLAMMATION

DEFINITION   The body's response to injury, infection, or foreign matter that results in pain, redness, swelling, and sometimes impaired function of the affected area (in this case, the breast). This is also known as **mastitis**.

ASK ABOUT

Onset.
Extent of redness and involvement.

ASSESSMENT

EMERGENT CARE NEEDED?

Are any of the following present?

Sudden bilateral red streaks with fever, aching, chills, etc.

IF YES,   *Seek emergency care now.*

PROMPT CARE NEEDED?

Are any of the following present?

Unilateral red streaks.

Symptoms of infection (fever, aching, chills, etc.).

IF YES,   *Seek medical care within 4 hours.*

SELF-CARE INFORMATION

Feed the baby at least 10 times per 24 hours.

Soften breasts between feedings with gentle hand expression.

Finish the full course of treatment prescribed (unless told to stop by a healthcare provider).

Continue nonprescription anti-inflammatory pain relief as recommended.

Continue to monitor for symptoms of recurring breast infection (redness, heat, fever, chills, pain).

IMPORTANT CONDITIONS TO REPORT

Worsening of symptoms.
Persistence of symptoms.
Recurrence of symptoms.

NOTES

Mothers with mastitis should continue to breastfeed. There is no reason to cease breastfeeding.

The symptoms listed previously may also indicate infection. Mastitis can have both inflammatory and infectious causes.

See also Acute infection; Bilateral mastitis; Breast infection; Mastitis

➤ BREAST, INSUFFICIENT GLANDULAR TISSUE

DEFINITION   A rare condition in which women have an inadequate amount of milk-making tissue in the breasts. This may be congenital or the result of trauma or surgery to the chest. Asymmetry between the breasts may be a hallmark of this condition.

ASK ABOUT

Onset.
Age of the baby.

ASSESSMENT

PROMPT CARE NEEDED?

Are any of the following present?

Failure of breastfed baby to grow adequately.

IF YES,   *Seek medical care today and call lactation care provider today.*

ROUTINE CARE NEEDED?

Are any of the following present?

Reported asymmetry with no concerns about milk supply or infant growth.

IF YES,   *Call lactation care provider.*

SELF-CARE INFORMATION

Practice skin-to-skin contact in the first hour and frequently thereafter.

Feed the baby at the first sign of hunger cues (signs that say "feed me" include hand-to-face or hand-to-mouth movements, lip smacking, seeking with lips, rooting, and head bobbing).

Feed the baby at least 10 times per 24 hours.

Listen for signs of the baby swallowing.

Allow the baby to end feedings.

Expect at least three infant stools per 24 hours after the first 4 days of life.

Good positioning and attachment are crucial.

If the baby is fed away from the breast, hand express or pump milk or both to maintain supply.

IMPORTANT CONDITIONS TO REPORT

Feeding or stooling expectations are not met.

NOTES

Growth of the baby should be closely followed even after the early weeks by the pediatric healthcare provider.

One sign of possible insufficient glandular tissue is marked asymmetry of the breasts. This may indicate problems with glandular tissue in both breasts. If the mother reports that she had an implant in one breast only, inquire about the reason for this surgery. If the surgery was to correct breast asymmetry, there may be increased concern regarding the mother's ability to make a full milk supply. Marked asymmetry may indicate insufficient glandular tissue in both breasts. Milk transfer and infant growth should be monitored closely.

See also Asymmetric breasts; Insufficient milk supply

➤ BREAST LUMPS

DEFINITION Hard, knotty areas inside the breast. In the lactating breast, these are commonly due to overfull milk ducts and alveoli or exterior pressure on the milk-making cells due to restrictive clothing, bras, etc. These are called "**plugged ducts.**" Lumps may also be fibroadenomas, fibrocystic changes, **abscesses**, and, rarely, cancerous tumors.

ASK ABOUT

Onset.

Location of lumps.

Whether unilateral or bilateral.

ASSESSMENT

PROMPT CARE NEEDED?

Are any of the following present?

Presence of a lump that has not responded to changes in feeding position and frequency for 24–48 hours.

Symptoms of inflammation or infection (fever, redness, malaise, chills, achiness) in the mother.

Concerns about breastfeeding.

IF YES, *Seek medical care within 4 hours and call lactation care provider today.*

SELF-CARE INFORMATION

Check for and remove any restrictive clothing.

Practice good attachment:

Watch the baby for hunger cues and offer the breast as soon as cues are seen.

Place the baby so that his or her nose is opposite the nipple.

Wait for the baby to open his or her mouth wide (greater than a 140° angle).

Pull the baby in so that his or her chin touches the breast first, and the nipple enters the mouth along the top of the tongue; this should result in a wide-open mouth full of breast tissue.

The baby's lips should be flanged outward. The mouth should be open to 140°–160°.

The baby's lips should look off center when compared with the areola; the bottom lip should be farther away from the nipple than the top lip.

Try nursing the baby in positions where the baby's chin points toward the lumpy area.

Massage the affected areas gently during nursing.

Consider warm soaks before feedings and cool gel packs on affected areas between feedings.

Monitor body temperature.

Watch for signs of infection.

Some mothers find manual massage of the area helps the lump to dislodge and move out of the breast. Others prefer warmth, such as a warm, wet towel.

IMPORTANT CONDITIONS TO REPORT

Worsening of symptoms.

Persistence of symptoms—call if lumps do not resolve in 24–48 hours.

Symptoms of infection.

NOTES

Lumps that do not resolve (after making changes in feeding pattern and position) within 48 hours should be assessed by the mother's medical care provider.

See also **Breast abscess; Breast infection; Breast inflammation; Mastitis**

➤ BREAST MASSAGE

DEFINITION   Gentle stroking technique used to encourage milk to flow from the breast.

NOTES

Care should be taken to avoid bruising the sensitive tissue of the lactating breast.

A technique called **alternate breast massage** is used during breastfeeding with sleepy or inefficient feeders, especially those who are premature or have low muscle tone. When the suckling baby pauses, the mother gently but firmly massages and compresses the breast the baby is attached to, thereby increasing the flow of milk and starting the suckling again.

See also **Alternate breast massage**

➤ BREASTMILK, ABNORMAL SECRETION

DEFINITION   Production of milk from the breast that is outside normal expectations. This condition, also called galactorrhea, can include production of milk by women who are neither pregnant nor lactating, as well as both excessive and inadequate amounts of milk produced during lactation.

ASK ABOUT

Onset.

ASSESSMENT

PROMPT MEDICAL CARE NEEDED?

Are any of the following present?

Less than 1 stool per 24 hours in a breastfed newborn.

Refusal to feed for longer than 6 hours in a newborn infant.

Baby who cries inconsolably.

IF YES,   *Seek medical care within 4 hours.*

Are any of the following present?

Production of milk in a nonlactating, nonpregnant woman.

IF YES,   *Call primary care provider today.*

PROMPT LACTATION CARE NEEDED?

Are any of the following present?

Concern about inadequate milk supply.

Concern about overabundant milk supply.

Fewer than three stools daily in a breastfed newborn.

Less than 0.5 oz gain daily by breastfed newborn.

Excessively large or frequent stools in a breastfed baby.

Recurrent engorgement or mastitis.

Colic symptoms in the baby.

IF YES,   *Call pediatric and lactation care providers today.*

SELF-CARE INFORMATION

Frequency of feeding and amount of milk removal drives milk supply. The cause of milk production above that should be investigated.

IMPORTANT CONDITIONS TO REPORT

Worsening of symptoms.

Continuation of symptoms.

Ongoing concerns.

NOTES

Because production of milk relies on many different body systems in both the mother and the baby, any milk supply problem requires consideration of maternal and infant factors. Occasionally, medical factors such as endocrine imbalance require evaluation.

It is common for mothers to continue to produce milk for prolonged periods after weaning.

See also Galactorrhea; Insufficient milk supply; Milk production; Overactive let-down reflex

➤ BREASTMILK, ENVIRONMENTAL CONTAMINANTS

DEFINITION   All foods, including breastmilk, may contain traces of chemical contaminants present in the environment. Breastmilk is one of the easiest and least painful body tissues to sample. For this reason, it is used to monitor population exposure to chemicals. Low-level exposure to contaminants should not contraindicate breastfeeding. The greatest exposure for the baby is during pregnancy.[79]

ASK ABOUT

Known contaminant exposure.

Age of the baby.

ASSESSMENT

EMERGENT CARE NEEDED?

Sudden exposure of the mother to toxic chemical.

IF YES, *Seek emergency care now.*

PROMPT CARE NEEDED?

History of past high level exposure to toxic chemicals in a breastfeeding woman.

IF YES, *Seek medical care today.*

ROUTINE CARE NEEDED?

General questions about environmental exposure.

IF YES, *Call lactation care provider today.*

IMPORTANT CONDITIONS TO REPORT

Known history of environmental or workplace exposure to toxic chemicals.
Any negative effects of past exposure.

NOTES

Women who know they have been exposed to specific chemicals or pollutants should consult with their physician regarding analysis of the contaminant content of their milk.

Researchers have looked for negative effects of background toxin exposure via breastmilk and found only benefits for breastfed babies, as compared with formula-fed babies.

See also Pesticides and pollutants in breastmilk

Footnote

[79]Lawrence, R. A., & Lawrence, R. M. (2011). *Breastfeeding: A guide for the medical profession* (7th ed.). St. Louis, MO: Elsevier/Mosby, p. 396.

➤ BREASTMILK FOR PRETERM INFANTS

DEFINITION   A preterm infant is any infant born before 37 weeks' gestation. Multiple pregnancy (e.g., twins) accounts for 15% of all premature births.

SELF-CARE INFORMATION

Express milk via hand expression for the first few days, then add pumping with a double-pumping kit and hospital grade pump eight or more times daily followed by hand expression while the baby is hospitalized.

Ask the baby's nurse for instructions for the collection and storage of milk.

Ask how soon the mother can hold the baby skin to skin (kangaroo care).

Premature babies can learn to breastfeed. Seek skilled lactation help.

NOTES

The preterm infant may require specialized care in a nursery until closer to the due date when his or her organ systems have developed enough to sustain life without specialized support. Depending on the extent of prematurity, this may take weeks or months.

Mothers of premature infants should begin expressing milk as soon as possible and do so regularly in order to increase the supply for the growing baby.

For about the first 30 days after she gives birth, the mother of the premature baby will produce milk that is higher in some of the components the baby needs.

See also Preterm milk

➤ BREASTMILK JAUNDICE

See Jaundice; Late onset jaundice

➤ BREASTMILK SECRETION

DEFINITION   Within the mammary gland, the production of a complete food for human infants.

The hormonal changes of pregnancy and birth trigger milk production in the breast. The first milk, called **colostrum**, begins in mid-pregnancy. Some mothers see dried yellowish secretions on their nipples in this phase.

Following birth of the baby and complete birth of the placenta, the breasts begin to produce mature milk. Increase in breast fullness, prominence of veins, and slight fever around days 2–5 postpartum indicate the production of mature milk.

To facilitate milk making, babies should be breastfed in response to hunger cues, at least 10 times per 24 hours. Frequent nipple stimulation and milk removal stimulate the hormones **prolactin** and **oxytocin** that control the manufacture and release of milk.

There is no known limit to the amount of milk that a woman can make. Case studies of mothers producing enough milk for quadruplets have been published. This is possible due to the supply and demand nature of milk production.

Some nursing mothers produce too little or too much milk. Refer to a lactation care provider for evaluation of milk supply questions. Occasionally medical factors such as endocrine imbalance may require evaluation.

Secretion of milk may happen outside of pregnancy and lactation in response to hormonal changes, pituitary conditions, and drug side effects. This condition, called **galactorrhea**, requires medical evaluation.

See also Feeding cues; Galactorrhea; Insufficient milk supply

➤ BREAST PADS

DEFINITION   Cloth or paper placed inside the bra to absorb leaked milk. Pads may be reusable or disposable.

SELF-CARE INFORMATION

Choose soft, absorbent pads.

Replace damp pads with fresh ones frequently to avoid irritation.

Avoid waterproof or plastic-lined pads.

Pads may be easily made by cutting appropriately sized circles out of new cloth diapers (edge stitching is recommended to hold the pad together in the wash).

Many baby supply, breast pump, and nursing bra companies carry pads designed for breastfeeding mothers. Caution mothers to change pads frequently and to avoid water-proof pads.

➤ BREAST PAIN

DEFINITION   Uncomfortable sensations in the breast. Pain is not an expected part of breastfeeding and indicates need for feeding evaluation.

There can be many reasons for pain in the breast including breast infection or inflammation, clogs, or cysts. Poor latch-on or positioning is a common reason for pain.

ASK ABOUT

Onset.
Location of pain.
Whether unilateral or bilateral.

ASSESSMENT

PROMPT MEDICAL CARE NEEDED?

Are any of the following present?

Constant pain.

Pain combined with color change of nipple(s).

Pain with visible fissure or bleeding of the nipple.

IF YES,   *Seek medical care within 4 hours.*

PROMPT LACTATION CARE NEEDED?

Are any of the following present?

Pain with feeding.

Pain between feedings.

IF YES,   *Seek lactation care within 4 hours.*

ROUTINE CARE NEEDED?

Are any of the following present?

Brief pain at beginning of feeding.

Mild recurrent pain.

IF YES,   *Call lactation care provider today.*

SELF-CARE INFORMATION

Practice skin-to-skin contact in the first hour and frequently thereafter.

Feed the baby at the first sign of hunger cues (signs that say "feed me" include hand-to-face or hand-to-mouth movements, lip smacking, seeking with lips, rooting, and head bobbing).

Feed the baby at least 10 times per 24 hours.

Listen for signs of the baby swallowing.

Allow the baby to end feedings.

Expect at least three infant stools per 24 hours after the first 4 days of life until 1 month of age.

Good positioning and attachment are crucial to prevent or reduce nipple pain.

IMPORTANT CONDITIONS TO REPORT

Symptoms worsen or persist.

Signs of infection.

Feeding or stooling expectations are not met.

NOTES

Breastfeeding should not be painful. Advise mothers to seek medical or lactation care for breast pain.

See also Latch-on; Nipple pain

➤ BREAST, PREPARATION FOR BREASTFEEDING DURING PREGNANCY

DEFINITION   The best preparation for breastfeeding is reading and learning about breastfeeding and connecting with community breastfeeding groups and resources.

No physical preparation is suggested for breastfeeding. Outdated practices such as toughening up nipples by brushing, toweling, or pulling are no longer recommended and may actually cause damage to the skin or trigger uterine contractions.

➤ BREAST PUMP

DEFINITION   A device designed to remove milk from the lactating breast.

SELF-CARE INFORMATION

A breast pump cannot tell you how much milk you are making.

If you have concerns about milk supply, please call or see a lactation care provider.

Problems with pumps should be reported to the manufacturer and the U.S. Food and Drug Administration (FDA). The FDA's Manufacturer and User Facility Device Experience Database (MAUDE) contains prior complaints filed about pumps. Visit http://www.accessdata.fda.gov/scripts/cdrh/cfdocs/cfMAUDE /search.CFM for more information.

A plethora of breast pumps are available. Styles, intended uses, and costs vary widely. There is no one pump that works best for all mothers. It is not appropriate to mix one manufacturer's pump kits with another manufacturer's pump, unless recommended by the manufacturer.

Pumps can be rented or purchased from representatives of various companies.

Most pumps (with the exception of rental grade models) are not intended to be shared between women. It is possible for the interior part of these pump motors to be contaminated with microorganisms.

Women will sometimes request a breast pump when they have doubts about their milk supply. Pumps should not be used to quantify or give reassurance about a woman's milk supply. Refer a woman to a lactation care provider if she has concerns about her milk supply.

See also Automatic electric breast pumps; Battery-operated breast pump; Hand expression of breastmilk; Manual pump

➤ BREAST, RASH AND SKIN LESIONS

DEFINITION   Red bumps or infected patches of skin on the breast or nipple can reflect infectious or allergic conditions. Because of the serious nature of some infectious conditions, including herpes, women reporting rashes or lesions on the breast should be seen immediately by medical personnel.

ASK ABOUT

Onset.
Age of the baby.
Known history of herpes lesions or other skin conditions.

ASSESSMENT

EMERGENT CARE NEEDED?

Are any of the following present?

History of herpes lesions on the nipple or breast.
Rash or lesions plus fever, aching, chills, malaise in mother or baby.
Rash or lesion on the breast with a history of herpes elsewhere on the mother or partner's body.

IF YES,   *Seek emergency care now.*

PROMPT CARE NEEDED?

Are any of the following present?

Pain during breastfeeding.
Trauma to nipple or breast from feeding.

IF YES,   *Call lactation care provider now.*

SELF-CARE INFORMATION

Practice good attachment:

Watch for feeding cues and offer the breast as soon as cues are seen.
Wait for the baby to open his or her mouth wide (greater than a 140° angle).
Pull the baby in so that his or her chin touches the breast first, and the nipple enters the mouth along the top of the tongue; this should result in a wide-open mouth full of breast tissue.

Lips should be flanged outward.

The baby's lips should look off center when compared with the areola; the bottom lip should be farther away from the nipple than the top lip.

IMPORTANT CONDITIONS TO REPORT

History of other skin conditions.

Known skin reactions.

NOTES

Rash or lesions may appear on the nipple and breast for several reasons, including eczema, psoriasis, topical allergy or sensitivity, poison ivy, chicken pox, poor latch, trauma, damage from nipple shields, **abscess**, or **blebs**.

   Emergency differential diagnosis is crucial in women with history of herpes lesions on the nipple. As herpes can be fatal to the newborn, breastfeeding should be discontinued on the affected nipple until differential diagnosis is obtained. *Active herpes or chicken pox lesions on the nipple and breast are potentially life threatening for the baby.* Herpes lesions elsewhere on the body do not contraindicate breastfeeding. However, parents should practice very careful hand-washing techniques to avoid touching lesions and then touching the baby.

See also Bleb; Blisters on nipple or breast; Contraindicated conditions; Nipple pain

➤ BREAST REDUCTION

DEFINITION   A procedure that decreases the size of the breast by removing fat and glandular tissue from the breast. Reduction surgery is likely to alter a woman's ability to make milk.

ASK ABOUT

Onset.

Type of procedure.

ASSESSMENT

PROMPT MEDICAL CARE NEEDED?

Are any of the following present?

Inadequate stooling pattern (less than three stools daily) in newborn period after 4th day.

Inadequate weight gain (less than 0.5 oz daily) in the early months.

Inadequate feeding (fewer than 10 times daily in the newborn period).

IF YES,   *Call pediatric care provider now.*

PROMPT LACTATION CARE NEEDED?

Are any of the following present?

Concerns about milk supply.

Concerns about infant weight gain.

IF YES,   *Call lactation care provider today.*

SELF-CARE INFORMATION

Monitor the baby's feeding, stooling, and urination daily.

Practice skin-to-skin contact in the first hour and frequently thereafter.

Feed the baby at the first sign of hunger cues (signs that say "feed me" include hand-to-face or hand-to-mouth movements, lip smacking, seeking with lips, rooting, and head bobbing).

Feed the baby at least 10 times per 24 hours.

Listen for signs of the baby swallowing.

Allow the baby to end feedings.

Expect at least three infant stools per 24 hours after the first 4 days of life.

Good positioning and attachment are crucial to prevent or reduce nipple pain.

If the baby is fed away from the breast, hand express or pump milk to maintain supply.

IMPORTANT CONDITIONS TO REPORT

Inadequate feeding (fewer than 10 feedings daily in the newborn).

Inadequate stooling pattern (fewer than three stools daily after 4th day).

Ongoing concerns.

It is not possible to predict the degree of lactation success prenatally. Women who are interested in breastfeeding should be supported to do so with ongoing, proactive monitoring of milk transfer and the baby's growth.

Surgical techniques that include complete removal of the nipple are more likely to impact innervation of the nipple (and thus the production of appropriate hormones through neuroendocrine pathways). Postsurgical nipple sensation may indicate the extent to which innervation has been altered.

Pedicle techniques that preserve nipple attachment may have a lesser impact on potential for milk production.

See also Breast surgery; Insufficient milk supply

➤ BREAST REFUSAL

DEFINITION   Sudden rejection of the breast by the baby.

ASK ABOUT

Onset.
Age of the baby.

ASSESSMENT

EMERGENT CARE NEEDED?

Are any of the following present?

Extreme lethargy or irritability in the baby.

Sudden change in the baby's muscle tone (extremely floppy or stiff).

Sudden disinterest in feeding.

Inability to wake baby.

Baby does not calm, even with cuddles.

IF YES,   *Seek emergency care now.*

PROMPT CARE NEEDED?

Are any of the following present?

Refusal to feed.

Repeated refusal of one breast.

IF YES, *Call lactation care provider today.*

SELF-CARE INFORMATION

Express milk from the refused breast(s) as many times daily as the baby would generally nurse.

Practice skin-to-skin contact with the baby, particularly at sleepy times.

Do not force the baby to the breast.

Make sure the baby is adequately fed (give expressed milk via cup, spoon, or dropper).

IMPORTANT CONDITIONS TO REPORT

Persistent or recurrent refusal.

Presence of ear infection or teething.

NOTES

Rarely, babies experience life-threatening infections or events that cause extreme lethargy and disinterest in feeding. They may be suddenly floppy or stiff. These symptoms indicate a medical emergency.

Occasionally, babies suddenly refuse to nurse from one or both breasts. This is often considered a **nursing strike**, rather than weaning. Typically it is an indication that something is troubling the baby. Troubles can range from stuffy nose, teething, and ear infection to a negative reaction to mother–baby separation or family stress. Strategies for overcoming a nursing strike include not forcing nursing, offering lots of cuddling and holding, having the mom lie down beside a sleepy baby and offering the breast, having the mom and baby take a bath together, and applying peer pressure by bringing the baby in contact with other nursing babies. When nursing strike persists, the baby should be examined to rule out ear infection or other contributing factors.

The mother may need assistance with expressing milk to continue her milk supply during this phase. She may be helped by exploring her reaction to the baby's refusal to nurse.

A mother whose baby refuses the same breast consistently and without explanation should be referred for breast evaluation and should be routinely monitored for breast cancer. Cancer has been diagnosed as late as 5 years after persistent breast refusal. This phenomenon is referred to as **Goldsmith's sign**.[80]

See also Goldsmith's sign; Nursing strike; Refusal of infant to breastfeed

Footnote

[80]Saber, A., Dardik, H., Ibrahim, I. M., & Wolodiger, F. (1996). The milk rejection sign: A natural tumor marker. *The American Surgeon, 62,* 998–999.

➤ BREAST SHELLS

DEFINITION   Hard plastic devices designed to be worn between the breast and the bra in order to surround the nipples with air and to hold clothing away from the breast.

NOTES

Mothers who request breast shells may be experiencing nipple or breast pain and should be referred to the lactation care provider for evaluation.

Breast shells have been recommended for women with inverted nipples. However, research does not support claims that these devices alter nipple inversion.

Repeated use of breast shells has been associated with increased risk of mastitis, perhaps due to the pressure placed on the breast.

See also **Breast pain; Inverted nipples; Nipple pain**

➤ BREAST STIMULATION

DEFINITION   Massage and stroking of the breast to trigger the flow of milk by increasing the hormones of lactation.

NOTES

Nursing babies are the best breast stimulators.

When mothers are separated from their babies, gentle manual stimulation of the breast and nipple may assist with milk collection.[81]

See also **Alternate breast massage; Hand expression of breastmilk; Milk production**

Footnote

[81]Jones, E., Dimmock, P. W., & Spencer, S. A. (2001). A randomised controlled trial to compare methods of milk expression after preterm delivery. *Archives of Disease in Childhood, Fetal & Neonatal Edition, 85*(2), F91–F95.

➤ BREAST STORAGE CAPACITY

DEFINITION   Referring to the potential milk-holding space within the breast.

NOTES

Research has identified a wide range of internal storage capacity among women.[82] Storage capacity may be the controlling factor in frequency of feeding, as mothers with larger capacity may be able to go longer between feedings.

Women with small breasts may be told that they will have trouble making enough milk. Research does not support this belief. Fat deposits are the major contributor to breast size.

Mothers should be encouraged to follow the baby's **feeding cues** to determine feeding frequency, rather than any external schedule. Signs that say "feed me" include hand-to-face or hand-to-mouth movements, lip smacking, seeking with lips, rooting, and head bobbing. Crying is a late indicator of hunger and should not be used to determine feeding needs.

See also Feeding cues; Milk production

Footnote

[82]Cregan, M. D., & Hartmann, P. E. (1999). Computerized breast measurement from conception to weaning: Clinical implications. *Journal of Human Lactation, 15*(2), 89–96.

➤ BREAST STRUCTURE

DEFINITION   Refers to the tissues within the breast that contribute to the production of milk.

Internal breast structure involved in making milk includes millions of clusters of **alveoli** or milk-making cells connected via ductules and **ducts** that carry milk to pores in the nipples. The average breast is thought to have nine ducts connecting to separate **lobes** of milk-making tissue, articulated with nine pores in the surface of the nipple.[83]

External breast structure includes the breast, nipple, areola (circle of dark pigment surrounding the nipple), and **Montgomery's glands** (sebaceous and alveolar tissue providing lubrication and protection to the nipple–areolar complex).

The breast is supported by **Cooper's ligaments**.

Milk is manufactured with nutrients carried to the breast through the arteries, arterioles, and capillaries of the intercostal (rib cage area) and thoracic arteries. Extensive lymphatic drainage of the breast helps maintain the health of mammary tissue. Sensation of the nipples and breasts is provided through extensive branching of the fourth, fifth, and sixth intercostal nerves.

Breast tissue tends to extend into the axillary (armpit) area.

Normal variations in breast structure include size and number of the breasts, nipples, areola, and Montgomery's glands. Women may have extra accessory breast or nipple tissue anywhere on the ventral surface of their trunk, as well as in the axillary, groin, and upper thigh area.

Women with small breasts may be told that they will have trouble making enough milk. Research does not support this at all. Fat deposits are the major contributor to breast size.

See also Milk production

Footnote

[83]Ramsay, D. T., Kent, J. C., Hartmann, R. A., & Hartmann, P. E. (2005). Anatomy of the lactating human breast redefined with ultrasound imaging. *Journal of Anatomy, 206*(6), 525–534.

➤ BREAST SURGERY

DEFINITION   Surgical procedures of many types, including breast **biopsy, abscess drainage, augmentation,** or **reduction**, may impact breastfeeding.

NOTES

Medical and lactation evaluation are indicated for breastfeeding women who have had breast surgery.

See also Augmentation surgery; Biopsy, breast; Breast augmentation; Breast reduction

➤ BREATHING, SUCKING, SWALLOWING

DEFINITION   These three reflexes must be coordinated in order for feeding to be successful.

ASK ABOUT

Gestational age of the baby at birth.

ASSESSMENT

PROMPT CARE NEEDED?

Are any of the following present?

Sputtering, choking, or gagging at the breast in the newborn.

IF YES,   *Call pediatric care provider and lactation care provider now.*

NOTES

Newborn babies who are unable to coordinate breathing, sucking, and swallowing should be referred for immediate medical evaluation. If untreated, babies may be at risk for aspiration.

Coordination of the suck, swallow, and breathe reflexes is thought to occur around 32 weeks' gestation, although it has been observed as early as 28 weeks in some babies.

In the older baby, problems with these reflexes may reflect nasal congestion, gastroesophageal reflux, overabundant milk supply, or overactive milk ejection. Routine medical and lactation evaluation is indicated.

See also Uncoordinated suckling; Weak suck

➤ BRONCHUS-ASSOCIATED LYMPHOID TISSUE (BALT)

DEFINITION   Immunologically active tissue found within the lungs.

NOTES

The breast is thought to act as an extension of bronchus-associated lymphoid tissue (BALT). When a pathogen is breathed into the lung, BALT tissue responds by triggering the production of an immunoglobulin to attach the pathogen. The breast may also respond to the BALT trigger by manufacturing and releasing appropriate immuno-globulins to fight the organism through the milk.

See also Bioactive components of breastmilk

➤ BURPING

DEFINITION   Referring to the practice of placing the baby upright after feeding (or between sides when breastfeeding) and patting baby's back gently to encourage the release of air from the stomach.

NOTES

Babies who take in a lot of air with their milk may need help with burping after feeding. Babies who feed calmly at the breast, without periods of crying or gasping, may not need to be burped. Mothers who work diligently at burping with no success may feel frustrated. In this event, they should be relieved of burping duty.

Babies who spit up routinely should be gently burped or held in an upright position after feeding to assist them in removing gas from their stomachs with minimal milk loss.

➤ CABBAGE LEAVES FOR ENGORGEMENT

DEFINITION   The use of cabbage leaves in the bra or a preparation of cabbage leaves applied to the breast has been suggested as a treatment for breast engorgement. Research has not identified any difference between cabbage leaves and cool gel packs in reducing engorgement.[84]

Cabbage has been acknowledged as a carrier of *Listeria monocytogenes*, which is associated with serious infection, listeriosis. Therefore, in the event that cool applications are preferred by the mother, cool gel packs are recommended rather than cabbage.

See also Engorgement

Footnote

[84]Mangesi, L., & Dowswell, T. (2010). Treatments for breast engorgement during lactation. *Cochrane Database of Systematic Reviews (Online)*, (9), CD006946. doi:10.1002/14651858.CD006946.pub2

➤ CAFFEINE

DEFINITION A chemical alkaloid with central nervous system stimulant properties. Caffeine is found in coffee beans, tea leaves, and cacao, among other plants. Breastfeeding mothers should moderate their caffeine usage. Caffeine use can result in physical dependence.

Caffeine is considered usually compatible with breastfeeding. Hale lists caffeine as an L2 (safer) drug.[85]

Mothers of premature babies and babies with cardiac problems should limit caffeine intake and should report what they do consume to baby's pediatric care provider. This is due to the routine practice of giving caffeine to premature babies in order to treat apnea.

Asthmatic women who take theophylline may need to be monitored for cumulative effects of this drug in combination with any dietary caffeine.

Rarely, mother's caffeine consumption may cause irritability or sleeplessness in her baby.

Caffeine content of coffee, tea, soda, and chocolate varies widely with brand and brewing method.

See also Medications

Footnote

[85]Hale, T. W. (2010) Medications and mothers milk (14th ed.). Amarillo, TX: Hale Publishing, p. 150.

➤ CALCIUM

DEFINITION   An important mineral for bone health, proper functioning of heart, muscles, nerves, and blood clotting. The recommended dietary allowance for calcium in lactating women older than 19 years of age is 1,000 mg per day. Women younger than 18 years require 1,300 mg.

It is not possible to increase the calcium content of a mother's milk by increasing her calcium intake.

Extra calcium during lactation will not prevent bone loss, which is recovered during weaning.[86] However, calcium is an important mineral for women to consume throughout their life in order to preserve bone density and health.

Women who entered pregnancy with osteoporosis or other bone density problems and women who do not consume dairy foods should be evaluated by their healthcare provider or dietary counselor during this time.

The following table provides the calcium content averages of various foods:

Selected Calcium-Rich Foods	Calcium (mg)
Low-fat yogurt, 8 oz	400
Sardines with bones, 3 oz	345
Low-fat milk, 8 oz	300
Cheddar cheese, 1 oz	200
Collards, ½ c	180
Tofu (with calcium sulfate), 4 oz	145
Kale, ½ c	100
American cheese, 1 oz	100

See also Bone loss; Bone mineral density (BMD); Osteoporosis

Footnote

[86]Kalkwarf, H. J. (2004). Lactation and maternal bone health. *Advances in Experimental Medicine and Biology, 554,* 101–114.

➤ CALORIC DENSITY OF BREASTMILK

DEFINITION The number of calories per unit of measure. Human milk is considered to average around 20 calories per ounce, although there is a range of published values, reflecting the difficulty of finding representative samples of milk. Fat content in milk varies throughout the day and within each feeding, depending on diurnal variation as well as how full the breast is and how well the baby or pump is eliciting the milk ejection reflex, which flushes fat down through the breast.

NOTES

Women may question the nutrient, fat, or caloric content of their milk. It is very rare for the nutrient composition of human milk to be inadequate. Routine testing of the fat or other content of milk is not recommended, due to diurnal variation and the difficulty of collecting a representative sample.

Evaluation of baby's growth, stooling pattern, feeding frequency, milk transfer, and feeding mechanics should occur when doubts arise about milk adequacy.

See also Weight gain, baby–high; Weight gain, baby–low

➤ CALORIC INTAKE OF BABY

DEFINITION The amount of energy, as measured by kilocalories, consumed by the infant daily. The Dietary Reference Intakes (DRI) for infants between 0 and 6 months are 570 kcals for males and 520 kcals for females. The DRI for infants between 6 and 12 months are 743 kcals for males and 676 kcals for females.

NOTES

When babies are allowed to feed in response to hunger cues, breastmilk typically provides adequate calories for the baby. When feedings are shortened by the mother, are infrequent (fewer than 10 times per 24 hours), or are delayed or missed through pacifier use, babies may not have an opportunity to remove an adequate amount of milk from the breast. Ongoing inadequate milk removal will decrease overall milk production.

It is very rare for the caloric composition of human milk to be inadequate. Routine testing of the fat or other content of milk is not recommended, due to diurnal variation and the difficulty of collecting a representative sample.

Evaluation of the baby's growth, stooling pattern, feeding frequency, milk transfer, and feeding mechanics should occur when doubts arise about milk adequacy.

See also Caloric density of breastmilk; Weight gain, baby–high; Weight gain, baby–low

➤ CALORIC INTAKE OF MOTHER

DEFINITION   The amount of energy, as measured by kilocalories, consumed by the mother daily. The recommended dietary intake for breastfeeding women is 500 additional calories daily during lactation than they consumed to maintain their weight before pregnancy.

NOTES

Nutrient-rich foods such as fresh fruits, vegetables, whole grains, and lean protein are the backbone of a healthful diet.

Postpartum weight loss is a goal of most women. Encourage nursing mothers to lose weight gradually while consuming a healthful diet, in order to maintain their energy levels. Moderate dieting has no effect on nutrient composition of milk. Extreme dieting may deplete women's energy stores but rarely affects milk production. Similarly, research indicates that increasing calories has no effect on milk production.

Research studies have demonstrated no negative effect for infant growth when breastfeeding mothers lost weight gradually (less than 1–2 lb per week on average).

See also Weight loss, mother

➤ CANCER OF THE BREAST

DEFINITION   Malignant growth within the tissues of the breast. Unexplained and unusual lumps in the lactating breast must be examined by a healthcare provider.

NOTES

While masses in the lactating breast are often associated with plugged milk ducts, other types of growths, including cancerous ones, are possible. When lumps in the breast do not move or resolve within 48 hours, a complete breast evaluation should be performed. Women who have previously been diagnosed and treated for breast cancer can breast-feed. Those who have had past breast surgery may experience decreased milk production in the segments of the breast that were surgically involved.

When cancer is identified in the lactating breast, weaning is generally indicated because of the nature of the drugs and other therapies used to treat cancer.

Breastfeeding reduces the risk of developing breast cancer in the mother and possibly the child.

See also Abrupt weaning; Biopsy, breast; Breast lumps; Breast refusal; Breast surgery; Goldsmith's sign

➤ CANDIDIASIS

DEFINITION   Overgrowth of *Candida albicans* or other common fungi.

Symptoms of yeast infection of the breast include red, shiny-looking skin on the nipple or areola, flaky skin, and sharp, itching pain that persists between feedings. Infant symptoms of yeast overgrowth or thrush include white patches of growth on the inner buccal surface (cheek) or tongue, and occasionally pain on latch. Infants may also have diaper-area yeast overgrowth.

ASK ABOUT

Onset.
Medications taken in the past month.

ASSESSMENT

PROMPT CARE NEEDED?

Are any of the following present?

Sharp, itching, persistent nipple pain (during as well as between feedings).

Flaky, shiny, or itchy skin on the nipple surface.

Presence of white patches in the infant's mouth.

A baby with a yeast infection in the diaper area.

IF YES,   *Call the mother's and baby's healthcare providers today.*

ROUTINE CARE NEEDED?

Are any of the following present?

Nipple pain during feeding.

> **IF YES,**   *Call lactation care provider today.*

SELF-CARE INFORMATION

Finish all medications prescribed.

If administering nystatin suspension to the infant, pour a dose into a clean cup or spoon. Half of the dose should be used for each side of the mouth. Suspension may be applied with a cotton swab. A clean swab should be used for each application. Take care not to introduce used swabs into the bottle of suspension.

If the baby uses artificial nipples, pacifiers, etc., these should be boiled at least daily and replaced after completion of yeast treatment.

The mother and baby should be treated simultaneously regardless of which one is symptomatic.

IMPORTANT CONDITIONS TO REPORT

Persistent symptoms after completion of a course of treatment.

Recurrent symptoms.

> **NOTES**
>
> *Candida* overgrowth may follow or increase after antibiotic treatment.
>
> Recommended treatment for candidiasis is a topical antifungal agent.
>
> If symptoms are not relieved by topical treatment, feeding evaluation should occur to rule out positioning or attachment problems contributing to pain.
>
> The healthcare provider's evaluation should rule out other conditions resulting in redness and pain, including **eczema**, reaction to surface allergens, trauma, **Raynaud's phenomenon**, concomitant bacteria, and infection.
>
> Subsequent treatment with oral antifungal agents may resolve symptoms.
>
> Lactation evaluation should rule out contributing problems with latch or distortion of the nipple in the baby's mouth.

See also Nipple pain; Yeast infection; Thrush

➤ CARDIAC PROBLEMS

DEFINITION   Referring to diseases and disorders of the heart and circulatory system.

ASK ABOUT

Onset.

History of heart problems.

ASSESSMENT

EMERGENT CARE NEEDED?

Are any of the following present?

A bluish tinge to the baby's mouth and lips during feeding.

Bluish hands and feet after hospital discharge.

Difficulty breathing.

Difficulty swallowing.

IF YES,   *Seek emergency care now.*

PROMPT CARE NEEDED?

Are any of the following present?

Breastfeeding baby diagnosed with cardiac problems.

IF YES,   *Call lactation care provider today.*

IMPORTANT CONDITIONS TO REPORT

Worsening, persistence, or recurrence of symptoms.

NOTES

Women with cardiac problems may breastfeed their babies. Any medications taken should be evaluated for their transfer into milk and effect on the baby using Lact Med or another drug resource.

Babies with cardiac problems benefit from receiving their mother's milk. They may have problems sustaining attachment to the breast, and suckling may be weak and ineffective.

However, breastfeeding is less physiologically stressful than bottle feeding. Heart, oxygen saturation, and respiratory rates are more optimal during breastfeeding than while bottle feeding.

Mothers may benefit from pumping or expressing milk after feeding to maintain an adequate milk supply.

A lactation care provider should evaluate effective positions and techniques for babies diagnosed with cardiac problems.

See also Medication resources (inside back cover)

➤ CARIES, NURSING-BOTTLE

DEFINITION   Decay of the teeth caused by the presence of sugary fluids in the mouth during bed and nap time.

NOTES

This phenomenon rarely happens with children falling asleep at the breast due to the different fluid dynamics of breastfeeding.

Breastfed children with strong family history of excess caries may be at greater risk for developing caries while nursing.

See also Nursing bottle caries

➤ CAROLINA GLOBAL BREASTFEEDING INSTITUTE (CGBI)

DEFINITION   Breastfeeding institute that "was established in 2006 in the Department of Maternal and Child Health of the UNC Gillings School of Global Public Health, and serves as the first such Public Health Breastfeeding Center of its kind. Situated in an academic home, we offer a comprehensive program of research, service to the greater community, and education. CGBI furthers statewide, national, and global health through increased understanding and support for breastfeeding, with attention to associated child survival, growth and development, and maternal reproductive health and survival. Our activities seek to promote increased quality of care and create an optimal breastfeeding norm."[87(p1)]

NOTES

Email: cbi@unc.edu.

Web: cgbi.sph.unc.edu/

CGBI disseminates information about breastfeeding through workshops, newsletters, research, and its website.

Footnote

[87]Carolina Global Breastfeeding Institute. (2012). Vision, mission, and policies. Retrieved from http://cgbi.sph.unc.edu/about-the-institute/vision-mission

➤ CASEIN

DEFINITION   The tough, curd-like protein fraction of all mammalian milk. (Whey is the name for the more liquid proteins in milk.)

NOTES

The casein–whey ratio of human milk is typically 40–60 as compared with cow's milk at 80–20. This difference is thought to account for some of the difficulty in digesting cow's milk and cow's milk–based formulae as well as for the colic related to cow's milk feeding. (Many cow's milk-based formulae have been chemically altered to reduce the casein–whey ratio.)

See also Colic

➤ CCK

See Cholecystokinin

➤ CDC

See DHHS/Centers for Disease Control and Prevention

➤ CELIAC DISEASE

DEFINITION   Celiac disease is a permanent intolerance of gluten, a protein found in wheat, rye, barley, and possibly oats. This autoimmune disease causes damage to the intestinal wall and interferes with nutrient absorption.

Mothers and babies with this disorder can breastfeed.

NOTES

Because celiac disease is a genetic disorder, children of mothers with this disorder are at greater risk. People with celiac disease are at increased risk for developing diabetes and other autoimmune diseases.

Research has shown that the risk of developing celiac disease is reduced when babies are still breastfeeding at the time of introduction of gluten in the baby's diet.[88] In children who have inherited celiac disease, extended breastfeeding may delay the development of celiac disease and reduce its severity.

See also Autoimmune diseases

Footnote

[88]Ivarsson, A., Hernell, O., Stenlund, H., & Persson, L. A. (2002). Breast-feeding protects against celiac disease. *American Journal of Clinical Nutrition, 75,* 914–921.

➤ CENTERS FOR DISEASE CONTROL AND PREVENTION

See DHHS/Centers for Disease Control and Prevention (CDC)

➤ CENTRAL NERVOUS SYSTEM (CNS)

DEFINITION   Referring to the brain and spinal cord.

➤ CEREALS FOR BABY

DEFINITION   Referring to pulverized grain foods prepared for babies. Often these cereals are iron enriched.

NOTES

Historically, iron fortified cereal was typically the first cereal to be introduced to infants of any age. Recent research suggests that early introduction of cereals (before 4 months of age) may trigger eczema, celiac disease, and type 1 diabetes in genetically susceptible children.

The recommendation is to begin family foods around 6 months, especially foods rich in zinc and iron. Parents should be encouraged to delay introducing their baby to cereal and other solid foods until 6 months of age.

See also Baby food; Complementary feeding; Mixed feeds; Solid foods for breast-fed babies

➤ CERTIFIED LACTATION COUNSELOR (CLC)

DEFINITION Breastfeeding care provider who has completed a course of study resulting in certification as a lactation counselor.

See also Academy of Lactation Policy & Practice; International Board Certified Lactation Consultant (IBCLC); International Board of Lactation Consultant Examiners (IBLCE); International Lactation Consultant Association (ILCA)

➤ CESAREAN BIRTH

DEFINITION Delivery of a baby via surgical incision made through the abdomen and uterus.

ASK ABOUT

Date of cesarean.
Age of the baby.
Feeding status.

ASSESSMENT

EMERGENT CARE NEEDED?

Are any of the following present?

The baby refuses to feed for more than 6 hours.

An exclusively breastfed baby stools less than once daily in the newborn period.

Extreme **lethargy** or **irritability** in the baby.

Sudden change in the baby's muscle tone (extremely floppy or stiff) or repetitive jerking movements (e.g., seizure activity).

The baby shows sudden disinterest in feeding.

Unable to wake the baby.

Does not calm, even with cuddles.

IF YES,   *Call pediatrician now.*

PROMPT CARE NEEDED?

Are any of the following present?

Difficulty finding comfortable feeding positions after surgery.

Concerns about adequacy of milk supply.

Concerns about adequacy of infant growth.

IF YES,   *Call lactation care provider today.*

SELF-CARE INFORMATION

Practice skin-to-skin contact in the first hour and frequently thereafter.

Feed the baby at the first sign of hunger cues (signs that say "feed me" include hand-to-face or hand-to-mouth movements, lip smacking, seeking with lips, rooting, and head bobbing).

Feed the baby at least 10 times per 24 hours.

Listen for signs of the baby swallowing.

Allow the baby to end feedings.

Expect at least three infant stools per 24 hours after the first 4 days of life.

Good positioning and attachment are crucial to prevent or reduce nipple pain.

If feedings are missed, hand express or pump milk to maintain supply.

IMPORTANT CONDITIONS TO REPORT

Ongoing difficulty with breastfeeding.

Ongoing concerns about infant growth.

NOTES

Mothers and babies who experience cesarean birth have greater risk of being separated in the hospital, as well as experiencing delayed skin-to-skin contact, delayed breastfeeding initiation, delayed development of mature milk, and early supplementation. Mothers should be monitored to ensure they are healing well after surgery and receiving appropriate pain relief.

A wide range of drugs are used to relieve pain. An up-to-date drug reference should be consulted to determine the safety and possible side effects of individual drugs.

Newborn and premature babies are at greater risk of side effects due to limited ability to clear drugs from their systems.

Face-to-face lactation counseling can assist mothers in finding comfortable breastfeeding positions and learning their babies' feeding cues.

See also Analgesia; Anesthesia; Childbirth

➤ CGBI

See Carolina Global Breastfeeding Institute (CGBI)

➤ CHEMICAL CONTAMINANTS IN BREASTMILK

DESCRIPTION Concern about presence of toxins and environmental pollutants in mothers milk.

NOTES

All foods, including breastmilk, may contain traces of chemical contaminants present in the environment. Breastmilk is one of the easiest and least painful body tissues to sample. For this reason, it is used to monitor population exposure to chemicals. Low-level exposure to contaminants should not contraindicate breastfeeding. The greatest exposure for the baby is during pregnancy.

ASK ABOUT

Known contaminant exposure.

Age of the baby.

ASSESSMENT

EMERGENT CARE NEEDED?

> Sudden exposure of mother to toxic chemical.

> **IF YES,**   *Seek emergency care now.*

PROMPT CARE NEEDED?

> History of high-level exposure to toxic chemicals in a breastfeeding woman.

> **IF YES,**   *Seek medical care today.*

ROUTINE CARE NEEDED?

> General questions about environmental exposure.

> **IF YES,**   *Call lactation care provider today.*

IMPORTANT CONDITIONS TO REPORT

Known history of environmental or workplace exposure to toxic chemicals.

Any negative effects of past exposure.

NOTES

Women who know they have been exposed to specific chemicals or pollutants should consult with their physician regarding need for analysis of the contaminant content of their milk.

Many researchers have looked for negative effects of background toxin exposure via breastmilk and have found no negative effects when outcomes are compared to those of formula-fed babies.

See also Medication resources (inside back cover); Pesticides and pollutants in breastmilk

➤ CHEMOTHERAPY

DEFINITION   Drugs and chemical agents used to destroy cancer cells. These drugs are typically contraindicated in breastfeeding as they may be toxic to the infant.

NOTES

An up-to-date drug reference should be consulted to determine the safety and possible side effects of individual drugs.

Mothers who must undergo **abrupt weaning** to begin cancer treatment or receive surgery or radiation may benefit from practical and emotional support from lactation and medical care providers.

See also Abrupt weaning; Breast cancer; Medication resources (inside back cover)

➤ CHICKEN POX, MOTHER-TO-CHILD TRANSMISSION

DEFINITION   Referring to the characteristic lesions resulting from infection with varicella-zoster, a virus of the herpes family. This highly infectious virus is passed via droplet and direct contact with lesions. Exposure can be dangerous for the newborn. If the mother is judged safe to be with her infant and she has no lesions on the breast area, breastfeeding is considered safe.

ASK ABOUT

Onset.
Age of baby.
Infection of any household members.

ASSESSMENT

EMERGENT CARE NEEDED?

Are any of the following present?

Eruption of chicken pox in a newborn infant.
Presence of chicken pox lesions on the breast and nipple area.

IF YES,   *Call pediatrician now.*

Mothers and other family members who are infected in the early perinatal period may infect their infants by passing droplets and allowing infant contact with lesions. Infection risk may be decreased by administering varicella-zoster immunoglobulin (VZIG) to the infant.

If a breastfeeding mother with chicken pox is separated from her baby, she should be encouraged to express or pump her milk eight or more times daily to maintain her milk supply. If she has no lesions on the breast or nipple area, her milk may be given to the baby. Careful hand washing should be practiced to avoid involving the breast or collected milk.

If only siblings are infected, the baby and the mother should be isolated and continue breastfeeding.

See Lawrence & Lawrence[89] for a detailed guidance for varicella-zoster exposure in the peripartum.

See also Acute infection

Footnote

[89]Lawrence, R. A., & Lawrence, R. M. (2011). *Breastfeeding: A guide for the medical profession* (7th ed.). St Louis: Elsevier/Mosby, p. 453.

➤ CHILD

DEFINITION   A young person up to the age of puberty.

➤ CHILDBIRTH

DEFINITION   The process of giving birth to a baby.

Several maternity care practices increase the chances of breastfeeding success, including:

Prenatal childbirth and breastfeeding education.

Nurturing, supportive care during the birth process.

Use of nonpharmacologic pain relief methods (massage, hydrotherapy, acupressure, hypnotherapy, etc.) during labor.

Immediate and ongoing skin-to-skin contact with the infant after delivery.

Continuous rooming in.

Ongoing education and support while the mother and her baby learn how to breastfeed, including feeding cues, comfortable positioning and latch, how to express milk, and how to find breastfeeding support after discharge.

Avoidance of unnecessary supplementation, use of bottles, use of pacifiers, etc.

See also Analgesia; Anesthesia; Cesarean birth; Doula; Epidural anesthesia

➤ **CHILD SPACING**

DEFINITION   Intentional or natural delay in the period of time between sequential births.

Women who are exclusively breastfeeding a young baby are likely to experience a lack of menses (**amenorrhea**). Women may be amenorrheic for more than 1 year while breastfeeding.

Birth intervals of 2 years or more are recommended to allow time for mother's body to recover and replenish nutrient stores.

Women who wish to become pregnant again may wish to breastfeed less intensively to trigger resumption of their menses. Nutritionally appropriate foods should be offered to the baby when mother begins to **wean**.

See also Amenorrhea; Birth interval; Lactational amenorrhea method (LAM); Weaning

➤ CHLAMYDIA

DEFINITION   A sexually transmitted infection caused by *Chlamydia trachomatis.* Symptoms in women may include redness of the vagina, discomfort, and vaginal discharge. Pelvic inflammatory disease may result from infection. Mothers with this condition may breastfeed.

NOTES

Newborns may contract *Chlamydia trachomatis* through the birth process, resulting in chlamydial conjunctivitis or pneumonia. *C. trachomatis* has not been known to pass through the milk of an infected mother. Weaning and mother–baby separation are not indicated.

An up-to-date drug reference should be consulted to determine the safety and possible side effects of drugs.

See also Medication resources (inside back cover)

➤ CHOANAL ATRESIA

DEFINITION   A congenital condition marked by blockage or narrowing of the nasal airway. Babies born with this condition may have difficulty breathing and coordinating breastfeeding with breathing.

ASSESSMENT

EMERGENT CARE NEEDED?

Are any of the following present?

Newborn baby unable to breathe while feeding.

Newborn breastfeeding baby breaking suction every few seconds to breathe.

Blue tinged lips and mouth during feeding.

IF YES,   *Seek emergency care now.*

PROMPT CARE NEEDED?

Are any of the following present?

Breastfeeding mother of baby with known or diagnosed choanal atresia.

> **IF YES,**   *Call lactation care provider today.*

IMPORTANT CONDITIONS TO REPORT

Ongoing feeding difficulties.

NOTES

Surgery is often performed to open up the nasal airway. Until surgery is performed, babies may have difficulty feeding at the breast. Babies with this condition are at risk for aspiration.

When feeding at the breast is not possible, mothers can be helped to express their milk to be fed to baby. After corrective surgery, babies may be fed at the breast.

See also Breast pump; Hand expression of breastmilk

➤ CHOCOLATE

DEFINITION   Foods made from the cacao seed. Moderate chocolate intake is compatible with breastfeeding. Chocolate contains small amounts of theobromine, a mild stimulant similar to caffeine.

NOTES

The American Academy of Pediatrics has warned of increased irritability and bowel movements with consumption of more than one pound of chocolate daily by the mother.[90]

See also Maternal diet, Medication resources (inside back cover)

Footnote

[90]AAP Committee on Drugs. (2001). The transfer of drugs and other chemicals into human milk. *Pediatrics, 108,* 782.

➤ C-HOLD

DEFINITION   Referring to a previously recommended breastfeeding technique in which the breast was supported by the mother's hand with the thumb resting above the nipple, and the remainder of the hand below the nipple, thus making the shape of the letter *C*. The most effective latch is achieved by allowing the breast to stay in its natural position and bringing the baby to the breast.

NOTES

In supporting the breast, it is crucial that the mother's fingers are held beyond the areas of the breast where the baby's lips should seal.

The mother's hand should not change the natural way the breast falls, but merely support the breast in its natural shape so that its weight is off the baby's chin and milk can flow directly from the alveoli to the baby.

If support is needed for larger breasts, a rolled towel placed under the breast may be helpful.

See also Cigarette hold

➤ CHOLECYSTOKININ (CCK)

DEFINITION   A hormone produced in the gut wall in response to the presence of fat and protein rich-food passing from the stomach to the small intestine. The presence of CCK causes the gallbladder to contract, sending bile to the duodenum to emulsify and aid in the digestion of fats and fat-soluble vitamins. CCK also triggers production of pancreatic enzymes that digest protein.

> **NOTES**

The presence of CCK in the gut is thought to give an overall sense of satiety or fullness, along with temporary sedation.

➤ CHOLERA

DEFINITION   An acute infectious disease caused by *Vibrio cholerae*. Symptoms of cholera are excessive and watery diarrhea, vomiting, cramping of the muscles, and mineral imbalance. Breastfeeding greatly reduces the risk of cholera infection. When a mother is infected with cholera, breastfeeding may continue.

➤ CHRONIC ILLNESS

DEFINITION   Diseases or disorders that reoccur or last for a long time. Breastfeeding is known to reduce the severity or risk of developing several chronic illnesses, including eczema, asthma, diabetes, multiple sclerosis, and celiac disease.

> **NOTES**

While breastfeeding is universally recommended, parents with a family history of chronic illness should be strongly encouraged to consider breastfeeding to decrease their child's risk.

Exclusive breastfeeding (offering no food or drink other than breastmilk to the young baby) offers the highest level of protection against chronic diseases.

➤ CIGARETTE HOLD

DEFINITION   Referring to a previously recommended breastfeeding technique in which the breast and nipple are held between the mother's index and middle fingers, as a smoker might hold a cigarette. This position can be difficult for breastfeeding, as the mother's fingers may be in the way of the baby's mouth. The most effective latch is achieved by allowing the breast to stay in its natural position and bringing the baby to the breast.

NOTES

The mother's fingers may compress the breast tissue, possibly restricting the flow of milk or causing local tissue injury.

The mother's hand should not change the natural way the breast falls, but merely support the breast in its natural shape so that its weight is off the baby's chin and milk can flow directly from the alveoli to the baby.

See also C-hold

➤ CIMS

See Coalition for Improving Maternity Services (CIMS)

➤ CIRCUMCISION

DEFINITION   The cultural or religious practice of removing the foreskin of the penis.

NOTES

After circumcision, breastfeeding babies should be offered skin-to-skin contact and the breast for comfort as well as nourishment. Breastfeeding has been demonstrated to reduce pain.

Feeding problems seen following circumcision should be referred for medical evaluation.

➤ CIRCUMORAL CYANOSIS

DEFINITION   A state where the skin and mucous membranes around the mouth turn purplish-blue, reflecting lack of oxygenation in the blood.

ASK ABOUT

Onset.
Medical conditions of the baby.

ASSESSMENT

EMERGENT CARE NEEDED?

Are any of the following present?

Circumoral cyanosis during feeding or at other times.
Cyanosis of the hands and feet beyond the first few days of life. (Remember, acrocyanosis is common and normal in newborns.)

IF YES, *Seek medical care now.*

IMPORTANT CONDITIONS TO REPORT

Medications used.

See also Acrocyanosis; Cyanosis

➤ CLC

See Certified lactation counselor (CLC)

➤ CLEFT LIP AND PALATE (CL/CP)

DEFINITION Congenital disruption of the formation of structures of the mouth and face, resulting in crevices in oral structures.

NOTES

Clefts may occur on one (unilateral) or both (bilateral) sides of the mouth.

Cleft lip (CL) can occur with or without clefts of the palate.

Cleft palate (CP) can involve the hard and/or soft palate (the roof of the mouth) and the alveolar (gum) ridge.

Palate clefts can also occur under the skin, with a coverage of intact skin. This is called a submucosal cleft.

The severity of the cleft will control the difficulty of feeding.

ASK ABOUT

Type and location of cleft.

ASSESSMENT

EMERGENT CARE NEEDED?

Are any of the following present?

Choking spells or dusky color of skin during feeding sessions.

IF YES,   *Seek medical care now.*

PROMPT CARE NEEDED?

Are any of the following present?

Learning to breastfeed a baby with CL/CP.

Problems breastfeeding a baby with CL/CP.

IF YES,   *Call lactation care provider today.*

SELF-CARE INFORMATION

With unilateral cleft lip, hold the baby in an upright or semiupright position for feeding.

Compress the breast gently into the baby's mouth to assist in milk removal.

Pump or hand express after feedings and store the collected milk to be fed to the baby.

A dental device called an "obturator" may make breastfeeding easier for babies with hard palate clefts.

Severe clefts may make it impossible to feed at the breast until repair surgery is completed. However, mothers should be encouraged to express their milk and feed it to their babies with a cleft palate feeder.

Breastmilk offers protection against ear infection, which babies with clefts are more prone to develop.

Alternate breast massage may increase milk flow for inefficient feeders.

See also Alternate breast massage; Obturator, palatal; Palate, abnormal.

➤ CLENCHING OR CLAMPING ONTO THE NIPPLE/AREOLA

DEFINITION Painful pressure applied by the baby's mouth on the nipple or areola. Clenching or clamping may indicate pain, excessive rate of flow, or inappropriate latch technique. Clenching and clamping can cause pain and trauma to the nipple.

ASK ABOUT

Onset.
Age of the baby.
Presence of nipple trauma.

ASSESSMENT

PROMPT CARE NEEDED?

Are any of the following present?

Persistent clenching or clamping.

Nipple pain on feeding.

Excessive stooling (more than six times per day).

Fussy, gassy baby.

Baby has difficulty managing excessive milk flow (sputters at the breast)

IF YES, *Call lactation care provider today.*

SELF-CARE INFORMATION

Practice good attachment:

Watch for feeding cues and offer the breast as soon as cues are seen.

Wait for the baby to open his or her mouth wide (greater than a 140° angle).

Pull the baby in so that his or her chin touches the breast first, and the nipple enters the mouth along the top of the tongue; this should result in a wide-open mouth on the breast.

The baby's lips should be flanged outward.

The baby's lips should look off center when compared with the areola; the bottom lip should be farther away from the nipple than the top lip.

Try the Australian posture.

IMPORTANT CONDITIONS TO REPORT

Ongoing pain.

NOTES

Occasionally babies compress the nipple when there is a high rate of flow or a powerful letdown reflex. A lactation care provider can assist mothers with this problem.

See also Australian posture; Nipple pain

➤ CLICKING SOUNDS DURING BREASTFEEDING

DEFINITION Noises such as suction breaks or tongue clicks that occur during feeding. Clicking indicates that there is open space inside the baby's mouth. This is most often due to poor positioning and attachment but may just be the sound the baby makes while nursing.

ASK ABOUT

Onset.

Age of the baby.

ASSESSMENT

EMERGENT CARE NEEDED?

Are any of the following present?

Extreme **lethargy** or **irritability** in the baby.

Sudden change in baby's muscle tone (extremely floppy or stiff) or repetitive jerking movements (e.g., seizure activity).

Baby shows sudden disinterest in feeding.

Inability to wake baby.

Baby doesn't calm, even with cuddles.

IF YES,   *Seek emergency care now.*

PROMPT MEDICAL CARE NEEDED?

Are any of the following present?

Low urinary and/or bowel output.

Nasal regurgitation.

Tight lingual frenulum with feeding difficulty.

Cyanosis and/or choking during feeding.

IF YES,   *Seek medical care within 4 hours.*

PROMPT LACTATION CARE NEEDED?

Are any of the following present?

Tight lingual frenulum in breastfeeding baby (tongue-tied baby).

Nipple or breast pain.

History of recurrent breast infection.

Milk supply problems.

Poor growth of a breastfed infant.

Clicking sounds that do not resolve with changes in positioning.

IF YES,   *Call lactation care provider today.*

ROUTINE CARE NEEDED?

Are any of the following present?

Ongoing problems with clicking.

IF YES,   *Call lactation care provider today.*

SELF-CARE INFORMATION

Practice good attachment:

Watch for hunger cues and offer the breast as they are seen.

Place baby so that nose is opposite nipple.

Wait for the baby to open his or her mouth wide (greater than a 140° angle).

Pull the baby in so that his or her chin touches the breast first, and the nipple enters the mouth along the top of the tongue; this should result in a wide-open mouth on the breast.

The baby's lips should be flanged outward.

The baby's lips should look off-center when compared with the areola; the bottom lip should be farther away from the nipple than the top lip.

NOTES

Presence of these sounds indicates need for lactation evaluation.

See also Ankyloglossia; Cleft lip and palate (CL/CP)

➤ CLOGGED DUCTS

DEFINITION   The milk ducts of the breast can become clogged. The mother may experience breast tenderness and feel a lump at the site of the clog.

ASK ABOUT

Age of the baby.

Location of the lump.

Tenderness around the lump.

When the lump was first noted.

ASSESSMENT

PROMPT CARE NEEDED?

Are any of the following present?

Temperature higher than 101°F (38.5°C).

Reddened area on the breast.

Identified lump or lumps on the breast that persist and do not move for more than 48 hours.

IF YES, *Call obstetric care provider now and call lactation care provider now.*

ROUTINE CARE NEEDED?

Are any of the following present?

Identified lump or lumps on the breast which persist for more than 48 hours with no other symptoms.

IF YES, *Call obstetric care provider and call lactation care provider today.*

SELF-CARE INFORMATION

Plugged ducts in the breast should move and disappear within 48 hours. If not, consult a physician for further evaluation.

Some mothers find manual massage of the area helps the plug to dislodge and move out of the breast. Others prefer warmth, such as a warm, wet towel.

Nursing the baby frequently on the affected breast will help to drain it.

Changing the baby's position can help to move the plug.

Try to understand why the plug happened. Could it be caused by an underwire bra or car seat belt applying pressure on the breast? Then, avoid the cause so that plugs do not reoccur. For example, wear a bra without underwires and use a seat belt pad to cushion the part that goes over the breast.

IMPORTANT CONDITIONS TO REPORT

Temperature higher than 101°F (38.5°C).

Reddened area on the breast.

NOTES

New mothers are not protected from breast cancer. Prompt evaluation is warranted if a lump does not move in 48 hours.

See also Breast infection; Breast inflammation; Breast lumps; Breast pain; Mastitis

➤ CLOSET NURSING

DEFINITION   Breastfeeding a baby or child secretly, usually due to fear of disapproval of continued breastfeeding.

SELF-CARE INFORMATION
Long-term breastfeeding is a great gift to baby's health.
Seek mother-to-mother support via La Leche League or other peer support network.

NOTES

Prolonged breastfeeding offers health benefits to child and mother. According to the American Academy of Pediatrics, breastfeeding should be continued for at least the first year of life and beyond for as long as mutually desired by mother and child.[91(p.e827)]
International health authorities recommend at least 2 years of nursing.

See also Breastfeeding during pregnancy; Tandem nursing; Weaning

Footnote
[91]AAP Section on Breastfeeding. (2012). Breastfeeding and the use of human milk. *Pediatrics*, *129*(3), e827–e841. doi:10.1542/peds.2011-3552

➤ CLOTHING, BREASTFEEDING

DEFINITION Clothing specially designed for the nursing mother, including bras, shirts, and dresses designed to provide easy, comfortable access to the breast while protecting modesty.

NOTES

Breastfeeding clothing is available from a number of retail establishments. A quick Internet search for breastfeeding clothing will identify multiple options.

See also Bras

➤ CLUSTER FEEDING

DEFINITION The tendency of young babies to have a cycle of short, closely spaced feedings interspersed with periods of rest or sleep. This means babies may nurse four or five times in 3 hours, rest for 3 hours, and then nurse again four to five times in 3–4 hours. This is a typical pattern that is associated with good milk production and growth.

NOTES

Although 10–12 feedings are expected in 24 hours, they are rarely evenly spaced throughout 24 hours. Mothers should be encouraged to respond to feeding cues, supporting a clustered feeding pattern. This allows babies to maximize the amount of milk produced.

➤ CLUTCH POSTURE

DEFINITION Another name for the football posture. A breastfeeding posture in which the baby is tucked under the mother's arm, with its feet behind her back, and attaches to the breast next to her arm. The mother supports the baby's torso with her forearm, holding the baby's neck in the palm of her hand.

NOTES

This is a good position for mothers recovering from cesarean delivery, those with large breasts, and premature babies.

See also Cradle posture; Football posture

➤ CMV

See Cytomegalovirus (CMV)

➤ CNS

See Central nervous system (CNS)

➤ COALITION FOR IMPROVING MATERNITY SERVICES (CIMS)

DESCRIPTION   "CIMS is a non-profit corporation comprised of our governing and administrative bodies (its Leadership Team and committees), annual members who make formal commitments of support and participation, and the broader community of childbirth organizations, birth professionals, advocates and consumers working towards evidence-based maternity care consistent with the ten steps defined in the MFCI."[92(p1)]

NOTES

The Coalition for Improving Maternity Services
Email: info@motherfriendly.org
Website: www.motherfriendly.org
   CIMS administers the Mother-Friendly Childbirth Initiative (MFCI).

Footnote

[92]Coalition for Improving Maternity Services. (n.d.) Meet CIMS. Retrieved from http://www.motherfriendly.org/coalition

➤ COBEDDING

DEFINITION   The practice of a parent or parents sleeping in the same bed with their baby. The AAP's Task Force on Sudden Infant Death (2011) states that "Room-sharing without bedsharing is recommended—There is evidence that this arrangement decreases the risk of SIDS by as much as 50%."[93(p1033)] The AAP's Section on Breastfeeding (2012) recommends that mothers and babies sleep in close proximity to one another, noting also that:

> Meta-analyses with a clear definition of degree of breastfeeding and adjusted for confounders and other known risks for sudden infant death syndrome (SIDS) note that breastfeeding is associated with a 36% reduced risk of SIDS. Latest data comparing any versus exclusive breastfeeding reveal that for any breastfeeding, the multivariate odds ratio (OR) is 0.55 (95% confidence interval [CI], 0.44–0.69). When computed for exclusive breastfeeding, the OR is 0.27 (95% CI, 0.27–0.31). A proportion (21%) of the US infant mortality has been attributed, in part, to the increased rate of SIDS in infants who were never breastfed. That the positive effect of breastfeeding on SIDS rates is independent of sleep position was confirmed in a large case-control study of supine-sleeping infants.[94]

SELF-CARE INFORMATION

Many authorities have expressed concern about the relationship between SIDS and cobedding. UK UNICEF has given the following guidelines for safer cosleeping:

- "Do not sleep with your baby when you have been drinking any alcohol or taking drugs (legal or illegal) that might make you sleepy.
- Do not sleep with your baby if you or anyone else in the bed is a smoker.
- Do not put yourself in the position where you could doze off with your baby on a sofa/armchair"[95(p1)]

See also Cosleeping; Sudden infant death syndrome (SIDS)

Footnotes

[93]AAP Task Force on Sudden Infant Death Syndrome, & Moon, R. Y. (2011). SIDS and other sleep-related infant deaths: Expansion of recommendations for a safe infant sleeping environment. *Pediatrics*, *128*(5), 1030–1039. doi:10.1542/peds.2011-2284

[94]AAP Section on Breastfeeding. (2012). Breastfeeding and the use of human milk. *Pediatrics*, *129*(3), e827–e841. doi: 10.1542/peds.2011-3552

[95]UNICEF UK Baby Friendly Initiative. (2011). Caring for your baby at night: A guide for parents. Retrieved from http://www.unicef.org.uk/Documents/Baby_Friendly/Leaflets/caringatnight_web.pdf

➤ COFFEE

DEFINITION   A beverage made from coffee beans that contains several aromatic and active chemicals, including caffeine, a CNS stimulant. Breastfeeding mothers should moderate their caffeine usage. Caffeine use is addictive.

NOTES

Caffeine is considered usually compatible with breastfeeding. Hale lists caffeine as an L2 (safer) drug.[96]

Mothers of premature babies and babies with cardiac problems should limit caffeine intake and should report what they do consume to the baby's pediatric care provider. This is due to the routine practice of giving caffeine to premature babies in order to treat apnea.

Asthmatic women who take theophylline may need to be monitored for cumulative effects of this drug in combination with any dietary caffeine.

Rarely, a mother's caffeine consumption may cause irritability or sleeplessness in her baby.

Caffeine content of coffee, tea, soda, and chocolate varies widely with brand and brewing method.

See also Caffeine; Medication resources (inside back cover)

Footnote

[96]Hale, T. W. (2012). Medications and mothers milk (15th ed., p. 172). Amarillo, TX: Hale Publishing.

➤ COLDS

DEFINITION   An acute viral infection characterized by inflammation of the upper respiratory tract, runny nose, and cough. Mothers and babies with colds should continue breastfeeding.

> **NOTES**
>
> Over-the-counter medications used to treat colds should be reviewed in a drug reference. In general, long-acting or extra-strength preparations should be avoided due to their long half-life in the body.
>
> Some antihistamine and decongestant drugs are noted to result in a dramatic decrease in milk supply during the time they are in circulation. Care should be taken to avoid these medications during lactation, particularly pseudoephedrine.
>
> If a breastfeeding mother and baby are receiving cold medication, care should be taken to avoid overdosing the baby.

See also Acute infection; Decongestants; Over-the-counter drugs

➤ COLIC, INFANTILE

DEFINITION   A condition of infancy described by the classic "rule of three": bouts of high-pitched crying lasting more than 3 hours per day, for more than 3 days per week, and for more than 3 weeks in a well-nourished, otherwise healthy baby.[97] Colic typically starts after 2 weeks of age and resolves by 4 months.

ASK ABOUT

Age of the baby.
Diet of the baby.
Weight gain of the baby.

ASSESSMENT

EMERGENT CARE NEEDED?

Are any of the following present?

Difficulty breathing.

IF YES,   *Seek emergency care now.*

Are any of the following present?

Hives.

Vomiting.

Diarrhea.

Blood in the stools.

Irritability and excessive crying.

IF YES,   *Seek medical care now.*

ROUTINE CARE NEEDED?

Are any of the following present?

Education needed about mixed feeding.

IF YES,   *Call lactation care provider today.*

IMPORTANT CONDITIONS TO REPORT

Signs of dehydration (scanty, dark urine).

Difficulty breathing.

Eczema.

Hives.

Vomiting.

Diarrhea.

Blood in the stools.

Irritability and excessive crying.

SELF-CARE INFORMATION

Solid foods do not help babies sleep through the night.

Try comfort techniques such as rocking, singing, skin-to-skin contact, bathing, seeking a quiet, calm environment, and going out for a walk.

NOTES

Medical evaluation should rule out organic problems such as rectal fissure, otitis media, and fractures.

This problem occurs evenly among exclusively breastfed, mixed fed, and formula fed infants, and is thus thought to have largely developmental causes.

In breastfed babies, a trial of removing dairy foods, especially liquid milk, from the mother's diet may be conducted for 10–14 days to determine if symptoms improve. If not, mothers should resume their normal diet.

See also Allergy in the breastfed infant

Footnote

[97]Wessel, M. A., Cobb, J. C., Jackson, E. B., Harris, G. S. Jr., & Detwiler, A. C. (1954). Paroxysmal fussing in infancy, sometimes called colic. *Pediatrics, 14,* 421–435.

➤ COLLECTION AND STORAGE OF BREASTMILK

DEFINITION Procedure by which milk is safely expressed and stored.

NOTES

Milk collection may be done by hand or pump expression or combination of both.

Begin all milk collection by washing hands, pump, and collection device carefully.

Massage breasts and stimulate nipples prior to expressing.

Label containers with date of expression and name of infant (if it will be used in a multichild setting).

Glass and hard plastic containers with tight lids are recommended. All containers should be food grade. Plastic bags designed for milk storage may be used, but it may be difficult to prevent spillage and puncture of these bags.

For the full-term, healthy baby, milk can be safely stored:[98]

Up to 4 hours at room temperature (66°–72°F), but it should be refrigerated immediately if possible (with a frozen gel pack in an insulated lunch bag or cooler if refrigerator is not available).

Three to five days in the refrigerator (32°–50°F).

Up to 3 months in the built-in freezer section (0°–32°F) of a refrigerator.

Up to 6 months in a deep freezer (-20°F or less).

Milk that will not be used fresh within 5 days should be frozen as soon as possible.

Thaw milk in its container.
Milk can be safely thawed by:

Placing frozen containers in the refrigerator overnight.

Holding frozen containers under lukewarm running tap water.

Placing frozen containers in lukewarm water.

Hot water is not recommended due to potential nutrient loss.
Milk should never be boiled or microwaved.
Milk does not need to be overly warm before being fed to the infant.
For the preterm or ill infant, request individual milk storage and handling guidelines from the hospital newborn intensive care unit.

See also Containers for milk storage; Storage of breastmilk; Thawing and warming frozen breastmilk

Footnote

[98]Cadwell, K., & Turner-Maffei, C. (2014). *Pocket guide for lactation management,* (2nd ed.). Burlington, MA: Jones & Bartlett Learning.

➤ COLOSTRUM

DEFINITION   Milk produced in the breast under the influence of the hormones of pregnancy. Colostrum is a yellowish, thick milk rich in immunoglobulins and other nutrients.

> **NOTES**
>
> The transition to mature milk begins with the delivery of the placenta. The composition of milk changes gradually from colostrum to transitional milk to mature milk over the next 2–4 days.
>
> When mothers report that their milk has not come in or changed by day 5 following delivery, lactation consultation is indicated.
>
> Prolonged production of colostrum may indicate retained placental fragments.
>
> It is normal to note some dried colostrum on the nipple or clothing during pregnancy.

See also Breastmilk secretion; Retained placental fragments

➤ COMFORT NURSING

DEFINITION   Offering the breast to calm an upset baby or child.

See also Nonnutritive suckling

➤ COMPLEMENTARY FEEDING

DEFINITION   A term used to indicate appropriate addition of solid foods to the baby's diet at around 6 months of age.

> **NOTES**
>
> The American Academy of Pediatrics (AAP), the United States Breastfeeding Committee (USBC), the United Nations Children's Fund (UNICEF), and the World Health Organization (WHO) recommend exclusive (full) breastfeeding for about the first 6 months of life.
>
> Researchers have shown that flavors from the foods the mother eats in pregnancy and during lactation pass into the milk. When foods taste familiar, the baby is more likely to accept them.
>
> In addition to age, signs of readiness may include increased interest in table foods, ability to sit, ability to pick up objects and put them in the mouth, and decreased tongue thrusting (automatically pushing foods out of the mouth with the tongue).

ASK ABOUT

Age of the baby.

Reason for wanting to start solid foods.

ASSESSMENT

PROMPT CARE NEEDED?

Are any of the following present?

Breastfed baby under 5 months of age.

Mother concerned about the baby's weight gain.

Decreased stooling or urination.

IF YES,   *Seek medical care today and call lactation care provider today.*

ROUTINE CARE NEEDED?

Are any of the following present?

Breastfed baby around 6 months of age.

Mother has questions about starting solids.

IF YES,   *Call lactation care provider today.*

SELF-CARE INFORMATION

Babies are not equally interested in starting solid foods; if the baby is not interested, wait a few days and try again.

When babies start solid foods around 6 months, they do not need to start with the semiliquid foods that were once popular recommendations for starting solids for younger babies. At the age of 6 months, babies are ready for foods with more texture, and complementary feeding can begin with appropriate family foods.[99]

IMPORTANT CONDITIONS TO REPORT

Difficulty breathing.

Difficulty swallowing.

Rapid progression of symptoms.

See also Allergy in the breastfed infant; Baby-led weaning; Solid foods for breastfed infants

Footnote

[99]Pan American Health Organization & World Health Organization. (2003). *Guiding principles for complementary feeding of the breastfed child.* Retrieved from http://whqlibdoc.who.int/paho/2003/a85622.pdf

➤ COMPONENTS OF BREASTMILK

DEFINITION Referring to the nutrients and other substances that constitute human milk. Breastmilk is a rich and changing mix of macronutrients and micronutrients, as well as immunoglobulins, white blood cells, minerals, growth factors, and enzymes.

NOTES

The nutrient and energy content of human milk is largely controlled by metabolic processes.

It is very rare for the nutrient composition of human milk to be inadequate. Routine testing of the fat or other content of milk is not recommended, due to diurnal variation and the difficulty of collecting a representative sample.

Evaluation of baby's growth, stooling pattern, and feeding frequency and mechanics should occur when doubts arise about milk adequacy.

See also Antibodies; Anti-infective agents in breastmilk; Anti-inflammatory agents in breastmilk

➤ CONCERNS ABOUT MILK SUPPLY

DEFINITION Concern about insufficient amount of milk produced by the breast.

ASK ABOUT

Onset.
Age of the baby.

ASSESSMENT

EMERGENT CARE NEEDED?

Are any of the following present?

Meconium bowel movements after 5 days of life.

Fewer than three bowel movements daily in a breastfed newborn after the first 2 days of life.

No urine in 6 hours.

Brick dust urine (uric acid crystals) after 2 days of life.

Dark-colored urine.

Fewer than four urinations daily in the breastfed newborn after day 5.

Noticeably sunken fontanelles (soft spot on top of head).

Decreased activity.

Baby below birthweight at 10–14 days.

Cessation of weight gain.

IF YES,   *Seek pediatric care now.*

PROMPT CARE NEEDED?

Are any of the following present?

Scanty or infrequent urination, fewer than six urinations per day after day 5 of life.

IF YES,   *Seek pediatric care today.*

Are any of the following present?

Identified milk supply problem.

Concern about possible milk supply problems.

IF YES,   *Call lactation care provider today.*

SELF-CARE INFORMATION

Ensure baby is feeding 10–12 times per 24 hours.

Express milk after feeding.

IMPORTANT CONDITIONS TO REPORT

Persistent problems.

Recurrent problems.

NOTES

Women typically have concerns about milk supply, many of which are not based in actual insufficiency. However, mothers with this concern should be carefully evaluated. Maternal, infant, and environmental factors all contribute to milk supply problems. Milk supply can be increased. This is accomplished by increasing stimulation and removal of milk from the breast.

See also Increasing milk supply

➤ CONSTIPATION

DEFINITION Delayed or infrequent passage of hard, dry stool. In the breastfed infant, more than three stools are expected daily. Fewer stools indicate need for evaluation of baby by the pediatric care provider.

ASK ABOUT

Onset.
Age of the baby.
Foods fed to the baby.

ASSESSMENT

EMERGENT CARE NEEDED?

Are any of the following present?

Fewer than one stool per day in breastfed newborn.

Lethargic baby of any age.

IF YES, *Seek emergency care now.*

PROMPT CARE NEEDED?

Are any of the following present?

Fewer than three stools per day in breastfed newborn.

Straining or grunting with stool.

IF YES, *Seek pediatric care now.*

ROUTINE CARE NEEDED?

Are any of the following present?

Concern about infrequent stooling in an older baby with adequate weight gain.

IF YES,   *Call pediatrician today.*

Are any of the following present?

Concern about stool changes in an older breastfeeding baby or after introduction of other foods to the baby.

IF YES,   *Call lactation care provider today.*

IMPORTANT CONDITIONS TO REPORT

No improvement of symptoms.
Ongoing problems with stooling.

NOTES

Constipation is not normal in the breastfeeding infant.

See also Botulism, infantile

➤ CONTAINERS FOR MILK STORAGE

DEFINITION   Safe vessels for preserving expressed milk.

NOTES

Glass and hard plastic containers with tight lids are recommended. All containers
should be food grade. Plastic bags designed for milk storage may be used. Prevent
spillage and puncture of bags.[100]

See also Collection and storage of breastmilk; Milk storage bags

Footnote

[100]Arnold, L. D. W. (2004). *Safe storage of expressed breastmilk for the healthy infant and child.* East Sandwich, MA: Health Education Associates.

➤ **CONTRACEPTION**

DEFINITION   Devices and drugs used to reduce fertility.

NOTES

Many contraceptive methods are compatible with breastfeeding, including all barrier methods (condoms, foam, diaphragms, and cervical caps), intrauterine devices (IUDs), and progestin-only hormonal methods.[101] Combined estrogen/progestin methods are generally not recommended as they may reduce milk supply and affect infant growth.

The **Lactational Amenorrhea Method (LAM)** is a form of natural family planning that is 98% effective in the first 6 months following the birth of a baby, so long as the mother's menses have not returned, her baby is exclusively breastfed, and there are no long periods of time between feedings, day and night. Once the baby is older than 6 months or any of the above criteria is no longer true, LAM is no longer effective and mothers should utilize other forms of birth control.

See also Amenorrhea; Birth interval; Lactational amenorrhea method (LAM); Natural family planning; Progestin-only contraceptives

Footnote

[101]Progestin-only injectibles are intended for use in breastfeeding women only after 6 weeks post-delivery or when full milk supply is developed. Use prior to that time may decrease milk supply due to high circulating progestin levels, simulating a state of pregnancy.

➤ **CONTRAINDICATED CONDITIONS**

DEFINITION   Diseases, conditions, or medications in the mother or infant that make it inadvisable to breastfeed.

NOTES

According to the Centers for Disease Control and Prevention, breastfeeding is *not* advisable if one or more of the following conditions is true:

1. An infant is diagnosed with galactosemia, a rare genetic metabolic disorder
2. The infant's mother:
   - Has been infected with the human immunodeficiency virus (HIV)
   - Is taking antiretroviral medications
   - Has untreated, active tuberculosis
   - Is infected with human T-cell lymphotropic virus type I or type II
   - Is using or is dependent upon an illicit drug
   - Is taking prescribed cancer chemotherapy agents, such as antimetabolites that interfere with DNA replication and cell division
   - Is undergoing radiation therapies; however, such nuclear medicine therapies require only a temporary interruption in breastfeeding.[102]

The AAP also recommends a temporary cessation of breastfeeding if the mother is diagnosed with untreated brucellosis.[103(p.e832)]

See also Contraindicated medications

Footnotes

[102]Centers for Disease Control and Prevention. (2009). *Breastfeeding—Diseases and conditions: When should a mother avoid breastfeeding?* Retrieved from http://www.cdc.gov/breastfeeding/disease/index.htm

[103]AAP Section on Breastfeeding. (2012). Breastfeeding and the use of human milk. *Pediatrics, 129*(3), e827–e841. doi:10.1542/peds.2011-3552

➤ CONTRAINDICATED MEDICATIONS

DEFINITION Drugs taken by the mother that make it inadvisable to breastfeed.

According to the American Academy of Pediatrics Section on Breastfeeding:

> Recommendations regarding breastfeeding in situations in which the mother is undergoing either diagnostic procedures or pharmacologic therapy must balance the benefits to the infant and the mother against the potential risk of drug exposure to the infant . . . In general, breastfeeding is not recommended when mothers are receiving medication from the following classes of drugs: amphetamines, chemotherapy agents, ergotamines, and statins.[104(p.e833)]

An up-to-date drug reference should be consulted to determine the safety and possible side effects of individual drugs.

Newborn and premature babies are at greater risk of drug side effects due to limited ability to clear drugs from their systems.

See also Contraindicated conditions; Medication resources (inside back cover)

Footnote

[104]AAP Section on Breastfeeding. (2012). Breastfeeding and the use of human milk. *Pediatrics*, *129*(3), e827–e841. doi:10.1542/peds.2011-3552

➤ COOPER'S LIGAMENTS

DEFINITION   Connective tissue within the breast that suspends the tissue.

➤ CORTICOSTEROIDS

DEFINITION   Hormones produced by the adrenal glands. These hormones are also synthesized and used as medications to reduce inflammation and treat many autoimmune disorders.

A wide range of corticosteroid preparations are in use. Potency varies widely. An up-to-date drug reference should be consulted to determine the safety and possible side effects of individual drugs.

Newborn and premature babies are at greater risk of drug side effects due to limited ability to clear drugs from their systems.

See also Medication resources (inside back cover)

➤ COSLEEPING

DEFINITION   The practice of a parent or parents sleeping in close proximity to their baby. Cosleeping does not necessarily denote bed sharing. Cosleeping is supportive of breastfeeding.

SELF-CARE INFORMATION

UK UNICEF has given the following guidelines for safer cosleeping:
- "Do not sleep with your baby when you have been drinking any alcohol or taking drugs (legal or illegal) that might make you sleepy
- Do not sleep with your baby if you or anyone else in the bed is a smoker
- Do not put yourself in the position where you could doze off with your baby on a sofa/armchair."[105(p1)]

AAP's Section on Breastfeeding (2012) states: "Mother and infant should sleep in proximity to each other to facilitate breastfeeding."[106(p e835)]

AAP's Task Force on Sudden Infant Death (2011) states that "Room-sharing without bedsharing is recommended—There is evidence that this arrangement decreases the risk of SIDS by as much as 50%."[107(p1033)]

See also Cobedding; Sudden infant death syndrome (SIDS)

Footnotes

[105]UNICEF UK Baby Friendly Initiative. (2011). Caring for your baby at night: A guide for parents. Retrieved May 14, 2012 from http://www.unicef.org.uk/Documents/Baby_Friendly/Leaflets/caringatnight_web.pdf

[106]AAP Section on Breastfeeding. (2012). Breastfeeding and the use of human milk. *Pediatrics, 129*(3), e827–e841. doi:10.1542/peds.2011-3552

[107]AAP Task Force on Sudden Infant Death Syndrome, & Moon, R. Y. (2011). SIDS and other sleep-related infant deaths: Expansion of recommendations for a safe infant sleeping environment. *Pediatrics, 128*(5), 1030–1039. doi:10.1542/peds.2011-2284

➤ COW'S MILK

DEFINITION The fluid produced by the mammary glands of the lactating cow. Cow's milk is not recommended for children younger than 1 year of age.

NOTES

Breastmilk and infant formula are the only appropriate milks for babies younger than 1 year old. While cow's milk–based formula is an appropriate substitute for breastmilk, unaltered cow's milk is not, as it may lead to mineral and nutrient imbalance and bleeding in the gut.[108]

Between 1 and 2 years of age, whole cow's milk may be offered to children. Low-fat and skim milk should not be offered until children are older than 2 years.

Concern about infant allergy is much more predominant than actual allergy. The American Academy of Pediatrics reports that the prevalence of infant cow's milk allergy is 2–3%. The overall prevalence of childhood food allergy is 4–6%.[109]

Counseling and education should include comfort techniques for the irritable baby and coping methods for parents.[110]

Breastfeeding babies may react to cow's milk protein in their mother's diet.

See also Allergy in the breastfed infant; Colic, infantile

Footnotes

[108]Greer, F. R., Sicherer, S. H., Burks, A. W., & and the Committee on Nutrition and Section on Allergy and Immunology. (2008). Effects of early nutritional interventions on the development of atopic disease in infants and children: The role of maternal dietary restriction, breastfeeding,

timing of introduction of complementary foods, and hydrolyzed formulas. *Pediatrics, 121*(1), 183–191. doi:10.1542/peds.2007-3022

[109]AAP Committee on Nutrition. (2000). Hypoallergenic infant formulas. *Pediatrics, 106*, 346.

[110]Ziegler, R. S. (2003). Food allergen avoidance in prevention of food allergy in infants and children. *Pediatrics, 111*, 1662–1671.

➤ CRADLE POSTURE

DEFINITION   A breastfeeding posture in which the baby is placed across the mother's lap and turned toward the mother. In this position, the weight of the baby is often carried on the arm of the mother on the same side as the breast that is being nursed. This position is also called the "Madonna" position.

➤ CREAMS AND OINTMENTS

DEFINITION   Topical preparations that have been made for several purposes, such as to protect the skin, to decrease itching, to clean the skin (antiseptics), and to moisturize the skin.

ASK ABOUT

Nipple discomfort.

ASSESSMENT

ROUTINE CARE NEEDED?
Are any of the following present?
Sore nipples.
Painful breastfeeding.
Skin rash, breakouts, or itching on the breast, areola, and nipple.

IF YES,   *Call lactation care provider today and call obstetric care provider today.*

IMPORTANT CONDITIONS TO REPORT

Symptoms worsen or persist.

Signs of infection.

Feeding or stooling expectations are not met.

SELF-CARE INFORMATION

Most ointments and creams are not intended for ingestion. When a mother puts an ointment or cream on her areola or nipple, her baby will be exposed to the ingredients during nursing.

Only use ointments and creams on the breast that are recommended for this purpose. Never use a product that has been prescribed for another problem.

Mothers can have reactions to ointments and creams. Report any changes immediately.

NOTES

Women with questions about creams may be experiencing nipple or breast pain. Women experiencing nipple pain may self-treat with inappropriate substances.

Women experiencing nipple pain should have a breastfeeding evaluation. Face-to-face counseling is effective in assessing and resolving nipple pain.

Women with a rash on the nipple area should be seen by a medical care provider to rule out herpes or other infection.

See also Breast pain; Herpes simplex virus; Nipple pain; Sore nipples

➤ CRIB DEATH

See Sudden infant death syndrome (SIDS)

➤ CROSS CRADLE POSTURE

DEFINITION A variation on the cradle or Madonna posture, where the mother's arms are switched so that the weight of the baby is supported by the opposite arm to the breast the baby is suckling. The mother supports the baby's back with her forearm, with her hand cradling the baby's neck. The other hand supports her breast if needed. Once the baby is successfully latched on, the mother can switch her arms to hold the baby in cradle.

> **NOTES**
>
> This position is helpful in the early postpartum period when the baby's head needs more support. It also helps mothers to remember to start feedings with the baby right in front of the nipple, rather than tucked in the crook of her arm (which is where women instinctively place the baby in the cradle or Madonna hold).

See also Cradle posture; Clutch posture; Football posture

➤ CROSS NURSING

DEFINITION   One woman breastfeeding another woman's baby. Cross nursing is not recommended due to fears of infection, which can pass from nurse to nursling or the reverse.

See also Wet nursing

➤ CRYING

DEFINITION   A behavioral state involving tears and other signs of distress. Crying is the most agitated state for babies. It does not have any positive effects on the baby's health.

ASK ABOUT

Onset.
Age of the baby.

ASSESSMENT

EMERGENT CARE NEEDED?

Are any of the following present?

Respiratory distress.

Lethargy or loss of muscle tone.

Fear that a parent will harm the crying baby.

Crying that does not respond to cuddles.

IF YES,   *Seek emergency care now.*

PROMPT CARE NEEDED?

Are any of the following present?

Projectile vomiting.

Fever.

Crying for longer than 3 hours.

IF YES,   *Seek medical care now.*

Are any of the following present?

Crying before or during feedings.

Intermittent crying.

Concern about foods mother is eating.

IF YES,   *Call lactation care provider today.*

SELF-CARE INFORMATION

Comfort techniques for irritable baby (rocking, singing, skin-to-skin contact, bathing, seeking quiet, calm environment, etc.).

NOTES

Infants have a predictable sequence of states of awareness including deep sleep, light sleep (with rapid eye movements), quiet alert, awake, active alert, and crying.

Light sleep, quiet alert, and awake states are the best times to initiate feeding. Crying is a late feeding cue.

Crying is a calorically expensive event for babies. Parents should be encouraged to comfort crying babies.

See also Allergy in the breastfed infant; Feeding cues

➤ CUP FEEDING

DEFINITION   An alternative feeding method for delivering liquid to infants. Cup feeding is the internationally recommended method of supplementing breastfed infants due to ease of cleaning the cup and the avoidance of introducing baby to an artificial nipple shape.

➤ CUSTODY

DEFINITION   Referring to legal custody shared between parents and the complications of meeting the needs of the breastfeeding baby in this situation.

ASK ABOUT

Age of the baby.
Length of mother–baby separation.

ASSESSMENT

PROMPT CARE NEEDED?

Are any of the following present?

The mother wishes to maintain milk supply during separation from her baby.

IF YES,   *Call lactation care provider today.*

SELF-CARE INFORMATION

Express milk on the same schedule the baby would normally feed during separation to maintain milk supply.
Monitor fullness of breasts closely.

NOTES

A compendium of state laws protecting breastfeeding, including some legislation regarding family law, is available on the U.S. Breastfeeding Committee's website at www.usbreastfeeding.org.

➤ CYANOSIS

DEFINITION   A state where the skin and mucous membrane turn purplish-blue, reflecting lack of oxygenation in the blood.

ASK ABOUT

Onset.
Medical conditions of the baby.

ASSESSMENT

EMERGENT CARE NEEDED?

Are any of the following present?

Circumoral cyanosis during feeding (cyanosis around the mouth) or at other times.

Cyanosis of the hands and feet beyond the first few days of life.
(Remember, acrocyanosis is common and normal in newborns.)

IF YES,   *Seek medical care now.*

IMPORTANT CONDITIONS TO REPORT

Medications used.

See also Acrocyanosis; Circumoral cyanosis

➤ CYSTIC BREASTS

DEFINITION   A common breast condition in women including variable lumpiness, tenderness, and palpable cysts (pockets of fluid). Symptoms may change during the menstrual period. This benign condition is compatible with breastfeeding.

New lumps in the breast should be medically examined to rule out **plugged ducts** and other problems.

See also Breast lumps; Fibrocystic breasts; Plugged breasts

➤ CYSTIC FIBROSIS

DEFINITION A chronic genetic disease that affects all the respiratory and digestive tracts, creating thick mucus that can cause obstruction leading to difficult respiration and digestion.

Infants and children with cystic fibrosis may have stunted growth and frequent infections. Breastfeeding is recommended for children with this condition, as it may boost their immune systems and decrease negative outcomes.

➤ CYTOKINE

DEFINITION A term for any of a number of immunoactive proteins, including interleukin, interferon, and others that are secreted by the cells of the immune system to regulate immune response.

➤ CYTOMEGALOVIRUS (CMV)

DEFINITION A virus of the herpes family that is widespread in the population and can be dormant in the body for years. CMV infection has no obvious symptoms, with rare exception of an illness similar to mononucleosis.

SELF-CARE INFORMATION

Practice routine, careful hand washing with soap and water, especially when handling children and diapers.

NOTES

CDC states:

> Although CMV can be shed in breast milk, infections that occur from breastfeeding usually do not cause symptoms or disease in the infant and there are no recommendations against breast feeding. Because CMV infection after birth may cause disease in very premature or low birth weight infants, mothers of these infants should consult their healthcare providers about breastfeeding.[111(p1)]

It is appropriate for mothers with CMV infection to breastfeed their full-term healthy babies.

AAP (2012) states that in the event that a mother with CMV infection has a preterm baby, "The value of routinely feeding human milk from seropositive mothers to preterm infants outweighs the risks of clinical disease, especially because no long-term neurodevelopmental abnormalities have been reported."[112(p.e833)] See the American Academy of Pediatrics' 2012 statement for more guidance.

Footnotes

[111]Centers for Disease Control and Prevention. (2010). Cytomegalovirus (CMV) and congenital CMV infection. Retrieved from http://www.cdc.gov/cmv/transmission.html

[112]AAP Section on Breastfeeding. (2012). Breastfeeding and the use of human milk. *Pediatrics, 129*(3), e827-e841. doi: 10.1542/peds.2011-3552

➤ DAIRY PRODUCTS FOR BABY

DEFINITION   Foods made from cow's milk. Cow's milk is not recommended for children younger than 1 year of age.

NOTES

Breastmilk and infant formula are the only appropriate milks for babies younger than 1 year. While cow's milk–based formula is an appropriate substitute for human milk, unaltered cow's milk is not, as it may lead to mineral and nutrient imbalance and bleeding in the gut.

Unless there is a family history of cow's milk allergy, babies may be introduced to small amounts of yogurt, cheese, and other dairy foods after 8 months of age.

Between 1 and 2 years of age, whole cow's milk may be offered to children. Low-fat and skim milk should not be offered until children are older than 2.

Concern about infant allergy is much more predominant than actual allergy. The American Academy of Pediatrics reports that the prevalence of infant cow's milk allergy is 2–3 %.[114] The overall prevalence of childhood food allergy is 4–6%.[115]

Breastfeeding babies may react to cow's milk protein in their mother's diet.

See also Allergy in the breastfed infant; Colic, infantile; Cow's milk

Footnotes

[114]AAP Committee on Nutrition. (2000). Hypoallergenic infant formulas. *Pediatrics, 106,* 346.

[115]Ziegler, R. S. (2003). Food allergen avoidance in prevention of food allergy in infants and children. *Pediatrics, 111,* 1662–1671.

➤ DANCER HAND POSITION

DEFINITION A technique used to assist the baby with low muscle tone or depressed reflexes in maintaining positioning at the breast. This technique keeps the weight of the breast off the baby's jaw and gives some support to the baby's facial muscles.

NOTES

In this position, the mother's hand slides up under the breast to hold the weight of the breast cupped in her hand. She supports the baby's chin and jaw with the web of tissue between her thumb and forefinger and uses her thumb and index finger to cup the baby's cheeks, giving support.

See also Down syndrome (DS); Uncoordinated suckling

➤ DAY CARE

DEFINITION   A substitute care provider or group of providers who care for a child while the parents go to work or school. Breastfeeding mothers should be supported in expressing and collecting their milk to be given to babies in day care.

ASK ABOUT

Onset of separation.
Age of the baby.

ASSESSMENT

ROUTINE CARE NEEDED?

Are any of the following present?

Mother–baby separation anticipated.
Mother wishes to express milk for baby.

IF YES,   *Call lactation care provider today.*

SELF-CARE INFORMATION

Frequent milk expression is ideal.

IMPORTANT CONDITIONS TO REPORT

Decreasing milk supply.
Questions about collection and storage.

See also Decrease in milk supply; Working women

➤ DECONGESTANTS

DEFINITION   A category of drugs used to decrease nasal mucous membrane and sinus congestion.

NOTES

Pseudoephedrine, a commonly used decongestant, has been noted to reduce milk production by 24% with a single dose. For this reason, Lawrence & Lawrence (2011) advise that "breastfeeding women should not take decongestants and should rely instead on saline nose drops and moisture (vaporizers) for relief of upper respiratory symptoms."[116(pp390–391)]

Footnote

[116]Lawrence, R. A., & Lawrence, R. M. (2011). *Breastfeeding: A guide for the medical profession* (7th ed.). St. Louis, MO: Elsevier/Mosby.

➤ DECREASE IN MILK SUPPLY

DEFINITION   Insufficient amount of milk produced by the breast. Maternal, infant, and environmental factors all contribute to milk supply problems.

ASK ABOUT

Onset.
Age of the baby.

ASSESSMENT

EMERGENT CARE NEEDED?

Are any of the following present?

Meconium bowel movements after 5 days of life.

Fewer than three bowel movements daily in breastfed newborn after the first 2 days of life.

No urine in 6 hours.

Brick dust urine (uric acid crystals) after 2 days of life.

Dark-colored urine.

Fewer than four urinations daily in the breastfed newborn after day 5.

Noticeably sunken fontanelles (soft spot on top of head).

Decreased activity.

Baby below birthweight at 10–14 days.

Cessation of weight gain.

IF YES, *Seek medical care within 4 hours.*

PROMPT CARE NEEDED?

Are any of the following present?

Scanty urination.

IF YES, *Call pediatric care provider today.*

Are any of the following present?

Identified milk supply problem.

Concern about possible milk supply problem.

IF YES, *Call lactation care provider today.*

SELF-CARE INFORMATION

Ensure baby is feeding 10–12 times per 24 hours.

Express milk after feeding.

IMPORTANT CONDITIONS TO REPORT

Persistent problems.

Recurrent problems.

Milk supply can be increased. This is accomplished by increasing stimulation and removal of milk from the breast.

Mothers of hospitalized infants and employed mothers may experience a decrease in milk supply when pumping.

Concerns about milk supply always warrant evaluation.

See also Increasing milk supply

➤ DECREASING SUPPLEMENTAL FORMULA

DEFINITION   Reducing the amount of formula used as breastmilk supply increases. Decreases in supplemental formula should be made gradually and with careful monitoring to ensure adequate growth and nutrition of the baby.

ASK ABOUT

Reason for supplementation.
Age of baby.

ASSESSMENT

PROMPT CARE NEEDED?

Are any of the following present?

Desire to begin decreasing formula supplementation.

Continued decrease in supplementation.

IF YES,   *Call lactation care provider today.*

SELF-CARE INFORMATION

Ensure adequate breast stimulation by expressing milk every time baby
   is supplemented.

Bring baby to a pediatric care provider for frequent weight checks.

IMPORTANT CONDITIONS TO REPORT
Decrease in stooling pattern of the baby.
Concerns about milk production.

NOTES

Decrease in supplementation should not be made without review and approval of the medical care provider who ordered supplementation.

See also **Milk transfer, estimating; Test weighing**

➤ DEEP BREAST PAIN

DEFINITION   Uncomfortable sensations in the breast. Pain is not an expected part of breastfeeding and indicates need for feeding evaluation.

ASK ABOUT

Onset.
Location of pain.
Whether pain is unilateral or bilateral.

ASSESSMENT

PROMPT CARE NEEDED?
Are any of the following present?
Persistent deep pain with feeding.
Persistent deep pain between feedings.
Constant deep pain.
Pain combined with color change of nipple(s).
Pain with visible fissure or bleeding of the nipple(s).

IF YES,   *Call lactation care provider today.*

NOTES

Breastfeeding should not be painful. Advise mothers to seek medical or lactation care for breast pain.

There can be many reasons for pain in the breast, including breast infection or inflammation, clogs, or cysts. Poor latch-on or positioning can also cause pain.

Pinched nerves and lymphatic congestion may contribute to deep pain.

Candida infection has been suggested as a cause of deep pain. However, research has not confirmed this suggestion.[117] Research shows bacteria is found more often in the ducts and milk of women with deep breast pain.[118]

See also Breast pain; Latch-on; Mastitis; Sore nipples

Footnotes

[117]Hale, T. W., Bateman, T. L., Finkelman, M. A., & Berens, P. D. (2009). The absence of *Candida albicans* in milk samples of women with clinical symptoms of ductal candidiasis. *Breastfeeding Medicine: The Official Journal of the Academy of Breastfeeding Medicine, 4*(2), 57–61. doi:10.1089/bfm.2008.0144

[118]Eglash, A., Plane, M. B., & Mundt, M. (2006). History, physical and laboratory findings, and clinical outcomes of lactating women treated with antibiotics for chronic breast and/or nipple pain. *Journal of Human Lactation: Official Journal of International Lactation Consultant Association, 22*(4), 429–433. doi:10.1177/0890334406293431

➤ DEHYDRATION

DEFINITION   Depletion of the water stores in the body, due to a number of causes including lack of adequate fluid intake, diarrhea, and vomiting. Infants and young children can become dehydrated quickly. Severely dehydrated women may make less milk, but mild dehydration has little effect on milk production and content.

ASK ABOUT

Onset.

Age of the baby.

ASSESSMENT

EMERGENT CARE NEEDED?

Are any of the following present?

Meconium bowel movements after 5 days of life.

Fewer than three bowel movements daily in breastfed newborn after the first 2 days of life.

No urine in 6 hours.

Brick dust urine (uric acid crystals) after 2 days of life.

Dark-colored urine.

Fewer than four urinations daily in the breastfed newborn after day 5.

Noticeably sunken fontanelles (soft spot on top of head).

Decreased activity.

Baby below birthweight at 10–14 days.

Cessation of weight gain.

Diarrhea or vomiting lasting more than a few hours.

> **IF YES,**   *Seek medical care within 4 hours.*

PROMPT CARE NEEDED?

Are any of the following present?

Scanty urination.

> **IF YES,**   *Call pediatric care provider today.*

SELF-CARE INFORMATION

Ensure baby is feeding 10–12 times per 24 hours.

Practice skin-to-skin care as much as possible.

IMPORTANT CONDITIONS TO REPORT

Persistent problems.

Recurrent problems.

➤ DEPARTMENT OF HEALTH & HUMAN SERVICES (DHHS)

DESCRIPTION   Government agency that is "the principal agency for protecting the health of all Americans. It is comprised of the Office of the Secretary (18 Staff Divisions) and 11 Operating Divisions."[119]

NOTES

DHHS
Web: www.hhs.gov/
  Through several of its divisions, HHS promotes healthy behaviors including breast-feeding.

Footnote

[119]U.S. Department of Health and Human Services. (2012). Home. Retrieved from http://www.hhs.gov/

➤ DEPRESSION

DEFINITION   Symptoms of depression are not unusual for women during the early days after giving birth. Depending upon the population studied, between 5 and 25% of women experience depression during this period.[120]

ASK ABOUT

Onset.
Age of the baby.
History of depression.

ASSESSMENT

EMERGENT CARE NEEDED?

Are any of the following present?

Suicidal thoughts.

Thoughts of harming the baby.

IF YES, *Seek emergency care now.*

PROMPT CARE NEEDED?

Are any of the following present?

Persistent sadness.

Inability to function.

IF YES, *Seek medical care within 4 hours.*

ROUTINE CARE NEEDED?

Are any of the following present?

Ongoing breastfeeding in a woman with depression.

IF YES, *Call lactation care provider today.*

SELF-CARE INFORMATION

Mood swings are normal in the postpartum period but may become more severe. Seek support.

Practice skin-to-skin contact in the first hour and frequently thereafter.

Feed the baby at first sign of hunger cues (signs that say "feed me" include hand-to-face or hand-to-mouth movements, lip smacking, seeking with lips, rooting, and head bobbing).

Feed the baby at least 10 times per 24 hours.

Listen for signs of the baby swallowing.

Allow the baby to end feedings.

Expect at least three infant stools per 24 hours after the first 4 days of life.

Good positioning and attachment are crucial to prevent or reduce nipple pain.

If feedings are missed, hand express or pump milk to maintain supply.

IMPORTANT CONDITIONS TO REPORT

Exacerbation of symptoms.

Nonresolution of symptoms.

History of depression, mood disorders, premenstrual syndrome, or thyroid disorders.

NOTES

Symptoms of depression can progress to other postpartum mood disorders. It is important to encourage mothers to report any worsening of symptoms.

Women who experienced depression during pregnancy and those with a prior history of depression, mood disorders, or premenstrual syndrome are at greater risk for postpartum depression.

Hypothyroidism, anemia, and other physical disorders share many symptoms with postpartum depression.

Many antidepressant medications are considered compatible with breastfeeding. Consult an up-to-date drug reference for more info. The Academy of Breastfeeding Medicine provides a protocol on use of antidepressant medications in breastfeeding women.[121]

The Edinburgh Scale of Postpartum Depression can be a helpful resource.[122]

See also Anemia; Baby blues; Hypothyroidism; Medication resources (inside back cover); Postpartum depression

Footnotes

[120]ABM Protocol Committee. (2008). ABM clinical protocol #18: Use of antidepressants in nursing mothers. *Breastfeeding Medicine: The Official Journal of the Academy of Breastfeeding Medicine, 3*(1), 44–52. doi:10.1089/bfm.2007.9978

[121]ABM Protocol Committee. ibid.

[122]Cox, J. L., Holden, J. M., & Sagovsky, R. (1987). Detection of postnatal depression. Development of the 10-item Edinburgh Postnatal Depression Scale. *The British Journal of Psychiatry: The Journal of Mental Science, 150*, 782–786. Tool accessible on the Web: http://www.fresno.ucsf.edu/pediatrics/downloads/edinburghscale.pdf

➤ DHA

See Docosahexaenoic acid

➤ DHHS

See Department of Health & Human Services (DHHS)

➤ DHHS/AGENCY FOR HEALTHCARE RESEARCH AND QUALITY

DESCRIPTION   Government agency whose mission "is to improve the quality, safety, efficiency, and effectiveness of health care for all Americans. As 1 of 12 agencies within the Department of Health and Human Services, AHRQ supports research that helps people make more informed decisions and improves the quality of health care services. AHRQ was formerly known as the Agency for Health Care Policy and Research."[123]

NOTES

Questions: https://info.ahrq.gov/app/answers/list
Web: http://www.ahrq.gov/

Footnote

[123]Agency for Healthcare Research and Quality. (2011). AHRQ at a glance. Retrieved from http ://www.ahrq.gov/about/ataglance.htm

➤ DHHS/CENTERS FOR DISEASE CONTROL AND PREVENTION

DESCRIPTION   Government agency whose mission is "Collaborating to create the expertise, information, and tools that people and communities need to protect their health—through health promotion, prevention of disease, injury and disability, and preparedness for new health threats."[124]

NOTES

Email: cdcinfo@cdc.gov
Web: www.cdc.gov/
    CDC provides surveillance, monitoring, and information about breastfeeding through the web portal www.cdc.gov/breastfeeding

Footnote

[124]Centers for Disease Control & Prevention. (2010). Vision, mission, core values, and pledge. Retrieved from http://www.cdc.gov/about/organization/mission.htm

➤ DHHS/FOOD AND DRUG ADMINISTRATION (FDA)

DEFINITION   Government agency that is "responsible for protecting the public health by assuring the safety, efficacy and security of human and veterinary drugs, biological products, medical devices, our nation's food supply, cosmetics, and products that emit radiation.

FDA is also responsible for advancing the public health by helping to speed innovations that make medicines more effective, safer, and more affordable and by helping the public get the accurate, science-based information they need to use medicines and foods to maintain and improve their health. FDA also has responsibility for regulating the manufacturing, marketing and distribution of tobacco products to protect the public health and to reduce tobacco use by minors.[125(p1)]

NOTES

U.S. Food and Drug Administration
Contact: www.fda.gov/AboutFDA/ContactFDA/default.htm
Web: www.fda.gov
    The FDA provides guidance on the safe use of breast pumps and tracks issues associated with pumps through the MAUDE database, found on its website. The FDA's Center for Food Safety and Applied Nutrition (CFSAN) is involved with infant formula safety.

Footnote

[125]Food and Drug Administration. (2010). About FDA: What we do. Retrieved from http://www.fda.gov/AboutFDA/WhatWeDo/default.htm

---

➤ DHHS/HEALTH SERVICES RESOURCES ADMINISTRATION (HRSA), MATERNAL CHILD HEALTH BUREAU

DESCRIPTION   Government agency whose mission "is to provide leadership, in partnership with key stakeholders, to improve the physical and mental health, safety and well-being of the maternal and child health (MCH) population which includes all of the nation's women, infants, children, adolescents, and their families, [i]ncluding fathers and children with special health care needs."[126](MCH Mission section)

NOTES

Maternal Child Health Bureau
Email: ask@hrsa.gov
Telephone: 888-ASK-HRSA
Web: http://mchb.hrsa.gov/
    MCHB administers the Title V program to coordinate, build capacity, and oversee the well-being of infants, children, and women at the state and community level.

Footnote

[126]Health Services Resources Administration, Maternal Child Health Bureau. (n.d.). About us. Retrieved from http://mchb.hrsa.gov/about/index.html

➤ DHHS/INDIAN HEALTH SERVICE

DESCRIPTION   A government agency that "is responsible for providing federal health services to American Indians and Alaska Natives. The provision of health services to members of federally-recognized tribes grew out of the special government-to-government relationship between the federal government and Indian tribes. This relationship, established in 1787, is based on Article I, Section 8 of the Constitution, and has been given form and substance by numerous treaties, laws, Supreme Court decisions, and Executive Orders. The IHS is the principal federal health care provider and health advocate for Indian people, and its goal is to raise their health status to the highest possible level. The IHS provides a comprehensive health service delivery system for approximately 1.9 million American Indians and Alaska Natives who belong to 564 federally recognized tribes in 35 states."[127(p1)]

NOTES

Email: webmaster@ihs.gov
Web: www.ihs.gov/
   IHS has a portal for its breastfeeding-related activities at http://www.ihs.gov /babyfriendly/

Footnote

[127]Indian Health Service. (n.d.). Indian Health Service introduction. Retrieved from http://www .ihs.gov/index.cfm?module=ihsIntro

➤ DHHS/OFFICE ON WOMEN'S HEALTH (OWH)

DESCRIPTION A government agency whose mission is "to provide leadership to promote health equity for women and girls through sex/gender-specific approaches. OWH achieves its mission and vision by developing innovative programs, educating health professionals, and motivating behavior change in consumers through the dissemination of health information."[128(p1)]

NOTES

Office on Women's Health
Web: http://womenshealth.gov/
   OWH provides breastfeeding information through a portal on its website at http ://womenshealth.gov/breastfeeding/. In addition, OWH convened the National Breastfeeding Awareness campaign and hosts a national breastfeeding information line for women at 800-994-WOMAN.

Footnote

[128]Office on Women's Health. (2010). About us. Retrieved from http://www.womenshealth.gov /about-us/mission-history-goals/index.cfm

➤ DIABETES

DEFINITION A chronic disease causing high levels of sugar in the blood. It is caused by too little insulin or resistance to insulin. There are three major types of diabetes:

Type 1, which is classically diagnosed in childhood. The pancreas makes little or no insulin, requiring daily injections of this hormone that regulates sugar metabolism.

Type 2, classically occurring in adulthood. The pancreas does not make enough insulin and/or the body's cells become resistant to the insulin in circulation. This type of diabetes may be managed by careful diet, and often with use of oral medications. Type 2 diabetes is becoming increasingly common.

Gestational diabetes is the condition of high blood sugar levels occurring during pregnancy in a woman without prior diabetes.

ASK ABOUT

Onset.

Type of diabetes.

ASSESSMENT

EMERGENT CARE NEEDED?

Are any of the following present?

Insulin shock in the breastfeeding woman.

IF YES,   *Seek emergency care now.*

PROMPT CARE NEEDED?

Are any of the following present?

Difficulty maintaining blood glucose levels during breastfeeding.

IF YES,   *Seek medical care today.*

ROUTINE CARE NEEDED?

Are any of the following present?

Ongoing breastfeeding in the diabetic woman.

IF YES,   *Call lactation care provider today.*

SELF-CARE INFORMATION

Women with diabetes are more prone to infection. Monitor breasts and nipples daily for any red, infected, or painful areas.

Women who are insulin dependent should be aware that less insulin may be required during breastfeeding—watch for signs of low blood sugar.

IMPORTANT CONDITIONS TO REPORT

Any symptoms of infection.

Difficulty regulating blood sugar.

Women with diabetes should be encouraged to breastfeed. Breastfeeding is known to reduce the risk of developing diabetes in susceptible individuals (e.g., children of diabetic mothers).

Research suggests that women who have experienced gestational diabetes are less likely to progress to diabetes if they breastfeed their babies.[129]

See also Autoimmune diseases

Footnote

[129]Kjos, S. L., Henry, O., Lee, R. M., Buchanan, T. A., & Mishell, D. R. (1993). The effect of lactation on glucose and lipid metabolism in women with recent gestational diabetes. *Obstetrics and Gynecology, 82*(3), 451–455.

➤ **DIARRHEA**

DEFINITION   Frequent loose, watery stools. Diarrhea is typically caused by a virus. Diarrhea can be serious in infants and young children, as they can become dehydrated quickly.

ASK ABOUT

Onset.
Age of the baby.

ASSESSMENT

EMERGENT CARE NEEDED?
   Are any of the following present?
      Diarrhea episodes in a baby younger than 3 months of age.
      Meconium bowel movements after 5 days of life.
      Fewer than three bowel movements daily in breastfed newborn after the first
        2 days of life.

No urine in 6 hours.

Brick dust urine (uric acid crystals) after 2 days of life.

Dark-colored urine.

Fewer than four urinations daily in the breastfed newborn after day 5.

Noticeably sunken fontanelles (soft spot on top of head).

Decreased activity.

Baby below birthweight at 10–14 days.

Cessation of weight gain.

IF YES, *Seek medical care within 4 hours.*

PROMPT CARE NEEDED?

Are any of the following present?

Scanty urination.

Sporadic diarrhea.

IF YES, *Call pediatric care provider today.*

SELF-CARE INFORMATION

Ensure baby is feeding 10–12 times per 24 hours.

Practice careful hand washing before and after handling the baby, changing diapers, and going to the bathroom.

IMPORTANT CONDITIONS TO REPORT

Persistent problems.

Recurrent problems.

NOTES

Diarrhea in the nursing mother is of concern for proper functioning of her body, but not for the manufacture of milk.

See also Acute infection; Blood in stool; Dehydration; Stooling patterns

➤ DIET OF THE MOTHER

DEFINITION   Referring to foods eaten by the mother on a daily basis.

NOTES

Mothers can produce enough milk, and milk of good quality, even when the mother's supply of nutrients is limited.[130] Rules about eating or not eating certain foods during lactation are not warranted, may be hard to follow, and may decrease the mother's enjoyment of breastfeeding. However, there may be individual cases where certain foods affect the baby. Most commonly, the mother's drinking of liquid cow's milk has been associated with colic symptoms in some babies. If this is the case, improvement may be seen after the mother eliminates cow's milk from her diet for at least a week. Mothers should seek further information about diet and breastfeeding on an individual basis.

See also Allergy in the breastfed infant; Macrobiotic diet of the mother; Maternal diet, vegetarian

Footnote

[130]National Academy of Sciences Subcommittee on Nutrition. (1991). *Nutrition during lactation.* Washington, DC: National Academy Press.

➤ DIETARY REFERENCE INTAKES (DRI)

DEFINITION   Values of the amount of nutrients needed by healthy people each day.

NOTES

This terminology replaces the concept of RDA (recommended dietary allowances), which offered population estimates of the amount of nutrients needed to avoid deficiency. The DRIs look at nutrient needs from the point of view of promoting health rather than avoiding deficiency. DRIs for infants, children, and lactating women may be found through the USDA's website.[113]

Footnote

[113]USDA, National Agricultural Library. (2012, May 22). DRI tables. Retrieved from http://fnic.nal.usda.gov/dietary-guidance/dietary-reference-intakes/dri-tables

➤ DIMPLED NIPPLE

DEFINITION   A condition in which the center of the nipple is retracted toward the chest wall. This condition may affect one or both nipples and may be cause for pain in the breastfeeding woman.

ASK ABOUT

Onset of nipple condition.

ASSESSMENT

EMERGENT CARE NEEDED?

Are any of the following present?

Sudden occurrence of dimpled nipples.

IF YES,   *Seek medical care today.*

PROMPT CARE NEEDED?

Are any of the following present?

Preexisting dimpled nipple with pain.

Ongoing problems with dimpled nipple.

IF YES,   *Call lactation care provider today.*

SELF-CARE INFORMATION

Keep the area around the dimpled nipple dry, changing pads frequently.

IMPORTANT CONDITIONS TO REPORT

Worsening of condition.

Symptoms of infection.

NOTES

Suddenly occurring dimpled nipples should be examined to rule out cancer.

See also Inverted nipples

➤ DISABILITIES, MOTHERS WITH

DEFINITION   Referring to mothers living with a physical or mental challenge.

ASK ABOUT

Type of disability.
Age of the baby.

ASSESSMENT

PROMPT CARE NEEDED?

Are any of the following present?

Mother with disabilities learning to breastfeed.
Ongoing breastfeeding support needed.

IF YES,   *Call lactation care provider today.*

SELF-CARE INFORMATION

Set up a feeding station in the home where nonperishable snacks, drinks of water, baby changing equipment, hand wipes, and a telephone can be at the ready.

IMPORTANT CONDITIONS TO REPORT

Concern about feeding adequacy or comfort.

NOTES

Breastfeeding is often an ideal feeding choice for mothers with disabilities, as it requires little preparation for feeding.

➤ DISCHARGE FROM NIPPLE

DEFINITION   Visible evidence of blood or other secretion from the nipple.

ASK ABOUT

Onset.
Age of the baby.
History of trauma or surgery to the breast.

ASSESSMENT

EMERGENT CARE NEEDED?

Are any of the following present?

Persistent bleeding from nipple after or between feedings.

Symptoms of infection (redness or pus at the site of bleeding, fever, chills, achiness, or malaise).

Appearance of nipple discharge in nonpregnant, nonlactating women.

IF YES, *Seek medical care within 4 hours.*

PROMPT CARE NEEDED?

Are any of the following present?

Sporadic bleeding after, between, or during feedings.

Pain on latch.

IF YES, *Call lactation care provider today.*

SELF-CARE INFORMATION

Practice good attachment:

Watch for feeding cues and offer the breast as soon as they are seen.

Wait for the baby to open his or her mouth wide (greater than a 140° angle).

Pull the baby in so that his or her chin touches the breast first, and the nipple enters the mouth along the top of the tongue; this should result in a wide-open mouth on the breast.

The baby's lips should be flanged outward and make a seal on the breast.

The baby's lips should look off center when compared with the areola; the bottom lip should be farther away from the nipple than the top lip.

IMPORTANT CONDITIONS TO REPORT

Any substance or item being used to decrease pain.

Worsening symptoms.

Persistent symptoms.

See also Bleeding, breast; Nipple pain; Intraductal papilloma

➤ DISTRACTIBILITY

DEFINITION A characteristic of babies older than 4 months whose attention is easily diverted away from feeding at the breast.

SELF-CARE INFORMATION
Try feeding the baby in a dark, quiet room.

➤ DIURNAL VARIATION

DEFINITION Changes that happen on a daily cycle. For example, prolactin levels appear to be naturally higher during the night and lower during the day.

➤ DOCOSAHEXAENOIC ACID (DHA) IN BREASTMILK

DEFINITION A long-chain polyunsaturated fatty acid (LCPUFA) found naturally in human milk. These fatty acids assist in the development of nerve and brain tissue.

NOTES

While LCPUFAs have been added to formula in recent years, there is no clear evidence of beneficial outcomes in children who have consumed them.[131,132] Supplements are also being marketed for mothers to consume during pregnancy and lactation, also with little evidence of efficacy.[133]

See also Arachidonic acid (AA, also ARA); Fat in breastmilk; LCPUFAs

Footnotes

[131]Schulzke, S. M., Patole, S. K., & Simmer, K. (2011). Longchain polyunsaturated fatty acid supplementation in preterm infants. *Cochrane Database of Systematic Reviews (Online)*, (2), CD000375. doi:10.1002/14651858.CD000375.pub4

[132]Simmer, K., Patole, S. K., & Rao, S. C. (2011). Longchain polyunsaturated fatty acid supplementation in infants born at term. *Cochrane Database of Systematic Reviews (Online)*, (12), CD000376. doi:10.1002/14651858.CD000376.pub3

[133]Dziechciarz, P., Horvath, A., & Szajewska, H. (2010). Effects of n-3 long-chain polyunsaturated fatty acid supplementation during pregnancy and/or lactation on neurodevelopment and visual function in children: A systematic review of randomized controlled trials. *Journal of the American College of Nutrition*, 29(5), 443–454.

➤ DONOR MILK

DEFINITION Excess milk obtained from breastfeeding mothers. In the United States, donor milk should be obtained only from a member milk bank of the Human Milk Banking Association of North America or a state-licensed milk bank.

NOTES

Informal donation of milk from one mother to another cannot be condoned, as it is possible to pass infectious agents through the milk.

Donor milk from a recognized human milk bank will have gone through several different screening processes (history and serology of the donor, bacteriology of the milk before and after heat treatment, etc.) and will be heat treated to remove most pathogens.

The uses of donor milk are many, including providing nourishment to preterm or chronically ill infants, such as those with feeding intolerance, malabsorption, cardiac problems, metabolic problems, and diarrhea.

Use of donor milk in preterm infants is thought to reduce the risk of necrotizing enterocolitis.

A prescription is necessary in order for donor milk to be dispensed from the milk bank.

There is a processing cost associated with obtaining donor milk; this fee may be waived or reduced if it is cost prohibitive.

Human Milk Banking Association of North America (HMBANA)

Web: www.hmbana.org

See also Cross nursing; Milk banks

➤ DOUBLE PUMPING

DEFINITION A system that allows both breasts to be pumped simultaneously. Double pumping generally takes less time and may stimulate more milk production. This technique is particularly helpful for mothers of preterm or ill babies and others who are separated from their babies routinely.

NOTES

Double pump kits can be purchased. All rental grade electric pumps are available with double pump kits. Some personal use pumps are available with double pump kits.

➤ DOULA

DEFINITION A person who accompanies the family during the peripartum period, offering support and nurturing care as the mother gives birth and develops a relationship with her new baby. Doula care has been shown to reduce the risk of prolonged labor, need for analgesia, and cesarean birth. Doula care has also been shown to increase exclusive breastfeeding.

NOTES

Doulas can be found by contacting:

ALACE (The Association of Labor Assistants & Childbirth Educators)

Email: info@alace.org

Web site: www.alace.org

DONA (Doulas of North America)

Email: doula@dona.org

Web: www.dona.org

➤ DOWN SYNDROME (DS)

DEFINITION A congenital genetic disorder that usually results in mild to moderate mental retardation and other conditions, including decreased muscle tone, and sometimes heart defects and gastrointestinal problems. Babies with Down syndrome benefit from breastfeeding, as do mothers with this syndrome.

ASK ABOUT

Age of the baby.

ASSESSMENT

EMERGENT CARE NEEDED?

Are any of the following present?

Circumoral cyanosis (blue tinge around lips).

Vomiting in the newborn with DS.

| IF YES, | *Seek emergency care now.* |

PROMPT CARE NEEDED?

Are any of the following present?

Beginning breastfeeding with DS baby.

Difficulty with breastfeeding DS baby.

| IF YES, | *Call lactation care provider today.* |

ROUTINE CARE NEEDED?

Are any of the following present?

Ongoing feeding concerns with DS baby.

| IF YES, | *Report to lactation care provider.* |

SELF-CARE INFORMATION

Because of the baby's low muscle tone, milk expression may be required after feeding to maximize milk removal (which will increase milk manufacture).

Feeding cues may be more subtle; ensure that the baby is feeding 10–12 times per 24 hours.

Avoid pacifier and bottle nipple use.

Practice continuous, uninterrupted skin-to-skin contact in the first hour and frequently thereafter.

IMPORTANT CONDITIONS TO REPORT

Vomiting.

Feeding difficulties.

Growth and development of babies with DS should be closely monitored. Vomiting in babies with DS in the newborn period is of special concern because of the increased risk of intestinal obstruction.

See also Breast pump; Dancer hand position; Hand expression of breastmilk; Muscle tone of infant

➤ DRI

See Dietary Reference Intakes

➤ DRUGS

DEFINITION   Prescription and over-the-counter medications and supplements that a breastfeeding mother may consume.

NOTES

Many factors influence whether a drug the mother takes will be found in her milk, the amount of the drug that is found in the milk, and the effect of the drug on the baby. Some drugs can also affect the milk supply.

ASK ABOUT

Age of the baby.
Weight of the baby.
History of taking a drug (i.e., was the drug taken during pregnancy?).
How long the drug will be taken.

ROUTINE CARE NEEDED?

Are any of the following present?

Questions about drug compatibility with lactation.

IF YES,   *Consult up-to-date drug references and call lactation provider today.*

SELF-CARE INFORMATION

Do not self-medicate while breastfeeding without discussing the drug with your healthcare provider. This includes prescription, over-the-counter, and street drugs, as well as herbs, tinctures, vitamins, minerals, and other nutritional supplements.

Tell every healthcare provider that you are breastfeeding.

If you are prescribed a drug that is not compatible with breastfeeding, ask if there is an alternative drug that is.

IMPORTANT CONDITIONS TO REPORT

Any changes in the baby's behavior or appearance.

Any changes in your milk supply.

NOTES

An up-to-date drug reference should be consulted to determine the safety and possible side effects of individual drugs.

Newborn and premature babies are at greater risk of drug side effects due to limited ability to clear drugs from their systems.

See also Drugs, contraindicated

➤ DRUGS, CONTRAINDICATED

DEFINITION   Drugs taken by the mother that make it inadvisable to breastfeed.

NOTES

Occasionally drugs taken by the mother may make it inadvisable to breastfeed. According to the American Academy of Pediatrics Section on Breastfeeding:

> Recommendations regarding breastfeeding in situations in which the mother is undergoing either diagnostic procedures or pharmacologic therapy must balance the benefits to the infant and the mother against the potential risk of drug exposure to the infant . . . In general, breastfeeding is not recommended when mothers are receiving medication from the following classes of drugs: amphetamines, chemotherapy agents, ergotamines, and statins.[134(p.e833)]

An up-to-date drug reference should be consulted to determine the safety and possible side effects of individual drugs.

Newborn and premature babies are at greater risk of drug side effects due to limited ability to clear drugs from their systems.

See also Medication resources (inside back cover)

Footnote

[134]AAP Section on Breastfeeding. (2012). Breastfeeding and the use of human milk. *Pediatrics, 129* (3), e827-e841. doi: 10.1542/peds.2011-3552

➤ DRY-UP MEDICATION

DEFINITION   Medications such as bromocriptine (Parlodel) that were once used to dry up the milk of women who did not wish to breastfeed. Several deaths were attributed to bromocriptine use. This drug is no longer approved for use as dry-up medication.

NOTES

Hale lists bromocriptine as a category L5 (contraindicated) drug.[135]

See also Weaning

Footnote

[135]Hale, T. (2012). *Medications and mothers' milk* (15th ed., p. 151). Amarillo, TX: Hale Publishing.

➤ DUCTS

DEFINITION   The tubes within the breast that carry milk from the alveoli through the breast tissue and out through the nipple pores.

See also Plugged ducts

➤ EAR INFECTION

DEFINITION   An infection or inflammation of the middle ear, also called "otitis media." The inflammation may begin with an infection that causes a sore throat, cold, or other respiratory or breathing problem. Babies who are breastfed have a lower incidence of otitis media compared to babies who are not.

ASK ABOUT

Age of the baby.
History of sore throat, cold, or respiratory or breathing problem.
Change in breastfeeding behavior.

ASSESSMENT

PROMPT CARE NEEDED?

Are any of the following present?

Unusual irritability.
Difficulty sleeping.
Tugging or pulling at one or both ears.
Fever.
Fluid draining from one or both ears.

IF YES,   *Seek medical care today.*

PROMPT LACTATION CARE NEEDED?

Are any of the following present?

Difficulty breastfeeding.

Crying at the breast or pulling away and crying after a few sucks.

The baby has been treated for ear infection but continues to fret or cry at the breast.

IF YES,   *Call lactation care provider today.*

SELF-CARE INFORMATION

Even after the otitis media has resolved, the baby may be uncomfortable nursing or may remember the pain of nursing. Changing positions may help. If the problem persists, have the ears checked again by the pediatric healthcare provider.

Keep the breasts soft by expressing excess milk during the time the baby is not nursing well.

IMPORTANT CONDITIONS TO REPORT

Less urination or stooling.

Continued symptoms of otitis media after treatment.

Continued problems with breastfeeding after treatment is initiated.

See also Acute infection

➤ ECZEMA

DEFINITION   An allergic inflammation of the skin characterized by itching, redness, and scaling.

ASK ABOUT

Onset.

Age of the baby.

Medications used.

ASSESSMENT

PROMPT CARE NEEDED?

Are any of the following present?

Eczema on the breast.

Eczema on the baby.

Questions about medications.

IF YES,   *Seek medical care today.*

IMPORTANT CONDITIONS TO REPORT

Allergy and eczema in parents and siblings.

Infant symptoms of blood in stool, wheezing, hives, facial swelling, runny nose, vomiting, and irritability.

NOTES

Research has identified that exclusive breastfeeding reduces the risk of atopic eczema in susceptible children.

In adults, atopic eczema is typically treated with topical steroid creams. The specific cream indicated should be examined in an up-to-date drug reference to ensure it is safe for use by the breastfeeding mother.

Steroid cream use is of greater concern when the affected area is on the breast where the baby's mouth will be placed, as the baby will then absorb the steroid both through direct contact and through the milk.

In the breastfed baby, atopic eczema may be a symptom of food allergy, related to an allergen in food that the mother or baby is consuming. Mother and baby should avoid consuming offending allergens such as cow's milk, fish, eggs, peanuts, and tree nuts as directed by the healthcare provider.

Infantile symptoms of an allergic reaction include hives, facial swelling, runny nose, wheezing, eczema, vomiting, irritability (colic), blood in the stool, and anaphylaxis. Treatment centers on identification and avoidance of the proteins that are triggering the allergic reaction.

Babies born into allergic families are more likely to develop allergy, particularly those with two allergic parents or one allergic parent and an allergic sibling. Exclusive breastfeeding is the optimal feeding choice for these babies in particular.

Hypoallergenic formula is recommended when supplementing babies with documented allergy and has been suggested as a preferable supplemental formula in babies with a strong family history (biparental, parental, and/or sibling) of allergy.[136,137]

See also Allergy in the breastfed infant; Medication resources (inside back cover)

Footnotes

[136]AAP Committee on Nutrition. Hypoallergenic infant formulas. (2000). *Pediatrics, 106*, 348.

[137]Greer, F. R., Sicherer, S. H., Burks, A. W., & and the Committee on Nutrition and Section on Allergy and Immunology. (2008). Effects of early nutritional interventions on the development of atopic disease in infants and children: The role of maternal dietary restriction, breastfeeding, timing of introduction of complementary foods, and hydrolyzed formulas. *Pediatrics, 121*(1), 183–191. doi:10.1542/peds.2007-3022

➤ EDINBURGH POSTNATAL DEPRESSION SCALE (EPDS)

DEFINITION   The EPDS is a 10-point self-report scale designed to screen women for postpartum depression. Validation studies indicated that the EPDS is sensitive to the presence and changes in severity of depression over time.[138] Higher scores on the EPDS have been associated with lower breastfeeding initiation[139] and more breastfeeding problems.[140]

NOTES

The EPDS tool may be found on the Web at http://www.fresno.ucsf.edu/pediatrics /downloads/edinburghscale.pdf

Footnotes

[138]Cox, J. L., Holden, J. M., & Sagovsky, R. (1987). Detection of postnatal depression. Development of the 10-item Edinburgh Postnatal Depression Scale. *The British Journal of Psychiatry: The Journal of Mental Science, 150*, 782–786.

[139]Fairlie, T. G., Gillman, M. W., & Rich-Edwards, J. (2009). High pregnancy-related anxiety and prenatal depressive symptoms as predictors of intention to breastfeed and breastfeeding initiation. *Journal of Women's Health (2002), 18*(7), 945–953. doi:10.1089/jwh.2008.0998

[140]Watkins, S., Meltzer-Brody, S., Zolnoun, D., & Stuebe, A. (2011). Early breastfeeding experiences and postpartum depression. *Obstetrics and Gynecology, 118*(2 Pt 1), 214–221. doi:10.1097 /AOG.0b013e3182260a2d

➤ ELECTRONIC SCALES

DEFINITION   Sensitive weighing devices that can be used to monitor growth of infants, and when highly sensitive, can be used to estimate the amount of milk transferred from the breast to the baby during a feeding.

ASK ABOUT

Age of the baby.
Reason for needing the scale.

ASSESSMENT

EMERGENT CARE NEEDED?

Are any of the following present?

Newborn with greater than 10% weight loss.

Infant who does not wake for feedings.

Baby below birthweight at 10 days.

Cessation of weight gain.

Fewer than four bowel movements daily in breastfed newborn after first
  4 days of life.

Inadequate urination or dark urine.

No yellow stools by day 5.

IF YES,   *Seek medical care within 4 hours.*

PROMPT CARE NEEDED?

Are any of the following present?

Concerns about milk supply.

History of inadequate milk transfer.

Baby with a known diagnosis that could negatively impact milk supply
  (e.g., Down syndrome, clefts, prematurity).

Mother with a history of breast surgery.

Mother with two inverted nipples.

IF YES,   *Call lactation care provider today.*

ROUTINE CARE NEEDED?

Are any of the following present?

Scale rental with none of above indicators.

IF YES,   *Refer to scale manufacturer, distributor, or durable equipment sales or rental depot.*

SELF-CARE INFORMATION

Frequent feedings are the key to adequate milk production. Expect 10–12 feedings per 24 hours.

If using an electronic scale to estimate weight gain, be sure to weigh the baby before and after feedings wearing the same clothing, without changing the diaper.

Track intake over several feedings and average the results. The amount of milk consumed normally varies widely from feed to feed.

IMPORTANT CONDITIONS TO REPORT

Inadequate weight gain.

Ongoing concerns.

NOTES

Scales with breastmilk intake function can be rented from breast pump distributors.

See also Milk transfer, estimating; Test weighing; Weight gain, baby—low

➤ EMPLOYMENT

DEFINITION   Mothers who work for pay may do so away from home or in the home.

Mothers who are employed may be separated from their babies or have the babies nearby.

In the United States, more than half of the mothers with babies under the age of 1 year are employed.[141]

Amount of separation—hours per day, days per week.

Start date of work.

Age of the baby.

Mother's plans to continue breastfeeding.

Mother's plans to express milk.

Accommodations at work for expressing and saving milk.

How the baby will be fed away from the mother.

ASSESSMENT

ROUTINE CARE NEEDED?

Are any of the following present?

Information about managing work and breastfeeding.

IF YES,   *Call lactation care provider.*

SELF-CARE INFORMATION

Stress does not seem to affect milk supply, but frequent milk removal is needed to maintain or improve the milk supply.

Milk can be collected and frozen in the early weeks to supplement milk collected after the mother's return to work.

Milk supply is best maintained by hand expression or combining hand expression with pumping using a pump that is intended for that purpose along with breast-feeding.

Select child care facilities carefully.

Expressed milk is a raw food and should be refrigerated immediately if possible. Get information about storage, use, and feeding expressed milk from your lactation care provider.

The timing of return to work and the number of hours spent away from the baby affect the duration of breastfeeding more than the type of work a woman does.

IMPORTANT CONDITIONS TO REPORT

Problems with expressing milk (check that the equipment is working properly).

Breast problems.

Problems with the infant accepting expressed milk.

NOTES

The Affordable Care Act, passed by Congress in 2010, specifies that:

> Employers are required to provide "reasonable break time for an employee to express breast milk for her nursing child for 1 year after the child's birth each time such employee has need to express the milk." Employers are also required to provide "a place, other than a bathroom, that is shielded from view and free from intrusion from coworkers and the public, which may be used by an employee to express breast milk."[142](General Requirements section)

Ongoing support and help with problem solving may be needed after returning to work.

See also Collection and storage of breastmilk; Day care; Decrease in milk supply

Footnotes

[141]U.S. Department of Labor, Bureau of Labor Statistics. (2012, April 26). Employment characteristics of families summary. Retrieved from http://www.bls.gov/news.release/famee.nr0.htm

[142]U.S. Department of Labor. (2010, December). Wage and Hour Division (WHD)—fact sheet. Retrieved from http://www.dol.gov/whd/regs/compliance/whdfs73.htm

➤ ENDING A FEEDING

DEFINITION Babies make a seal at the breast with their lips and tongue. In addition, the chin is drawn into the breast and held there firmly during suckling. In order to take the baby off of the breast, the mother needs to break the seal. She can do this by inserting her clean finger into the corner of the baby's mouth or by pressing down onto her breast to break the seal.

SELF-CARE INFORMATION

Satisfied babies end feedings by themselves. The baby's hands are loose and his or her arms are heavy. Feedings should not be timed or routinely ended by the mother.

IMPORTANT CONDITIONS TO REPORT

Nipple pain.

The baby does not end feeding.

Deep breast pain.

The baby does not sustain a feeding.

➤ ENGORGEMENT

DEFINITION   Swelling in the breast associated with increase in the flow of blood and lymph to the breast, as well as the manufacture of milk. More common in the first days postpartum, engorgement may also occur whenever feedings are infrequent.

ASK ABOUT

Onset.

Age of the baby.

Feeding pattern.

ASSESSMENT

EMERGENT CARE NEEDED?

Are any of the following present?

Symptoms of infection (fever, aching, chills, and malaise).

Red streaks on the breast.

IF YES,   *Seek medical care within 4 hours.*

PROMPT CARE NEEDED?

Are any of the following present?

The baby is unable to latch onto the breast because it is too firm.

Engorgement is not resolving after latch-on.

IF YES,   *Call lactation care provider today.*

SELF-CARE INFORMATION

Consider soaking breasts in warm water before feedings or applying cool gel packs between feedings if that is comfortable for the mother.

Gently hand express to soften breasts before feedings.

Nonprescription anti-inflammatory agents may also be helpful.

IMPORTANT CONDITIONS TO REPORT

Lack of resolution in 24–48 hours.

Symptoms of infection (fever, chills, aching, redness, and malaise).

NOTES

Engorgement is best resolved by softening the breast so that the baby can latch onto the breast. Nursing the baby offers more relief than does hand expression or pumping.

See also Breast infection; Hand expression of breastmilk

➤ ENVIRONMENTAL CONTAMINANTS

DEFINITION Chemical contaminants present in the environment.

ASK ABOUT

Known contaminant exposure.

Age of the baby.

ASSESSMENT

EMERGENT CARE NEEDED?

Are any of the following present?

Sudden exposure of mother to toxic chemical.

IF YES, *Seek emergency care now.*

PROMPT CARE NEEDED?

Are any of the following present?

History of high level exposure to toxic chemicals in a breastfeeding woman.

IF YES,   *Call maternal medical care provider today.*

ROUTINE CARE NEEDED?

Are any of the following present?

General questions about environmental exposure.

IF YES,   *Call lactation care provider.*

IMPORTANT CONDITIONS TO REPORT

Known history of environmental or workplace exposure to toxic chemicals.
Any negative effects of past exposure.

NOTES

All foods, including breastmilk, may contain traces of environmental contaminants. Breastmilk is one of the easiest and least painful body tissues to sample. For this reason, it is used to monitor population exposure to chemicals. Low-level exposure to contaminants should not contraindicate breastfeeding. The greatest exposure for the baby is during pregnancy.[143]

Women who know they have been exposed to specific chemicals or pollutants should consult with their physician regarding analysis of the contaminant content of their milk. Several contaminants are addressed in the medication resources.

Many researchers have looked for negative effects of toxin exposure via breastmilk and have found only that there do not seem to be negative outcomes for breastfed babies, especially when health outcomes are compared to formula-fed babies.

See also Breastmilk, environmental contaminants; Medication resources (inside back cover); Pesticides and pollutants in breastmilk

Footnote

[143]Lawrence, R. A., & Lawrence, R. M. (2011). *Breastfeeding: A guide for the medical profession* (7th ed., p. 396). St. Louis: Elsevier/Mosby.

➤ ENZYMES IN BREASTMILK

DEFINITION　Proteins such as lipoprotein lipase and amylase found in human milk that assist in metabolism, digestion, and growth. Sometimes expressed milk will begin to break down during storage due to these enzymes, resulting in the milk smelling or tasting off or soapy. The milk has not gone bad. However, mothers have found that scalding milk decreases the enzymatic activity.

See also Rancid or soapy odor of frozen breastmilk

➤ EPDS

See Edinburgh Postnatal Depression Scale

➤ EPIDERMAL GROWTH FACTOR

DEFINITION　A component in human milk that triggers the growth of the skin cells lining the gastrointestinal and respiratory tracts.

➤ EPIDURAL ANESTHESIA

DEFINITION　Administration of drugs to the spinal cord to cause partial loss of sensation during childbirth and painful procedures.

SELF-CARE INFORMATION

When mothers receive pain medications during the birth process, extended skin-to-skin contact should be practiced immediately after birth and continued, uninterrupted, until the infant self-attaches for the first breastfeeding.

IMPORTANT CONDITIONS TO REPORT

Feeding difficulties.

NOTES

A number of drugs are used as epidural agents. An up-to-date drug reference should be consulted to determine the safety and possible side effects of individual drugs especially if the baby does not complete the expected nine stages before suckling and sleep.

Newborn and premature babies are at greater risk of side effects due to limited ability to clear drugs from their systems.

See also Analgesia; Anesthesia; Childbirth; Medication resources (inside back cover); Nine stages

➤ EPILEPSY

DEFINITION   A disorder of the electrical rhythm in the central nervous system, characterized by seizures. Mothers and babies with epilepsy can breastfeed.

IMPORTANT CONDITIONS TO REPORT

Any unusual symptoms in the baby of the epileptic mother.

NOTES

A number of drugs are used to treat epilepsy. An up-to-date drug reference should be consulted to determine the safety and possible side effects of individual drugs.

Newborn and premature babies are at greater risk of side effects due to limited ability to clear drugs from their systems.

Breastfeeding is thought to provide gradual withdrawal for the baby exposed to mother's epilepsy medications in utero.

See also: Medication Resources (inside back cover)

➤ EVERY MOTHER

DESCRIPTION   Organization whose mission is "to help every new mother reach her parenting goals through training, technical assistance, and breastfeeding promotion materials for breastfeeding educators, healthcare professionals, and mothers."[144]

NOTES

Email: info@everymother.org
Web: www.everymother.org/
    Every Mother achieves its mission through training programs, curriculum development, technical assistance, and resources and products to aid health professionals in serving new families.

Footnote

[144]Every Mother. (2007–2012). Our mission. Retrieved from http://www.everymother.org/about_us.php

➤ EXCLUSIVE BREASTFEEDING

DEFINITION   Giving no other food or drink to a breastfed infant.

NOTES

The American Academy of Pediatrics (AAP), the United States Breastfeeding Committee (USBC), the United Nations Children's Fund (UNICEF), and the World Health Organization (WHO) recommend exclusive (full) breastfeeding for about the first six months of life.

See also **Complementary feeding**

➤ EXERCISE

DEFINITION   Physical exertion.

Age of the baby.
Type and amount of exercise.
Prior cautions against exercise.

SELF-CARE INFORMATION

Moderate exercise does not decrease milk production.
Mothers may be more comfortable with a supportive (but not too constricting) bra.
Mothers may be more comfortable exercising after nursing, when the breasts are the most soft.
Mothers should be advised to discuss new physical activities with their healthcare providers.

NOTES

Bodily activity or exercise is a normal part of the life of lactating women around the globe. There is no reason for lactating women not to exercise in moderation during lactation, even women who have previously been sedentary. For comfort, mothers may want to select a well-fitting supportive bra that does not compress their breasts.

See also Maternal exercise

➤ EXPRESSION OF MOTHERS' MILK

DEFINITION Removal of milk from the breast via compression and vacuum. Expression may be accomplished by hand (manual expression) or pump.

ASK ABOUT

Reason mother plans to express milk.

ASSESSMENT

PROMPT CARE NEEDED?

Are any of the following present?

Imminent separation of mother and baby.

IF YES,   *Call lactation care provider today.*

ROUTINE CARE NEEDED?

Are any of the following present?

Desire to learn hand expression.

Desire to pump.

Questions about storage and handling of breastmilk.

Questions about donating milk to a milk bank.

IF YES,   *Call lactation care provider.*

SELF-CARE INFORMATION

Wash hands before beginning.

When baby is latched onto one breast, practice hand expression on the other breast.

Gently massage and then compress the breast with the thumb and pointer finger opposite each other on the areola. Repeat.

Your skill will improve with practice.

Store expressed milk in the refrigerator or in a cooler with ice packs, or the freezer if it will not be used within 48 hours.

Follow safe milk storage guidelines.

IMPORTANT CONDITIONS TO REPORT

Questions or problems with this technique.

See also Breast pump; Collection and storage of breastmilk

➤ FAILURE TO THRIVE (FTT)

DEFINITION A condition in which a child's size and growth rate is significantly below that of average children. There are multiple causes for FTT ranging from organic problems such as metabolic disorders, cerebral palsy, and organ defects, as well as psychological and social causes. FTT occurs in both formula-fed and breast-fed infants.

ASK ABOUT

Onset.
Age of the baby.
Feeding method.

ASSESSMENT

EMERGENT CARE NEEDED?

Are any of the following present?

Meconium bowel movements after 5 days of life. No yellow stools by day 5.

Fewer than three bowel movements daily in a breastfed newborn after the first 2 days of life.

No urine in 6 hours.

Brick dust urine (uric acid crystals) after 2 days of life.

Dark-colored urine.

Fewer than four urinations daily in the breastfed newborn after day 5.

Noticeably sunken fontanelles (soft spot on top of head).

Decreased activity.

Baby below birthweight at 10–14 days.

Cessation of weight gain.

IF YES,   *Seek medical care within 4 hours.*

PROMPT CARE NEEDED?

Are any of the following present?

Concern about inadequate infant growth.

IF YES,   *Call pediatric care provider today.*

Are any of the following present?
Diagnosed FTT in a breastfed child.

IF YES, *Refer to growth and nutrition department.*

Are any of the following present?
Continued breastfeeding in a child diagnosed with FTT.

IF YES, *Call lactation care provider today.*

SELF-CARE INFORMATION

Practice skin-to-skin contact in the first hour and frequently thereafter.
Watch for hunger cues (signs that say "feed me" include hand-to-face or hand-to-mouth movements, lip smacking, seeking with lips, rooting, and head bobbing).
Feed baby at first sign of hunger cues.
Expect 10–12 unscheduled feedings in 24 hours.
Allow the baby to end feedings.

IMPORTANT CONDITIONS TO REPORT

Infant disinterest in feeding.
Ongoing problems with milk supply.

NOTES

The use of the World Health Organization growth charts[145] is recorded by the American Academy of Pediatrics and the Center for Disease Control. These charts were standardized on breastfed babies. Breastfed babies are expected to begin slowing their rate of growth by 4–6 months.

See also Milk supply, inadequate

Footnotes

[145]World Health Organization. (2006). WHO child growth standards: Methods and development. Retrieved from http://www.who.int/childgrowth/standards/technical_report/en/index.html

➤ FASTING

DEFINITION   Going without food for periods of 6 hours or more. Fasting may be performed in preparation for certain medical tests (e.g., blood glucose) before surgery, as a religious observance (e.g., during Ramadan for Muslims), or as a misguided weight loss plan.

SELF-CARE INFORMATION

If fasting is considered for religious purposes, check with your religious leader. For example, in many areas, pregnant and breastfeeding women are exempted from the observance of the fast during Ramadan.

If fasting is recommended for a surgical procedure for the baby, ask the surgeon or anesthesiologist how long the baby should fast before surgery. Fasting is typically only recommended for 4 hours prior to surgery for breastfed infants.

NOTES

Fasting is not a recommended method for weight loss in breastfeeding women. Short-term fasting is not thought to have a negative effect on milk production. Breastfeeding women should continue to drink to satisfy thirst during a period of fasting (unless not allowed in the case of fasting before blood work or surgery).

See also Maternal diet

➤ FATHERS

DEFINITION   The father of the baby plays an important role in the mother's opinion of and success with breastfeeding. In two studies, fathers who attended prenatal classes designed to help then understand breastfeeding had babies who were breast-fed longer and more exclusively.[146,147]

Footnotes

[146]Pisacane, A., Continisio, G. I., Aldinucci, M., D'Amora, S., & Continisio, P. (2005). A controlled trial of the father's role in breastfeeding promotion. *Pediatrics*, *116*(4), e494–498. doi:10.1542/peds.2005-0479

[147]Susin, L. R. O., & Giugliani, E. R. J. (2008). Inclusion of fathers in an intervention to promote breastfeeding: Impact on breastfeeding rates. *Journal of Human Lactation: Official Journal of International Lactation Consultant Association, 24*(4), 386–392; quiz 451–453. doi:10.1177/0890334408323545

➤ FATIGUE, MATERNAL

DEFINITION   Exhaustion, weariness, or lack of energy. May be the result of lack of sleep. May also be associated with anemia, postpartum mood disorder, infection, underactive or overactive thyroid, pain, and the use of some drugs (including prescription drugs).

ASK ABOUT

Onset of symptom of fatigue.
Age of the baby.
Weight gain of the baby.
Medication and/or drugs used.

ASSESSMENT

EMERGENT CARE NEEDED?
Are any of the following present?

Fever.

Confusion.

Dizziness.

Blurred vision.

Swelling, weight gain, and little or no urine.

IF YES,   *Seek medical care now.*

PROMPT CARE NEEDED?

Are any of the following present?

Ongoing fatigue.

Sadness or depression.

Intolerance to cold.

Dry skin.

Headache.

Insomnia.

Constipation.

IF YES, *Seek medical care today.*

ROUTINE CARE NEEDED?

Are any of the following present?

Concern about frequency of nighttime and daytime nursings.

Concern about adequacy of milk supply.

IF YES, *Call lactation care provider.*

SELF-CARE INFORMATION

Although tiredness is common postpartum, fatigue should be investigated since it can be a nonspecific symptom of other problems.

IMPORTANT CONDITIONS TO REPORT

Fatigue that is not relieved by sleep.

See also Anemia; Hypothyroidism; Postpartum depression; Thyroid disease

➤ FAT IN BREASTMILK

DEFINITION   A calorie-rich nutrient in human milk. Fat is composed of fatty acids of different lengths. The naturally occurring, long-chain fats in human milk, especially DHA and ARA, are particularly noted for their beneficial effects on the growth of brain and nerve cells.

ASK ABOUT

Age of the baby.
Questions about milk supply.
Adequacy of growth.

ASSESSMENT

PROMPT CARE NEEDED?

Are any of the following present?
    Concern about inadequate infant growth.

IF YES,   *Call pediatric care provider today.*

Are any of the following present?
    Slow weight gain in a breastfed child.

IF YES,   *Call lactation care provider.*

SELF-CARE INFORMATION

Practice skin-to-skin contact in the first hour and frequently thereafter.
Watch for hunger cues (signs that say "feed me" include hand-to-face or hand-to-mouth movements, lip smacking, seeking with lips, rooting, and head bobbing).
Feed the baby at the first sign of hunger cues.
Expect 10–12 unscheduled feedings in 24 hours.
Allow the baby to end feedings.

IMPORTANT CONDITIONS TO REPORT

Infant disinterest in feeding.
Ongoing problems with milk supply.
The baby's inability to sustain a feeding.

NOTES

Fat content in milk varies throughout the day and within each feeding, depending on how full the breast is, as well as how well the baby, hand expression, or pump is eliciting the milk ejection reflex, which propels fat down through the breast.

It is very rare for the caloric composition of human milk to be inadequate.

Routine testing of the fat or other content of milk is not recommended, due to diurnal variation and the difficulty of collecting a representative sample.

See also Arachidonic acid (AA, also ARA); Caloric density of breastmilk; Docosahexaenoic acid (DHA) in breastmilk

➤ FAT-SOLUBLE VITAMINS IN BREASTMILK

DEFINITION   Organic chemicals required by the body in small amounts. Vitamins are divided into two groups: fat soluble and water soluble. Vitamins A, E, and K as well as precursors of D are the fat-soluble vitamins found in human milk.

NOTES

According to the American Academy of Pediatrics:

> Breastfed and partially breastfed infants should be supplemented with 400 IU/day of vitamin D beginning in the first few days of life. Supplementation should be continued unless the infant is weaned to at least 1 L/day or 1 qt/day of vitamin D–fortified formula or whole milk.[148(p1148)]

Footnotes

[148]Wagner, C. L., & Greer, F. R. (2008). Prevention of rickets and vitamin D deficiency in infants, children, and adolescents. *Pediatrics, 122*(5), 1142–1152. doi:10.1542/peds.2008-1862

➤ FDA

See DHHS Food and Drug Administration (FDA)

➤ FEEDING CUES

DEFINITION   Infant behaviors that indicate hunger and satiety (fullness). Adults can learn to read feeding cues to aid in breastfeeding and the overall development of the parent–child relationship.

SELF-CARE INFORMATION

Practice skin-to-skin contact in the first hour and frequently thereafter.

Keep the baby close to learn feeding cues.

Signs that say "feed me" include hand-to-face or hand-to-mouth movements, lip smacking, seeking with lips, rooting, and head bobbing.

Signs of fullness include removing the mouth from the nipple with relaxed body tone, falling asleep during feeding, and general bodily relaxation.

➤ FEEDING METHODS, ALTERNATE

DEFINITION   Ways of supplementing a breastfed baby that avoid introduction of a bottle.

ASK ABOUT

Reason for supplementation or alternate feeding.

ASSESSMENT

PROMPT CARE NEEDED?

Are any of the following present?

The baby is unable to withdraw sufficient milk from the breast.

IF YES,   *Seek medical care within 4 hours.*

Are any of the following present?

Need or desire to supplement the baby's diet.

IF YES,   *Call lactation care provider today.*

SELF-CARE INFORMATION

Clean devices carefully according to product literature.

IMPORTANT CONDITIONS TO REPORT

Difficulty with feeding method.

See also At-breast supplementation; Bottle feeding; Cup feeding; Feeding tube devices; Finger feeding; Gavage feeding; Tube feeding

➤ FEEDING PATTERN OF BREASTFED INFANTS

DEFINITION   The observed method or schedule of seeking nutrition. Observation of breastfed newborns indicates that while most babies nurse 10–12 times or more over 24 hours, they tend to do so in a clustered feeding pattern. That is, young babies tend to have a cycle of short, closely spaced feedings interspersed with periods of rest or sleep. This pattern is associated with good milk production and growth.

ASK ABOUT

Age of the baby.
Current feeding pattern.

ASSESSMENT

EMERGENT CARE NEEDED?

Are any of the following present?

Sudden disinterest in feeding.

Extreme lethargy in baby.

Sudden change in baby's muscle tone (extremely floppy or stiff).

IF YES,   *Seek emergency care now.*

PROMPT MEDICAL CARE NEEDED?

Are any of the following present?

    Meconium bowel movements after 5 days of life.

    Fewer than three bowel movements daily in a breastfed newborn after the first 2 days of life.

    No urine in 6 hours.

    Brick dust urine (uric acid crystals) after 2 days of life.

    Lack of yellow stools by day 5.

    Dark-colored urine.

    Fewer than four urinations daily in the breastfed newborn after day 5.

    Noticeably sunken fontanelles (soft spot on top of head).

    Decreased activity.

    Weight loss of more than 7% from birthweight[149(p.e835)]

    Baby below birthweight at 10–14 days.

    Cessation of weight gain.

    IF YES,   *Seek pediatric care within 4 hours.*

PROMPT LACTATION CARE NEEDED?

Are any of the following present?

    Fewer than eight feedings per day in a newborn.

    Concerns about adequacy of milk supply.

    Baby waking frequently at night to feed.

    IF YES,   *Call lactation care provider today.*

SELF-CARE INFORMATION

Practice skin-to-skin contact in the first hour and frequently thereafter.

Watch for hunger cues (signs that say "feed me" include hand-to-face or hand-to-mouth movements, lip smacking, seeking with lips, rooting, and head bobbing).

Feed the baby at the first sign of hunger cues.

Practice good attachment.

Expect 10–12 feedings per 24 hours (feedings may occur in clusters—three or four feedings in 2 hours, followed by a few hours of rest, then more clusters, rest, etc.).

Listen for signs of the baby swallowing.

Allow the baby to end feedings.

Expect at least three infant stools per 24 hours after the first 4 days of life and yellow stools by day 5.

Good positioning and attachment are crucial to prevent or reduce nipple pain.

If feedings are missed, hand express or pump milk or both to maintain supply.

IMPORTANT CONDITIONS TO REPORT

Inadequate feeding (fewer than 10 feedings daily in the newborn).

Inadequate stooling pattern (fewer than three stools daily) in the early weeks.

See also Cluster feeding

Footnotes

[149]AAP Section on Breastfeeding. (2012). Breastfeeding and the use of human milk. *Pediatrics*, *129*(3), e827–e841. doi:10.1542/peds.2011-3552

➤ FEEDING TUBE DEVICES

DEFINITION   Administration of extra fluids (expressed breastmilk or formula) to the baby through a tube. Tube devices may be attached to the breast (at-breast feeding), a finger (finger feeding), or inserted into the baby's stomach through the nose or mouth (gavage feeding).

ASK ABOUT

Reason for the device.

ASSESSMENT

PROMPT CARE NEEDED?

Are any of the following present?

The baby is unable to withdraw milk from the breast.

IF YES,   *Seek pediatric care within 4 hours.*

Are any of the following present?

        Need or desire to use a feeding tube device with a breastfed baby.

        Problems with a feeding tube device.

IF YES,   *Call lactation care provider today.*

SELF-CARE INFORMATION

Clean devices carefully according to product literature.

IMPORTANT CONDITIONS TO REPORT

Difficulty with feeding method.

NOTES

At-breast supplementation may be useful when a baby is not transferring an adequate amount of milk from the breast. This may be due to a temporary or permanent problem with milk supply on the part of the mother. It may also result from weak or inefficient suckling on the part of the baby, due to temporary or permanent conditions (e.g., prematurity, undernourishment, Down syndrome, cardiac problems).

    Gavage feeding is typically practiced in hospital settings and can be a supportive step toward full breastfeeding with the ill or premature baby.

See also At-breast supplementation; Bottle feeding; Cup feeding; Feeding methods, alternate; Finger feeding; Gavage feeding

➤ FENUGREEK

DEFINITION   An herb frequently used in teas and syrups. Fenugreek has been sold as a galactagogue (substance that increases milk), but there is currently little scientific evidence of this effect. Fenugreek may interfere with the absorption of any medication used concurrently,[150(p261)] and higher doses may cause hypoglycemia.[151(p407)]

Footnotes

[150]Skidmore-Roth, L. (2010). *Mosby's handbook of herbs & natural supplements.* St. Louis, MO: Elsevier/Mosby.

[151]Hale, T. (2012). *Medications and mothers' milk* (15th ed.). Amarillo, TX: Hale Publishing.

➤ FERTILITY

DEFINITION   Referring to a woman's ability to conceive and carry a child. Breastfeeding is associated with decreased fertility in the first 6 months following birth. This is due to amenorrhea, a period of cessation of menses (monthly flow of blood from the uterus).

ASK ABOUT

Age of infant.
Feeding pattern.

ASSESSMENT

PROMPT CARE NEEDED?

Are any of the following present?

Desire to extend lactational amenorrhea.

IF YES,   *Call lactation provider today.*

ROUTINE CARE NEEDED?

Are any of the following present?

Concern about prolonged lack of menses.
Concern about contraceptive usage.
Desire to conceive again.

IF YES,   *Schedule routine medical visit.*

SELF-CARE INFORMATION

Characteristics of breastfeeding thought to increase the chances of amenorrhea include having a baby younger than 6 months, **exclusive breastfeeding**, unrestricted feeding (at least 10 feedings per day), avoidance of pacifiers and bottles, and frequent nursing night and day. Once any of these criteria is no longer true, secure another family planning method.

IMPORTANT CONDITIONS TO REPORT

Past fertility problems.

Resumption of menstrual period.

NOTES

Women who continue to breastfeed exclusively during the first 6 months of their baby's life are likely to experience amenorrhea (that is, no menstrual period). Many breastfeeding women experience amenorrhea of a year or more, as long as they continue to breastfeed frequently.

Lactational amenorrhea method (LAM) is a form of natural family planning that is 98% effective in the first 6 months following the birth of a baby, so long as the mother's menses have not returned, her baby is exclusively breastfed, and there are no long periods of time between feedings, day and night. Once the baby is older than 6 months, or any of the above criteria is no longer true, LAM is no longer effective and mothers should utilize other forms of birth control.

See also Bellagio Consensus; Contraception; Lactational Amenorrhea Method (LAM); Menstrual cycle; Natural family planning

➤ FEVER

DEFINITION   Elevated body temperature is a sign of inflammation or infection. There is no reason to stop breastfeeding during a fever, except in the case of contraindicated infections.[152]

Fever can also follow epidural anesthesia and may occur during labor.

Fever in a breastfeeding woman may be a symptom of inflammatory process in the breast.

Onset.

Age of the baby.

ASSESSMENT

EMERGENT CARE NEEDED?

Are any of the following present?

About the baby:

Extreme **lethargy**.

Sudden change in muscle tone (extremely floppy or stiff).

Sudden disinterest in feeding.

Inability to wake baby.

Problems with breathing.

IF YES, *Seek emergency care now.*

PROMPT CARE NEEDED?

Are any of the following present?

About the mother:

Fever higher than 100°F (37.7°C).

Extreme breast discomfort.

Flu-like aching throughout the body.

Extreme exhaustion.

Visible or palpable breast **abscess**.

About the baby:

Extreme discomfort.

Fever higher than 100°F (37.7°C) in a baby younger than 3 months of age.

Vomiting and diarrhea that last for more than a few hours in a child of any age.

Rash accompanied by a fever.

A cold that gets worse and includes a fever.

Ear pain or drainage from an ear.

Sore throat or problems swallowing.

Sharp or persistent pains in the abdomen or stomach.

Fever and vomiting at the same time.

Not eating for more than a day in the older baby who is eating solid foods.

IF YES, *Seek medical care now.*

ROUTINE CARE NEEDED?

Are any of the following present?

Fever higher than 100°F (37.7°C) in an older baby or child.

Any cough or cold that does not get better in several days.

IF YES,   *Call pediatric care provider today.*

SELF-CARE INFORMATION

Feed the baby at least 10 times per 24 hours.

Soften the breasts between feedings with gentle hand expression.

Finish the full course of antibiotics prescribed (unless told to stop by a physician).

Continue nonprescription pain relief as recommended.

Continue to monitor for symptoms of recurring breast infection (redness, heat, fever, chills, pain).

IMPORTANT CONDITIONS TO REPORT

Symptoms worsen or persist.

Signs of infection.

NOTES

Rarely, babies experience life-threatening infections or events that cause extreme lethargy and disinterest in feeding. They may be suddenly floppy or stiff. These symptoms indicate a medical emergency, as they may reflect botulism, meningitis, or other life-threatening infection.

Many mothers experiencing **mastitis** may mistake symptoms of mastitis for flu. When a mother calls to ask for recommendations of safe flu medications, remember to ask her if she has any red, painful, hot spots on her breasts. See **Mastitis** for more information.

Few infections are incompatible with breastfeeding.

Infections in the breastfeeding mother that are not compatible with breastfeeding include **HIV**, **HTLV-1**, and active **herpes** lesion on the nipple and/or other area that will be in contact with the baby's mouth.[153]

Mothers with certain infections may breastfeed once a period of treatment is initiated. These infections include tuberculosis, brucellosis, hepatitis, and Lyme disease. The Centers for Disease Control and Prevention and state health departments can provide further information.

See also Breast infection; Mastitis

Footnotes

[152] Centers for Disease Control and Prevention. (2009). Diseases and Conditions. Retrieved from http://www.cdc.gov/breastfeeding/disease/index.htm

[153] AAP Section on Breastfeeding. (2012). Breastfeeding and the use of human milk. *Pediatrics, 129* (3), e827–e841. doi: 10.1542/peds.2011-3552

➤ FIBROADENOMA

DEFINITION   A benign tumor found in the breast. Fibroadenomas are compatible with breastfeeding.

SELF-CARE INFORMATION
Routine breast self-exam should be performed monthly.
Continue breast screening as recommended by medical care provider.

IMPORTANT CONDITIONS TO REPORT
New lumps.
Changes to existing lumps.

See also Breast lumps

➤ FIBROCYSTIC BREASTS

DEFINITION   A common breast condition in women including variable lumpiness, tenderness, and palpable cysts (pockets of fluid). Symptoms may change during the menstrual period. This benign condition is compatible with breastfeeding.

NOTES

New lumps in the breast should be medically examined to rule out **plugged ducts** and other problems.
Women who have experienced fibrocystic breasts may misdiagnose plugged ducts and other breastfeeding problems as fibrocystic changes.

See also Breast lumps; Plugged ducts

➤ FINGER FEEDING

DEFINITION   A feeding technique that includes taping or otherwise attaching a feeding tube to a parent's or healthcare provider's finger and inserting the finger into the baby's mouth. Expressed breastmilk or formula contained in the feeding syringe is then allowed to flow into the baby's mouth in response to suckling motions.

NOTES

Efficacy and safety of finger feeding have not been established.
   Finger feeding offers no known advantage to at-breast feeding or cup feeding. Whenever possible, infants requiring supplementation should be fed with an at-breast device to maximize stimulation of milk-making hormones.

➤ FLAT NIPPLES

DEFINITION   Nipples that appear level with surrounding tissue.

ASK ABOUT

Appearance of the nipple.
Change in the nipple appearance after feeding or pumping.
Action of the nipple when it is exposed to the cold.
Nipple changes during pregnancy and lactation.
Diagnosis of "flat" nipple.

ASSESSMENT

MEDICAL CARE NEEDED?

Are any of the following present?

Meconium bowel movements after 5 days of life.

No yellow stool by 5 days.

Fewer than three bowel movements daily in a breastfed newborn after the first 2 days of life.

No urine in 6 hours.

Brick dust urine (uric acid crystals) after 2 days of life.

Dark-colored urine.

Fewer than four urinations daily in the breastfed newborn after day 5.

Noticeably sunken fontanelles (soft spot on top of head).

Decreased activity.

Baby below birthweight at 10–14 days.

Cessation of weight gain.

IF YES,   *Seek pediatric care within 4 hours.*

PROMPT LACTATION CARE NEEDED?

Are any of the following present?

Poor feeding.

Poor milk transfer.

Inadequate weight gain.

Problems with latch-on.

Concern about milk supply.

IF YES,   *Call lactation care provider today.*

SELF-CARE INFORMATION

Training flat nipples to stand out during pregnancy has not been demonstrated to be effective. Most flat nipples evert with effective latch and suckling.

IMPORTANT CONDITIONS TO REPORT

Poor feeding.

Poor milk transfer.

Inadequate weight gain.

Problems with latch-on.

See also Milk transfer, estimating; Weight gain, baby—low

➤ FLUID NEEDS OF BREASTFEEDING MOTHER

DEFINITION   Amount of water and watery liquids required daily for lactation.

> **NOTES**

Mothers should drink to satisfy thirst during lactation for their own health.
    Only in severe dehydration would fluid status affect milk production.
    Research indicates that increasing maternal fluids has no effect on volume or composition of milk produced.

➤ FLU, MATERNAL

DEFINITION   Flu, or influenza, is a viral infection. This condition is compatible with breastfeeding.

SELF-CARE INFORMATION
Examine your breasts and nipples for any sign of inflammation.
Continue to breastfeed.

IMPORTANT CONDITIONS TO REPORT
Any redness, pain, or tenderness of the breast.
Symptoms of flu (fever, body aches, and chills) may also indicate breast inflammation or infection.

See also Fever; Mastitis

➤ FLUORIDE

DEFINITION   A compound of the trace mineral fluorine. Fluoride helps harden the teeth during formation and protects erupted teeth from decay.

> **NOTES**

According to the American Academy of Pediatrics:

> Supplementary fluoride should not be provided during the first 6 months of life. From 6 months to 3 years of age, the decision whether to provide fluoride supplementation should be limited to infants residing in communities where the fluoride concentration in the water is < 0.3 ppm.[154(p.e385)]

Footnotes

[154]AAP Section on Breastfeeding. (2012). Breastfeeding and the use of human milk. *Pediatrics*, *129*(3), e827–e841. doi: 10.1542/peds.2011–3552.

➤ FLUTTER SUCKING

DEFINITION   A light, fast sucking associated with little or no milk transfer. This phenomenon is also called nonnutritive suckling.

See also Nonnutritive suckling; Uncoordinated suckling

➤ FNS

See United States Department of Agriculture (USDA) Special Supplemental Food Program for Women, Infants, and Children

➤ FOOD ALLERGIES

DEFINITION   An abnormal immune reaction to substances that are eaten.

ASK ABOUT

Onset.
Age of the baby.
Known allergies.

ASSESSMENT

EMERGENT CARE NEEDED?

Are any of the following present?

Difficulty breathing.

Difficulty swallowing.

Swelling of the tongue.

IF YES, *Seek emergency care now.*

PROMPT CARE NEEDED?

Are any of the following present in the baby?

Swelling of the face, hands, or feet.

Persistent rash, headache, or fever.

Persistent diarrhea, nausea, or vomiting.

Bloody stool.

IF YES, *Seek pediatric care within 4 hours.*

ROUTINE CARE NEEDED?

Are any of the following present in the baby?

Suspected reaction to food.

Occasional nausea, vomiting, or diarrhea.

Persistent runny nose.

Wheezing.

Mild rash or itching.

IF YES, *Call pediatric care provider today.*

SELF-CARE INFORMATION

Monitor symptoms.

Possibility of developing allergy to other proteins.

Comfort techniques for irritable baby (rocking, singing, skin-to-skin contact, bathing, seeking quiet, calm environment, etc.).

IMPORTANT CONDITIONS TO REPORT

Family history of allergy.

Symptoms worsen, persist, or reoccur.

NOTES

If difficulty breathing or other extreme symptoms are reported, refer to emergency care immediately.

Babies born into allergic families are more likely to develop allergy, particularly those with two allergic parents or one allergic parent and an allergic sibling. Exclusive breastfeeding is the optimal feeding choice for these babies in particular. Should the baby develop allergy symptoms, the mother may be counseled to avoid consuming offending allergens such as cow's milk, fish, eggs, peanuts, and tree nuts.

Mothers who have not chosen breastfeeding may **relactate** for their allergic infant. Other allergic infants are fed hypoallergenic formula.

In the event that the allergic response is to a solid food, that food should not be fed to the baby and should be avoided by the breastfeeding mother until a medical care provider directs her to reintroduce the allergen.

Rarely, babies develop allergies to foreign protein fragments consumed by their breastfeeding mother. The most potent allergens in the United States diet include cow's milk, fish, eggs, peanuts, and tree nuts. Infantile symptoms of an allergic reaction include hives, facial swelling, runny nose, wheezing, eczema, vomiting, irritability (colic), blood in the stool, and **anaphylaxis**. Treatment centers on identification and avoidance of the proteins that are triggering the allergic reaction.

If supplementation is required, babies with documented allergy should be fed hypoallergenic formula identified by a medical care provider.

Concern about infant allergy is much more predominant than actual allergy. The American Academy of Pediatrics reports that the prevalence of infant cow's milk allergy is 2–3%.[155] The overall prevalence of childhood food allergy is 4–6%.[156]

Counseling and education should include comfort techniques for the irritable baby and coping methods for parents.

See also Atopic eczema

Footnotes

[155]AAP Committee on Nutrition. (2000). Hypoallergenic infant formulas. *Pediatrics, 106,* 346–349.

[156]Ziegler, R. S. (2003). Food allergen avoidance in prevention of food allergy in infants and children. *Pediatrics, 111,* 1662–1671.

➤ FOOD RESTRICTIONS POSTPARTUM

DEFINITION   The thought that certain substances should not be eaten by nursing mothers for fear that they will alter the quality or acceptability of their milk. There are no foods that should be universally forbidden during lactation. Mother's milk is indeed flavored by the foods she consumes, as is amniotic fluid.

IMPORTANT CONDITIONS TO REPORT

Concerns about an infant's behavior related to the mother's diet should be evaluated by infant's healthcare provider.

See also Food allergies; Maternal diet; Reaction to foods in the mother's diet

➤ FOOTBALL POSTURE

DEFINITION   Another name for the "clutch posture," a breastfeeding posture in which the baby is tucked under the mother's arm, with its feet behind her back, and attaches to the breast next to her arm. The mother supports the baby's torso with her forearm, holding the baby's neck in the palm of her hand.

NOTES

This is a good position for mothers recovering from cesarean delivery, those with large breasts, and premature babies.

See also Clutch posture; Cradle posture

➤ FOREMILK

DEFINITION   Refers to the milk that flows from the breast at the beginning of a feeding.

NOTES

There is an outdated belief that foremilk is always low in fat. Fat content in milk varies throughout the day and within each feeding, depending on how full the breast is, as well as how well the baby or pump is eliciting the milk ejection reflex, which flushes fat down through the breast.

There is no scientific evidence to support the common advice that mothers should keep the baby at the breast longer to get more hindmilk. The baby can regulate its caloric intake when allowed to feed and stop feeding according to its own feeding cues.

It is very rare for the caloric composition of human milk to be inadequate. Routine testing of the fat or other content of milk is not recommended, due to diurnal variation and the difficulty of collecting a representative sample.

See also Caloric density of breastmilk; Fat in breastmilk; Hindmilk

➤ FORMULA, INFANT

DEFINITION   A food patterned on breastmilk, which is the only suitable replacement for human milk in the first year of a baby's life. Formula may also be called artificial baby milks, manufactured baby milk, infant formula, artificial milks, formulated baby milks, or breastmilk substitutes. Formula may be used to supplement breastfeeding when desired by the mother or when medically indicated.

ASK ABOUT

Age of the baby.
Age of the baby when supplements were started.
Type of supplements.
How supplements are fed.
Amount of supplement per 24 hours.
Reactions from supplement.

ASSESSMENT

EMERGENT CARE NEEDED?

Are any of the following present?

Signs of dehydration (scanty, dark urine).

Difficulty breathing.

IF YES,   *Seek emergency care now.*

PROMPT CARE NEEDED?

Are any of the following present?

Eczema.

Hives.

Vomiting.

Diarrhea.

Blood in the stools.

Irritability and excessive crying.

Meconium bowel movements after 5 days of life.

No yellow stool by 5 days.

Fewer than three bowel movements daily in breastfed newborn after the first 2 days of life.

No urine in 6 hours.

Brick dust urine (uric acid crystals) after 2 days of life.

Dark-colored urine.

Fewer than four urinations daily in the breastfed newborn after day 5.

Noticeably sunken fontanelles (soft spot on top of head).

Decreased activity.

Baby below birthweight at 10–14 days.

Cessation of weight gain.

IF YES,   *Seek pediatric care within 4 hours.*

ROUTINE CARE NEEDED?

Are any of the following present?

Education needed about formula feeding.

Education wanted about decreasing amount of supplement.

Education wanted about increasing milk volume.

Concerns about milk supply.

IF YES,   *Call lactation care provider today.*

SELF-CARE INFORMATION

Complementary feedings are those that are added to breastfeeding.

IMPORTANT CONDITIONS TO REPORT

Ongoing symptoms.

NOTES

Formula is regulated by the FDA Center for Food Safety and Applied Nutrition (CFSAN). Visit http://www.fda.gov/Food/GuidanceComplianceRegulatoryInformation/Guidance Documents/InfantFormula/default.htm for more information.

For supplementation guidelines, consult a reference such as the Academy of Breast-feeding Medicine's protocol for supplementary feeding.[157]

See also Decreasing supplemental formula; Increasing milk supply

Footnotes

[157]ABM Protocol Committee. (2009). ABM clinical protocol #3: Hospital guidelines for the use of supplementary feedings in the healthy term breastfed neonate, revised 2009. *Breastfeeding Medicine: The Official Journal of the Academy of Breastfeeding Medicine, 4*(3), 175–182. doi:10.1089/bfm.2009.9991

➤ FORTIFICATION OF HUMAN MILK FOR PREMATURE INFANTS

DEFINITION   The practice of adding minerals and fats to expressed breastmilk to increase its nutrient content. Calcium, phosphorus, zinc, and iron are among the nutrients added.

NOTES

In the United States, commercially available "human milk" fortifiers may be made with cow's milk products or with human milk only.

Fortifiers are typically used only for very low birthweight infants in neonatal care unit settings.

See also Lactoengineering; Premature infant; Preterm milk properties

➤ FREEZING AND STORING HUMAN MILK

DEFINITION   Safe methods for preserving expressed milk.

Glass and hard plastic containers with tight lids are recommended. All containers should be food grade. Plastic bags designed for milk storage may be used, but it is important to prevent spillage and puncture of the bags.

Milk can be safely stored:[158]

Up to 4 hours at room temperature (66°–72°F), but should be refrigerated immediately if possible (with a frozen gel pack in an insulated lunch bag or cooler if a refrigerator is not available).

Three to five days in the refrigerator (32°–50°F).

Up to 3 months in the built-in freezer section (0°–32°F) of a refrigerator.

Up to 6 months in a deep freezer (-20°F or less).

Milk that will not be used fresh within 5 days should be frozen as soon as possible. Thaw milk in its container.

Milk can be safely thawed by:

Placing frozen containers in the refrigerator overnight.

Holding frozen containers under lukewarm running tap water.

Placing frozen containers in lukewarm water.

Hot water is not recommended due to potential nutrient loss.

Milk should never be boiled or microwaved.

Milk does not need to be overly warm before being fed to the infant.

See also Collection and storage of breastmilk; Milk storage bags

Footnote

[158]Cadwell, K., & Turner-Maffei, C. (2014). *Pocket guide for lactation management* (2nd ed.). Burlington, MA: Jones & Bartlett Learning.

➤ FRENOTOMY

DEFINITION   A procedure that releases the restriction of the frenulum, the tissue that holds the tongue to the bottom of the mouth.

➤ FRENULUM, LINGUAL

DEFINITION   The membrane attaching the tongue to the bottom of the mouth. When the frenulum is tight, it can restrict the movement of the tongue, resulting in breastfeeding problems for some mothers and babies.

ASK ABOUT

Age of the baby.
Appearance of tongue.

ASSESSMENT

PROMPT MEDICAL CARE NEEDED?

Are any of the following present?

Meconium bowel movements after 5 days of life.

Fewer than three bowel movements daily in a breastfed newborn after the first 2 days of life.

No yellow stool by day 5.

No urine in 6 hours.

Brick dust urine (uric acid crystals) after 2 days of life.

Dark-colored urine.

Fewer than four urinations daily in the breastfed newborn after day 5.

Noticeably sunken fontanelles (soft spot on top of head).

Decreased activity.

Baby below birthweight at 10–14 days.

Cessation of weight gain.

IF YES,   *Seek pediatric care within 4 hours.*

PROMPT LACTATION CARE NEEDED?

Are any of the following present?

Tight lingual frenulum in the baby.

Nipple or breast pain or damage.

History of recurrent mastitis.

Milk supply problems.

Poor growth of a breastfed infant.

IF YES,   *Call lactation care provider today.*

SELF-CARE INFORMATION

Practice skin-to-skin contact in the first hour and frequently thereafter.

Watch for hunger cues (signs that say "feed me" include hand-to-face or hand-to-mouth movements, lip smacking, seeking with lips, rooting, and head bobbing).

Feed the baby at the first sign of hunger cues.

Practice good attachment:

Offer the breast as soon as cues are seen.

Wait for the baby to open his or her mouth wide (greater than a 140° angle).

Pull the baby in so that his or her chin touches the breast first, and the nipple enters the mouth along the top of the tongue; this should result in a wide-open mouth full of breast tissue.

The baby's lips should be flanged outward and make a seal to the breast.

The baby's lips should look off center when compared with the areola; the bottom lip should be farther away from the nipple than the top lip.

IMPORTANT CONDITIONS TO REPORT

Unresolved symptoms.

Ongoing concerns.

Insufficient intake or output of the baby.

See also Nipple pain

➤ FREQUENCY OF FEEDINGS

DEFINITION   The number of feedings in a period of time. Expectation for breast-feeding is 10–12 feedings per 24 hours. Observation of breastfed newborns indicates that while most babies nurse 10–12 times per day, they tend to do so in a clustered feeding pattern. That is, young babies tend to have a cycle of short, closely spaced feedings interspersed with periods of rest or sleep. This pattern is associated with good milk production and growth.

ASK ABOUT

Age of the baby.
Current feeding pattern.

ASSESSMENT

EMERGENT CARE NEEDED?

Are any of the following present?

Sudden disinterest in feeding.
Extreme **lethargy** in the baby.
Sudden change in the baby's muscle tone (extremely floppy or stiff).
Difficulty breathing.

IF YES,   *Seek emergency care now.*

PROMPT MEDICAL CARE NEEDED?

Are any of the following present?

Meconium bowel movements after 5 days of life.
Fewer than three bowel movements daily in breastfed newborn after the first 2 days of life.
No yellow stool by 5 days.
No urine in 6 hours.
Brick dust urine (uric acid crystals) after 2 days of life.
Dark-colored urine.
Fewer than four urinations daily in the breastfed newborn after day 5.
Noticeably sunken fontanelles (soft spot on top of head).
Decreased activity.
Baby below birthweight at 10–14 days.
Cessation of weight gain.

IF YES,   *Seek pediatric care within 4 hours.*

PROMPT LACTATION CARE NEEDED?

Are any of the following present?

Fewer than eight feedings per day in a breastfed newborn.

Concerns about adequacy of milk supply.

IF YES,   *Call lactation care provider today.*

ROUTINE CARE NEEDED?

Are any of the following present?

Baby waking frequently at night to feed.

IF YES,   *Call lactation care provider.*

SELF-CARE INFORMATION

Practice skin-to-skin contact in the first hour and frequently thereafter.

Watch for hunger cues (signs that say "feed me" include hand-to-face or hand-to-mouth movements, lip smacking, seeking with lips, rooting, and head bobbing).

Feed the baby at the first sign of hunger cues.

Practice good attachment.

Expect 10–12 feedings per 24 hours (feedings may occur in clusters—three or four feedings in 2 hours, followed by a few hours of rest, then more clusters, rest, etc.).

Listen for signs of the baby swallowing.

Allow the baby to end feedings.

Expect at least three infant stools per 24 hours after the first 4 days of life.

Good positioning and attachment are crucial to prevent or reduce nipple pain.

If feedings are missed, hand express or pump milk to maintain supply.

IMPORTANT CONDITIONS TO REPORT

Inadequate feeding (fewer than 10 feedings daily in the newborn).

Inadequate stooling pattern (fewer than three stools daily).

See also Ankyloglossia; Cluster feeding; Feeding pattern of breastfed infants

➤ FTT

See Failure to thrive (FTT)

➤ FULL BREASTFEEDING

DEFINITION   A form of exclusive breastfeeding.

See also Exclusive breastfeeding

➤ G6PD

See Glucose-6-phosphate dehydrogenase deficiency (G6PD)

➤ GALACTAGOGUE

DEFINITION   Foods, herbs, and other substances thought to increase milk production. Requests from mothers for galactagogues indicate concern about milk supply.

ASK ABOUT

Onset.
Age of the baby.

ASSESSMENT

EMERGENT CARE NEEDED?

Are any of the following present?

Meconium bowel movements after 5 days of life.

Fewer than three bowel movements daily in breastfed newborn after the first 2 days of life.

No yellow stool by day 5.

No urine in 6 hours.

Brick dust urine (uric acid crystals) after 2 days of life.

Dark-colored urine.

Fewer than four urinations daily in the breastfed newborn after day 5.

Noticeably sunken fontanelles (soft spot on top of head).

Decreased activity.

Baby below birthweight at 10–14 days.

Cessation of weight gain.

IF YES, *Seek pediatric care within 4 hours.*

PROMPT CARE NEEDED?

Are any of the following present?

Scanty or infrequent urination.

IF YES, *Call obstetric care provider today.*

Are any of the following present?

Identified milk supply problem.

Concern about milk supply.

IF YES, *Call lactation care provider today.*

SELF-CARE INFORMATION

Ensure baby is feeding 10–12 times per 24 hours.

Express milk after feeding and give to baby.

Increasing feeding frequency and milk removal are the keys to increasing milk supply.

Breastfeed your baby at least 10 times per 24 hours.

If galactagogues are prescribed, follow instructions carefully.

Report any other medications, herbs, and dietary supplements you are using to everyone who prescribes for you and your baby.

IMPORTANT CONDITIONS TO REPORT

Persistent problems.

Recurrent problems.

Concerns about milk supply.

Jitteriness.

Insomnia.

Sedation.

Anxiety.

NOTES

There are no recommended drugs, foods, or herbs that have been shown to increase milk supply in well-done studies. Indeed, a review of the literature indicates current high-level evidence does not support claims that galactagogues increase milk volume.[159]

In addition, fenugreek, a herb commonly thought to increase milk supply, may interfere with the absorption of any medication used concurrently,[160(p261)] and higher doses may cause hypoglycemia.[161(p407)]

See also Increasing milk supply; Milk supply, inadequate; Milk transfer, estimating; Weight loss—baby

Footnotes

[159]Anderson, P. O., & Valdés, V. (2007). A critical review of pharmaceutical galactagogues. *Breastfeeding Medicine: The Official Journal of the Academy of Breastfeeding Medicine, 2*(4), 229–242. doi:10.1089/bfm.2007.0013

[160]Skidmore-Roth, L. (2010). *Mosby's handbook of herbs & natural supplements.* St. Louis, MO: Elsevier/Mosby.

[161]Hale, T. (2012). *Medications and mothers' milk* (15th ed.). Amarillo, TX: Hale Publishing.

➤ GALACTOCELE

DEFINITION   A milk retention cyst within the breast. Galactoceles are caused by blocked or blind milk ducts. This condition is compatible with breastfeeding. These cysts may be aspirated, but will refill. They do not move toward the nipple with breastfeeding or milk expression.

ASK ABOUT

Onset.

ASSESSMENT

PROMPT CARE NEEDED?

Are any of the following present?

Suspected galactocele—a lump that does not move in 24–48 hours with breastfeeding, hand expression, or pumping.

IF YES,   *Call obstetric care provider today.*

IMPORTANT CONDITIONS TO REPORT

Recurrence of symptoms.

See also Breast lumps

➤ GALACTOPOIESIS

DEFINITION   Maintenance of milk production in the breast. Galactopoiesis is sustained by frequent stimulation of the nipple and frequent removal of milk from the breast.

➤ GALACTORRHEA

DEFINITION   Production of milk from the breast that is outside normal expectations. This can include production of milk by women who are neither pregnant nor lactating, as well as excessive amounts of milk produced during lactation.

ASK ABOUT

Onset.

ASSESSMENT

PROMPT CARE NEEDED?

Are any of the following present?

Production of milk in a nonlactating, nonpregnant woman.

IF YES,   *Seek medical care today.*

Are any of the following present?

Concern about overabundant milk supply.

Excessively large or frequent stools in a breastfed baby.

Recurrent engorgement or mastitis.

Baby has difficulty managing excessive milk flow (sputters at the breast).

IF YES,   *Call lactation care provider today.*

SELF-CARE INFORMATION

Frequency of feeding and amount of milk removal drives milk supply.

IMPORTANT CONDITIONS TO REPORT

Worsening of symptoms.

Continuation of symptoms.

Ongoing concerns.

NOTES

Because production of milk relies on many different body systems in both the mother and baby, any milk supply problem requires consideration of maternal and infant factors. Occasionally medical factors such as endocrine imbalance may require evaluation.

➤ GALACTOSE

DEFINITION   A simple sugar that, when combined with glucose, creates lactose.

➤ GALACTOSEMIA

DEFINITION   A congenital inability to metabolize the simple sugar galactose due to an enzyme deficiency. This condition is the only infant medical contraindication to receiving breastmilk.

See also Metabolic disorder, galactosemia

➤ GALT

DEFINITION   Gut-associated lymphoid tissue. Immunologically active tissue found within the lining of the gastrointestinal tract.

NOTES

The breast is thought to act as an extension of gut-associated lymphoid tissue (GALT). When a pathogen enters the gut, GALT tissue responds by triggering the production of an immunoglobulin to attack the pathogen. The breast may also respond to the GALT trigger by manufacturing and releasing appropriate immunoglobulins to fight the organism through the milk.

See also Bioactive components of breastmilk

➤ GAS AND GASSY FOODS

DEFINITION   Referring to foods containing an abundance of indigestible carbohydrates (fiber) and the gas produced by the fermentation of carbohydrates in the gut. Foods that adults commonly find gassy include beans, cabbage, broccoli, cauliflower, and whole grain foods. There is little evidence that any vegetables mothers consume negatively affect their babies.

NOTES

Gas and flatulence are normal occurrences in the newborn, as in all humans. An infant's gas may carry the scent of aromatic oils in vegetables and other foods eaten by its mother; however, the oils do not contain fiber, and thus do not cause gastric distress in the infant.

Many mothers will put themselves on unnecessarily restrictive diets without seeking help for their baby's symptoms.

Clinicians should carefully evaluate the mother's concerns and the baby's symptoms to distinguish normal gas from colic or digestive difficulty.

See also Colic, infantile; Maternal diet

➤ GASTROESOPHAGEAL (GE) REFLUX

DEFINITION   Movement of stomach contents up into the esophagus and mouth. Gastroesophageal (GE) reflux in infants is not common in babies who are exclusively breastfed, except in babies who have been previously tube fed.[162] With GE reflux, the stomach contents move up out of the stomach and back into the esophagus. With GE reflux, babies vomit after eating. The vomiting happens most of the time and is not projectile (does not clear the chin).

ASK ABOUT

Age of the baby.
History of vomiting/description of vomiting.
History of weight gain or loss.
History of pneumonia or lung problems.
History of choking.

ASSESSMENT

EMERGENT CARE NEEDED?

Are any of the following present?

Difficulty breathing.

Choking.

Difficulty swallowing.

Rapid progression of symptoms.

IF YES,   *Seek emergency care now.*

PROMPT CARE NEEDED?

Are any of the following present?

Decrease in urination.

Decrease in stooling.

Meconium bowel movements after 5 days of life.

No yellow stool by day 5.

Fewer than three bowel movements daily in breastfed newborn after the first 2 days of life.

No urine in 6 hours.

Brick dust urine (uric acid crystals) after 2 days of life.

Dark-colored urine.

Fewer than four urinations daily in the breastfed newborn after day 5.

Noticeably sunken fontanelles (soft spot on top of head).

Decreased activity.

Baby below birthweight at 10–14 days.

Cessation of weight gain.

IF YES,   *Seek pediatric care within 4 hours.*

ROUTINE CARE NEEDED?

Are any of the following present?

Baby spits up regularly after nursing.

Weight gain is adequate.

Urination and stooling pattern is adequate.

IF YES,   *Call lactation care provider today.*

SELF-CARE INFORMATION

Many breastfed babies spit up frequently without any underlying medical cause. A baby who spits up often should be evaluated by his or her healthcare provider.

IMPORTANT CONDITIONS TO REPORT

Difficulty breathing.
Choking.
Difficulty swallowing.
Rapid progression of symptoms.
Decrease in urination.
Decrease in stooling.
Signs of dehydration.

See also Milk flow, too fast

Footnotes

[162]Heacock, H. J., Jeffery, H. E., Baker, J. L., & Page, M. (1992). Influence of breast versus formula milk on physiological gastroesophageal reflux in healthy, newborn infants. *Journal of Pediatric Gastroenterology and Nutrition, 14*, 41–46.

➤ GASTROINTESTINAL (GI)

DEFINITION   Pertaining to the organs of the digestive tract, including the stomach, small intestine, and large intestine.

➤ GASTROINTESTINAL (GI) INFECTION

DEFINITION   Establishment of virus, bacteria, or other organism in the digestive tract. Breastfeeding is compatible with GI infection and offers protection to the infant against common pathogens triggering GI infection.

SELF-CARE INFORMATION

Practice careful hand washing, especially when handling the baby and changing diapers.

See also Acute infection; Blood in stool; Diarrhea; Vomiting

➤ GASTROSCHISIS

DEFINITION A congenital defect in the abdominal wall, resulting in the protrusion of the intestines through skin. Babies with this condition can be fed breastmilk and go on to breastfeed after surgical repair.

➤ GAVAGE FEEDING

DEFINITION Delivering food to an infant through a tube that is inserted into the baby's stomach through the nose or mouth.

See also Feeding tube devices

➤ GEL PACKS

DEFINITION Devices containing gel matrix within a protective covering. Intended to be heated or chilled and worn next to the skin over an inflamed area to provide relief. Care should be taken to use gel packs at a comfortable temperature.

➤ GEL PADS

See also Glycerine gel pads; Hydrogel pads

➤ GENTIAN VIOLET

DEFINITION   A chemical dye used in laboratories. Also an antimicrobial and anti-fungal agent. Use of gentian violet has been reported as a treatment for candidiasis. This chemical is a powerful irritant to the skin and can cause tissue necrosis if not used in the proper dilution. Nausea, vomiting, and diarrhea have also been reported.[163(p467)]

NOTES

Hale rates gentian violet as an L3 (moderately safe) drug.[164(p510)]

See also Candidiasis; Thrush; Yeast infection

Footnotes

[163]Hale, T. (2012). *Medications and mothers' milk* (15th ed., p. 467, 510). Amarillo, TX: Hale Publishing.

[164]Hale, T. ibid.

➤ GI

DEFINITION   Gastrointestinal. Pertaining to the organs of the digestive tract, including the stomach, small intestine, and large intestine.

➤ GIGANTOMASTIA

DEFINITION   A rare condition of massive overgrowth of the breasts occurring during pregnancy. The breasts may increase to several times their prepregnancy size.

NOTES

With gigantomastia, serious problems can develop, including hemorrhage within the breast due to rapid change. Surgery may be required to stop hemorrhage.

Gigantomastia generally recedes after delivery but usually reoccurs with every subsequent pregnancy.

Breastfeeding is not contraindicated, as the condition typically reverses after delivery.

Breastfeeding women who experienced gigantomastia in pregnancy should receive ongoing lactation support.

➤ GILBERT'S SYNDROME

DEFINITION A common, mild, inherited liver disorder in which the liver does not efficiently process bilirubin. Bilirubin is produced by the breakdown of red blood cells. Illness, fasting, and stress may cause symptoms such as jaundice, fatigue, and weakness to appear.

NOTES

In the breastfed baby, Gilbert's syndrome may be confused with breastmilk jaundice. Gilbert's syndrome is compatible with lactation and breastfeeding.

See also Jaundice; Late onset jaundice

➤ GLANDULAR TISSUE, INSUFFICIENT

DEFINITION A rare condition in which women have an inadequate amount of milk-making tissue in the breast. This may be congenital, or the after effect of trauma or surgery to the chest. Asymmetry between the breasts may be a hallmark of this condition.

ASK ABOUT

Onset.
Age of the baby.

ASSESSMENT

EMERGENT CARE NEEDED?

Are any of the following present?

Meconium bowel movements after 5 days of life.

Fewer than three bowel movements daily in breastfed newborn after the first 2 days of life.

No yellow stool by day 5.

No urine in 6 hours.

Brick dust urine (uric acid crystals) after 2 days of life.

Dark-colored urine.

Fewer than four urinations daily in the breastfed newborn after day 5.

Noticeably sunken fontanelles (soft spot on top of head).

Decreased activity.

Baby below birthweight at 10–14 days.

Cessation of weight gain.

IF YES,   *Seek pediatric care within 4 hours.*

PROMPT MEDICAL CARE NEEDED?

Are any of the following present?

Failure of breastfed baby to grow adequately.

IF YES,   *Call pediatric care provider today.*

PROMPT LACTATION CARE NEEDED?

Are any of the following present?

Marked asymmetry of the breasts with concerns about milk supply or infant growth.

IF YES,   *Call lactation care provider today.*

ROUTINE LACTATION CARE NEEDED?

Are any of the following present?

Reported asymmetry with no concerns about milk supply or infant growth.

IF YES,   *Call lactation care provider.*

SELF-CARE INFORMATION

Practice skin-to-skin contact in the first hour and frequently thereafter.

Feed the baby at the first sign of hunger cues (signs that say "feed me" include hand-to-face or hand-to-mouth movements, lip smacking, seeking with lips, rooting, and head bobbing).

Feed the baby at least 10 times per 24 hours.

Listen for signs of the baby swallowing.

Allow the baby to end feedings.

Expect at least three infant stools per 24 hours after the first 4 days of life.

Good positioning and attachment are crucial.

If feedings are missed, hand express or pump milk to maintain supply.

IMPORTANT CONDITIONS TO REPORT

Feeding or stooling expectations are not met.

NOTES

The growth of the baby should be closely followed by a medical care provider.

One sign of possible insufficient glandular tissue is marked asymmetry of the breasts. This may indicate problems with glandular tissue in both breasts. If the mother reports that she had an implant in one breast only, inquire about the reason for this surgery. If the surgery was to correct breast asymmetry, there may be increased concern regarding the mother's ability to make a full milk supply. Marked asymmetry may indicate insufficient glandular tissue in both breasts.

See also **Asymmetric breasts; Insufficient milk supply**

➤ GLOBAL STRATEGY FOR INFANT AND YOUNG CHILD FEEDING

DEFINITION A World Health Organization document designed to improve child health through seamless integration of appropriate nutrition and feeding strategies.[165] The document identifies the responsibilities of governmental and nongovernmental organizations, health workers, and others in supporting optimal practices. Exclusive breastfeeding for the first 6 months of life, as well as continued breastfeeding with addition of appropriate complementary foods to 2 years and beyond is identified as a cornerstone of ideal infant feeding.

Footnote

[165]World Health Organization. (2003). *Global strategy for infant and young child feeding*. Geneva, Switzerland: World Health Organization. Retrieved from http://whqlibdoc.who.int/publications /2003/9241562218.pdf

➤ GLUCOSE-6-PHOSPHATE DEHYDROGENASE DEFICIENCY (G6PD)

DEFINITION A hereditary condition that decreases production of the enzyme G6PD.

NOTES

This deficiency results in red blood cell breakdown when an individual is exposed to certain drugs, foods, infection, and other stressors. This condition is more common among those of African and Mediterranean descent and among males.

Jaundice is a prominent symptom of G6PD, along with dark urine, enlarged spleen, fatigue, rapid heart rate, and others. In an infant, jaundice may be the first sign.

Infants with G6PD may be breastfed; however, this condition has sometimes been mistaken for breastmilk jaundice.

See also Jaundice

➤ GLYCERINE GEL PADS

DEFINITION Devices designed to give comfort to painful nipples. These gel matrix pads with a cloth backing are intended to be worn over the nipple. There is little research supporting claims that glycerin gel pads heal trauma to the nipple without improving the latch.[166]

ASK ABOUT

Nipple discomfort.

ASSESSMENT

PROMPT CARE NEEDED?

Are any of the following present?

Extreme nipple pain.

Bleeding from nipples.

Inability to breastfeed due to pain.

IF YES,   *Call lactation care provider immediately.*

ROUTINE CARE NEEDED?

Are any of the following present?

Feeding discomfort.

Trauma to nipple or breasts.

Misshapen nipple after feedings.

Visible fissures on nipples.

IF YES,   *Call lactation care provider today.*

SELF-CARE INFORMATION

Any substance that is applied to the nipple area will be consumed by the nursing baby. Do not apply any creams or ointments to the nipple area without getting your medical care provider's approval first.

Report nipple pain to the lactation care provider.

IMPORTANT CONDITIONS TO REPORT

Symptoms worsen or persist.

Signs of infection.

Feeding or stooling expectations are not met.

Women experiencing **nipple pain** may self-treat with gel pads and other substances rather than seek help to resolve the cause of the pain.

Women experiencing nipple pain should have a breastfeeding evaluation. Face-to-face counseling is effective in assessing and resolving nipple pain.

Any glycerine gel pads used should be approved for use in breastfeeding mothers.

Breast milk and Montgomery gland secretions provide natural antimicrobial lubrication of the nipple and areola.

See also Nipple pain; Sore nipples

Footnote

[166]Cadwell, K., Turner-Maffei, C., Blair, A., Brimdyr, K., & McInerney, Z. M. (2004). Pain reduction and treatment of sore nipples in nursing mothers. *The Journal of Perinatal Education: An ASPO/ Lamaze Publication*, *13*(1), 29–35. doi:10.1624/105812404X109375

➤ GOLDSMITH'S SIGN

DEFINITION   Consistent refusal to breastfeed on one breast without explanation. This indicates the need for routine breast evaluation. Cancer has been diagnosed as late as 5 years after persistent breast refusal.[167]

There are many common reasons for breast refusal. Cancer is an unusual, but possible, finding.

See also Breast cancer; Breast refusal; Refusal of infant to breastfeed

Footnote

[167]Saber, A., Dardik, H., Ibrahim, I. M., & Wolodiger, F. (1996). The milk rejection sign: A natural tumor marker. *The American Surgeon, 62,* 998–999.

➤ GRAVES' DISEASE

DEFINITION A type of thyroid disorder resulting in hyperthyroidism.

See also Hyperthyroidism

➤ GROWTH CHART

DEFINITION A document containing percentile curves showing the comparative height and weight of a population of babies of varying ages. These documents are used to track an individual baby's growth and evaluate that growth against the standards.

NOTES

Exclusively breastfed babies have a different growth pattern than mixed-fed and formula-fed babies. Exclusively breastfed babies grow faster in the first 4–6 months of age. The use of the World Health Organization growth charts[168] is recorded by the American Academy of Pediatrics and the Center for Disease Control and Prevention. These charts were standardized on breastfed babies. Breastfed babies are expected to begin slowing their rate of growth by 4–6 months. Both the CDC and the AAP recommend that the WHO growth charts that reflect the growth standard of breastfed babies are used. Changes in growth percentiles should be individually evaluated; such an occurrence may be an artifact of the charts. (Growth charts for breastfed babies that indicate both the CDC and WHO growth standards are available from Health Education Associates at www.healthed.cc.)

Footnote

[168] World Health Organization. (2012). The WHO Child Growth Standards. Retrieved from http ://www.who.int/childgrowth/standards/en/

➤ GUT-ASSOCIATED LYMPHOID TISSUE (GALT)

DEFINITION Immunologically active tissue found within the lining of the gastrointestinal tract.

The breast is thought to act as an extension of gut-associated lymphoid tissue (GALT). When a pathogen enters the gut, GALT tissue responds by triggering the production of an immunoglobulin to attack the pathogen. The breast may also respond to the GALT trigger by manufacturing and releasing appropriate immunoglobulins to fight the organism through the milk.

See also Bioactive components of breastmilk; Weight gain, low—baby

➤ HAIR CARE PRODUCTS

DEFINITION   Referring to dyes and "permanent" chemical applications to curl or relax curl. No evidence of harm to the breastfeeding infant exists. Application of these products is topical; rarely are chemicals absorbed into the skin.

➤ HAND EXPRESSION OF BREASTMILK

DEFINITION   A method of removing milk from the lactating breast that does not require any device with the exception of a hand and a bowl or jar to collect milk. Hand expression is a simple skill that should be taught to all breastfeeding mothers.

ASK ABOUT

The reason the mother plans to express milk.

ASSESSMENT

PROMPT CARE NEEDED?

Are any of the following present?

Imminent separation of the mother and her baby.

IF YES,   *Call lactation care provider today.*

ROUTINE CARE NEEDED?

Are any of the following present?

Desire to learn hand expression.

Desire to pump.

Questions about storage and handling of breast milk.

Questions about donating milk to a milk bank.

IF YES,   *Call lactation care provider.*

SELF-CARE INFORMATION

Wash hands before beginning.

When the baby is latched onto one breast, practice hand expression on the
other breast.

Gently massage and then compress the breast with the thumb and pointer finger
opposite each other on the areola; repeat.

Your skill will improve with practice.

Store expressed milk in the refrigerator or in a cooler with ice packs, or the freezer
if it will not be used within 48 hours.

Follow safe milk storage guidelines.

IMPORTANT CONDITIONS TO REPORT

Questions or problems with this technique.

See also Breast pump; Collection and storage of breastmilk

➤ HAND PUMP

DEFINITION   A device designed to remove milk from the breast. Manual pumps work
by hand pressure, squeezing a lever or contracting levers, or pulling out a cylinder to
generate pressure to operate the pump.

➤ HEADACHES

DEFINITION   The occurrence of painful pressure in the head during breastfeeding. Some women experience repeated headaches while breastfeeding. Headache may last only a few minutes and reoccur with subsequent feedings.

ASK ABOUT

Onset.
History of headache or migraine.

ASSESSMENT

EMERGENT CARE NEEDED?

Are any of the following present?

Sudden, severe pain.

Sudden weakness, tingling, or numbness on one side of the body.

Confusion.

Difficulty speaking.

Stiff neck and fever.

Persistent vomiting.

High fever.

Eye pain or visual blurring.

Persistent, unrelieved, severe pain.

IF YES,   *Seek emergency medical care now.*

ROUTINE CARE NEEDED?

Are any of the following present?

Pain during the first minutes of feeding.

No pain between feedings.

IF YES,   *Call lactation care provider today.*

SELF-CARE INFORMATION

Try a cool compress on the forehead before feedings.

Try an ice pack on the back of the neck at the beginning of a feeding.

Report any increase in symptoms to a healthcare provider.

NOTES

When other possible medical causes are ruled out, headache is considered to be a self-limited condition triggered by the hormone spikes of lactation. Lactational headache may be associated with Raynaud's phenomenon.

See also Raynaud's phenomenon/syndrome

➤ HEALTH EDUCATION ASSOCIATES

DESCRIPTION   An independent health publishing company, Health Education Associates, Inc. has been leading the patient education field by creating multi-ethnic pamphlets, in various reading levels. Books, modules, monographs, growth charts, breastfeeding assessment forms, and promotional items celebrating breastfeeding are also available.[169(p1)]

NOTES

Health Education Associates
Email: info@healthed.cc
Web: www.healthed.cc

Footnote

[169]Health Education Associates, Inc. (2010). Health Education Associates, Inc. Home page. Retrieved from http://www.healthed.cc

➤ HEALTHY CHILDREN PROJECT, INC.

DESCRIPTION   An institution that "is defining the field of research based breastfeeding education and ethical, evidence-based breastfeeding practice. Healthy Children is a non-profit 501(c)3 research and educational institution dedicated to improving child health outcomes through partnerships with public, private and non-profit agencies."[170](The Center for Breastfeeding section)

NOTES

Healthy Children Project
Email: info@healthychildren.cc
Web site: www.healthychildren.cc
   The Healthy Children Project offers several training programs (including the Certified Lactation Counselor, Advanced Issues in Lactation Consulting, and Maternal Infant Assessment courses), and educational materials for those who work in the fields of maternal child health and lactation. In addition, the Healthy Children Project conducts breastfeeding research and partners with Union Institute & University to provide bachelor's and master's degree curricula with a focus in lactation.

Footnote

[170]Healthy Children's Center for Breastfeeding. (2008–2009). The Center for Breastfeeding: A major focus of The Healthy Children Project. Retrieved from http://healthychildren.cc/index.cfm?show=about

➤ HEART PROBLEMS

DEFINITION   Referring to diseases and disorders of the cardiac and circulatory system.

ASK ABOUT

Onset.
History of cardiac problems.

ASSESSMENT

EMERGENT CARE NEEDED?

Are any of the following present?

A bluish tinge to the baby's mouth and lips during feeding.

Bluish hands and feet after hospital discharge.

Difficulty breathing.

Difficulty swallowing.

IF YES,   *Seek emergency care now.*

PROMPT CARE NEEDED?

Are any of the following present?

Breastfeeding baby diagnosed with cardiac problems.

IF YES,   *Call lactation care provider today.*

IMPORTANT CONDITIONS TO REPORT

Worsening, persistence, or recurrence of symptoms.

NOTES

Women with cardiac problems may breastfeed their babies. Any medications taken should be evaluated for their transfer into milk and effect on the baby using Lact Med or other drug resource. Babies with cardiac problems benefit from receiving their mother's milk. They may have problems sustaining attachment to the breast, and suckling may be weak and ineffective.

However, breastfeeding is less physiologically stressful than bottle feeding. Heart, oxygen saturation, and respiratory rates are lower while breastfeeding than while bottle feeding.

Mothers may benefit from pumping or expressing milk after feeding to maintain an adequate milk supply.

A lactation care provider should evaluate effective positions and techniques for babies diagnosed with cardiac problems.

➤ HEATING BREASTMILK

DEFINITION   Techniques used to safely warm milk for consumption by a baby.

NOTES

Thaw frozen milk in its container.
  Warm by:

   Holding container under lukewarm running tap water.

   Placing container in lukewarm water.

Hot water is not recommended due to potential nutrient loss.
  Milk should never be boiled or microwaved.
  Milk does not need to be overly warm before fed to infant.[171]

See also Collection and storage of breastmilk; Storage of breastmilk

Footnote

[171]Arnold, L. D. W. (2004). *Safe storage of expressed breastmilk for the healthy infant and child*. East Sandwich, MA: Health Education Associates.

➤ HEMORRHAGE, POSTPARTUM

DEFINITION   An abnormally high amount (generally more than 500 ml) of blood loss during or after delivery.

NOTES

Postpartum hemorrhage is of concern to breastfeeding because extreme blood loss can cause **Sheehan's syndrome**, an insult to the **pituitary gland**, and in turn the hormones of lactation (**prolactin** and **oxytocin**).
  Women affected by Sheehan's syndrome may be unable to make an adequate amount of milk.

Other symptoms of this syndrome include sudden onset of hypothyroidism, diabetes insipidus, and hair loss along with menstrual irregularities. Medical evaluation should include measurement of prolactin levels before and after sucklings. The extent to which women recover from Sheehan's syndrome is variable with the degree of infarct.[172(p562)]

Babies of mothers who suffered postpartum hemorrhage should be closely monitored for inadequate intake.

See also Sheehan's syndrome

Footnote

[172]Lawrence, R. A., & Lawrence, R. M. (2011). *Breastfeeding: A guide for the medical profession* (7th ed.). St. Louis, MO: Elsevier/Mosby.

➤ HEPATITIS

DEFINITION   Inflammation of the liver caused by a number of pathogens and substances. Of pertinence here are the common viruses hepatitis A, B, and C. Breastfeeding is compatible with hepatitis infection in the mother with a few qualifications:

Hepatitis A: Lawrence & Lawrence (2011) state: "no reason exists to interrupt breastfeeding with maternal HAV [Hepatitis A virus] infection. The infant should receive Ig [immunoglobulin] and HAV vaccine, administered simultaneously.[173(p431)]

Hepatitis B: CDC (2009) states:

All infants born to HBV-infected mothers should receive hepatitis B immune globulin and the first dose of hepatitis B vaccine within 12 hours of birth. The second dose of vaccine should be given at aged [sic] 1–2 months, and the third dose at aged [sic] 6 months. The infant should be tested after completion of the vaccine series, at aged [sic] 9–18 months (generally at the next well-child visit), to determine if the vaccine worked and the infant is not infected with HBV through exposure to the mother's blood during the birth process. However, there is no need to delay breastfeeding until the infant is fully immunized. All mothers who breastfeed should take good care of their nipples to avoid cracking and bleeding.[174](Hepatitis B section)

Hepatitis C: According to the CDC (2009):

> There is no documented evidence that breastfeeding spreads HCV. Therefore, having HCV-infection is not a contraindication to breastfeed. HCV is transmitted by infected blood, not by human breast milk. There are no current data to suggest that HCV is transmitted by human breast milk.[175](Hepatitis C section)

NOTES

Seek updates from the Centers for Disease Control and Prevention, as this is a rapidly expanding area of knowledge and research.

See also Acute infection

Footnotes

[173]Lawrence, R. A., & Lawrence, R. M. (2011). *Breastfeeding: A guide for the medical profession* (7th ed.). St. Louis, MO: Elsevier/Mosby.

[174]Centers for Disease Control and Prevention. (2009, October 20). Breastfeeding: Hepatitis B and C infections. Retrieved from http://www.cdc.gov/breastfeeding/disease/hepatitis.htm

[175]Centers for Disease Control and Prevention. (2009, October 20).

➤ HERBS

DEFINITION   Plants or parts of plants that can be valued for their medicinal qualities. Herbs can have powerful effects. As with some drugs taken by breastfeeding mothers, troubling effects have also been reported in breastfed babies whose mothers have taken certain herbs.

SELF-CARE INFORMATION

Tell all healthcare providers about any herbs and natural supplements you are taking.

Fenugreek has been sold as a galactagogue (substance that increases milk), but there is currently little scientific evidence of this effect. Fenugreek may interfere with the absorption of any medication used concurrently,[176(p261)] and higher doses may cause hypoglycemia.[177(p407)]

Investigate medicinal herbs with the same care you would with prescribed and over-the-counter medications.

IMPORTANT CONDITIONS TO REPORT

Any change in the baby's physical condition or behavior such as problems sleeping, vomiting, rash, or irritability.

See also Drugs; Medication resources (inside back cover); Over-the-counter (OTC) drugs

Footnotes

[176]Skidmore-Roth, L. (2010). *Mosby's handbook of herbs & natural supplements.* St. Louis, MO: Elsevier/Mosby.

[177]Hale, T. (2012). *Medications and mothers' milk* (15th ed.). Amarillo, TX: Hale Publishing.

➤ HERPES SIMPLEX VIRUS

DEFINITION   Infection with the herpes simplex 1 or 2 virus, characterized by lesions (blisters) on the skin surface. In the context of breastfeeding, the presence of herpes lesions on the nipple or parts of the breast that the baby's mouth will contact is of great concern, due to the life-threatening nature of herpes infection in the newborn. Herpes lesions elsewhere on the mother's body do not contraindicate breastfeeding; however, mother should be cautioned to cover lesions, avoid touching them, and practice careful hand washing.

ASK ABOUT

Onset.

Age of the baby.

Known history of herpes lesions or other skin conditions.

ASSESSMENT

EMERGENT CARE NEEDED?

Are any of the following present?

History of herpes lesions on the nipple or breast, or elsewhere on the mother's or partner's body, with:

- Blisters plus fever and aching.
- A baby with blisters, fever, and/or lethargy.

IF YES,   *Seek emergency care now.*

SELF-CARE INFORMATION

Wash your hands carefully, especially if you have a herpes outbreak.

Family members with cold sores should refrain from kissing the baby.

IMPORTANT CONDITIONS TO REPORT

Fever.

Signs of infection.

See also Acute infection; Blisters on nipple or breast

➤ HHS

See Department of Health & Human Services (DHHS)

➤ HIGHER ORDER MULTIPLES (HOM)

DEFINITION   Birth of three or more infants from the same pregnancy.

Mothers can breastfeed higher order multiples. Increased suckling, especially nursing two babies simultaneously, stimulates an increased supply of milk.

Multiples may be born prematurely, spend weeks or months in the hospital before discharge, and may not be discharged on the same day.

Mothers may express milk to be fed to hospitalized babies. Expression should start as soon after the babies are born as possible. Mothers should express milk eight or more times per day.

ASK ABOUT

Age of the babies.
Gestational age of babies at birth.

ASSESSMENT

ROUTINE CARE NEEDED?

Are any of the following present?

Strategies for managing the nursing of multiples.
Strategies for managing milk supply for multiples.
Questions about breastfeeding.
Problems with breastfeeding.

IF YES,   *Call lactation care provider today.*

SELF-CARE INFORMATION

Nursing babies simultaneously is helpful for building a milk supply, but may be difficult to manage at first. Ask for help with positioning.

At first, switch the babies from one breast to another. As the babies get older, they may prefer nursing on one breast or another.

Many mothers have found it helpful at first to write down who nursed when to ensure that each baby gets enough nourishment.

IMPORTANT CONDITIONS TO REPORT
Lethargy.
Decrease in urine and stools.
Change in breastfeeding behavior.
Problems with feeding.

See also Breast pump; Hospitalization; NICU, milk storage and handling in; Premature infant; Preterm milk

➤ HINDMILK

DEFINITION   The milk that flows from the breast at the end of a feed.

NOTES

The belief that hindmilk is always the richest milk is outdated. Fat content in milk varies throughout the day and within each feeding, depending on how full the breast is, as well as how well the baby, hand expression, or pump is eliciting the milk rejection reflex, which propels fat down through the breast.

There is no scientific evidence to support the common advice that mothers should keep the baby at the breast longer to get more hindmilk. The baby can regulate its caloric intake when allowed to feed and stop feeding according to its own feeding cues.

The caloric composition of human milk rarely is inadequate. Routine testing of the fat or other content of milk is not recommended, due to diurnal variation and the difficulty of collecting a representative sample.

See also Caloric density of breastmilk; Fat in breastmilk; Foremilk

➤ # HIV

See Human immunodeficiency virus (HIV)

➤ # HMBANA

See Human Milk Banking Association of North America (HMBANA)

➤ # HMHB

See National Healthy Mothers, Healthy Babies Coalition (HMHB)

➤ # HOM

See Higher order multiples (HOM)

➤ # HORMONAL CONTRACEPTIVE METHODS

DEFINITION   Drugs used to reduce fertility.

NOTES

Progestin-only hormonal methods are considered compatible with breastfeeding.

Combined estrogen/progestin methods are generally not recommended as they may reduce milk supply and affect infant growth.

Progestin-only injectibles are intended for use in breastfeeding women only after 6 weeks postdelivery or when full milk supply is developed. Use prior to that time may decrease milk supply due to high circulating progestin levels, simulating a state of pregnancy.

See also Birth control; Contraception; Oral contraceptives; Progestin-only contraceptives

➤ HORMONES

DEFINITION   A substance produced by cells that regulates or stimulates other cells and organs. Hormones are produced by several different endocrine glands in the body.

NOTES

Hormones are crucial to the production and flow of breastmilk. The alveolar cells produce droplets of milk in response to suckling and the resulting spike in blood levels of the hormone prolactin. The hormone oxytocin (which is secreted in response to nipple stretching, breast massage, and other stimuli) causes the myoepithelial bands around the alveoli to contract, squeezing the milk into the ducts, propelling it toward the nipple.

Synthetic hormones (e.g., cortisone, progestin, etc.) are used to treat hormone disorders and provide contraception.

See also Birth control; Hyperthyroidism; Hypothyroidism; Progestin-only contraceptives

➤ HOSPITALIZATION

DEFINITION   The effect of separation of mother and baby when required for medical purposes. Mother, baby, or both may be hospitalized. Breastmilk production can be supported during this time if breastfeeding is not possible due to separation. When possible, mothers and babies may be hospitalized together so that breastfeeding can continue.

ASK ABOUT

Onset.
Age of the baby.
Reason for hospitalization.

ASSESSMENT

PROMPT CARE NEEDED?

Are any of the following present?

Breastfeeding mother planning hospitalization.

IF YES,   *Call lactation care provider today.*

SELF-CARE INFORMATION

Express milk as much as possible to relieve pressure and maintain milk supply; aim to express milk as often as the baby would normally feed (at least eight times daily).

Store milk as appropriate (ask for storage guidelines if the baby is premature or ill).

Ask about medication compatibility and side effects.

Arrange for transport and feeding of expressed milk to the baby if the baby will be separated from the mother.

Ask when skin-to-skin contact and breastfeeding can resume.

IMPORTANT CONDITIONS TO REPORT

Discomfort.

Declining milk production.

See also Abrupt weaning; Breast pump; Hand expression of breastmilk; Separation of mother and baby

➤ HRSA

See DHHS/Health Resources Services Administration (HRSA), Maternal Child Health Bureau

➤ HTLV-I, HTLV-II

See Human T-cell lymphotropic virus I and human T-cell lymphotropic virus II (HTLV-I, HTLV-II)

➤ HUMAN IMMUNODEFICIENCY VIRUS (HIV)

DEFINITION   Human immunodeficiency virus (HIV) causes the life-threatening disease of the immune system, acquired immunodeficiency syndrome (AIDS). People with AIDS have increased susceptibility to infections and rare cancers including Kaposi sarcoma. HIV is transmitted primarily by exposure to contaminated body fluids, especially blood, semen, and potentially breastmilk.

ASK ABOUT

Onset.
Age of the baby.

ASSESSMENT

EMERGENT CARE NEEDED?

Are any of the following present?

Breastfeeding mother with concern about possibility of recently
contracting HIV.

Breastfeeding mother diagnosed with HIV.

Pregnant woman with concerns about possibility of recently contracting HIV.

Pregnant woman diagnosed with HIV.

Pregnant or breastfeeding woman taking antiretroviral medications.

IF YES,   *Seek medical care within 4 hours.*

ROUTINE CARE NEEDED?

Are any of the following present?

General questions about HIV.

IF YES,   *Call pediatric or obstetric care provider today.*

SELF-CARE INFORMATION

Know your HIV status.
Know your treatment options.
Know the HIV status of all sexual partners.
Practice safe sex.
Avoid dirty needles with intravenous drug use.

IMPORTANT CONDITIONS TO REPORT

Need for testing.

NOTES

In the United States, breastfeeding is contraindicated in women diagnosed as HIV positive or with **AIDS**. Women at high risk for HIV (e.g., women who are sex workers, women with an HIV-positive sexual partner, women using intravenous drugs, women whose sexual partners use intravenous drugs, and women who are raped or coerced to have sex) should receive ongoing testing and counseling regarding infant feeding.

See also Contraindicated conditions

➤ HUMAN MILK BANKING ASSOCIATION OF NORTH AMERICA (HMBANA)

DEFINITION   A "multidisciplinary group of health care providers that promotes, protects, and supports donor milk banking. HMBANA is the only professional membership association for milk banks in Canada, Mexico and the United States and as such sets the standards and guidelines for donor milk banking for those areas."[179(p1)]

NOTES

Human Milk Banking Association of North America (HMBANA)
Email: info@hmbana.org
Website: www.hmbana.org
  HMBANA develops standards for milk banking, provides a forum for information sharing among experts in the field, encourages research into the science of human milk, and facilitates communication among milk banks.

See also Donor milk; Milk banks

Footnote

[179]Human Milk Banking Association of North America. (n.d.). Mission/Description. Retrieved from https://www.hmbana.org/missiondescription

➤ HUMAN MILK FORTIFICATION

DEFINITION The practice of adding minerals, fats, and protein to expressed breast milk to increase its nutrient content. Calcium, phosphorus, zinc, and iron are among the nutrients added. In the United States, commercially available human milk fortifiers may be made with cow's milk products or with only human milk.

NOTES

Human milk fortification is typically used only for very low birthweight infants in neonatal care unit settings.

See also Lactoengineering; Premature infant; Preterm milk

➤ HUMAN T-CELL LYMPHOTROPIC VIRUS I AND HUMAN T-CELL LYMPHOTROPIC VIRUS II (HTLV-I, HTLV-II)

DEFINITION Infection with the human T-cell lymphotropic virus I or II (HTLV-I, HTLV-II). Breastfeeding is contraindicated in the mother with HTLV infection.

NOTES

HTLV infection is not common in the United States but may be found in intravenous drug users, people with **human immunodeficiency virus (HIV)**, and other emerging populations.

HTLV testing by enzyme-linked immunosorbent assay, or ELISA (as done by cord blood donation/storage companies), can yield false positives due to cross-reactivity with pregnancy antibodies. Confirmation by Western blot is indicated.

See also Contraindicated conditions

➤ HYDROGEL PADS

DEFINITION   Devices designed to give comfort to painful nipples. Hydrogel matrix pads with a cloth backing are intended to be worn over the nipple. There is little research supporting claims that hydrogel pads heal trauma to the nipple without improvements made to the latching process.[180]

ASK ABOUT

Nipple discomfort.

ASSESSMENT

PROMPT CARE NEEDED?

Are any of the following present?

Extreme nipple pain.

Bleeding from nipples.

Unable to breastfeed due to pain.

IF YES,   *Call lactation care provider now.*

ROUTINE CARE NEEDED?

Are any of the following present?

Feeding discomfort.

Trauma to nipples or breasts.

Misshapen nipple after feedings.

Visible fissures on nipples.

IF YES,   *Call lactation care provider today.*

SELF-CARE INFORMATION

Any substance that is applied to the nipple area will be consumed by the nursing baby. Do not apply any creams or ointments to the nipple area without getting your healthcare provider's approval first.

Report nipple pain to your lactation care provider.

IMPORTANT CONDITIONS TO REPORT

Symptoms worsen or persist.

Signs of infection.

Feeding or stooling expectations not met.

NOTES

Women experiencing **nipple pain** may self-treat with gel pads and other substances rather than seeking help to resolve the cause of the pain.

Women experiencing nipple pain should have a breastfeeding evaluation. Face-to-face counseling is effective in assessing and resolving nipple pain.

Any hydrogel pads used should be approved for use in breastfeeding mothers.

See also Nipple pain; Sore nipples

Footnote

[180]Cadwell, K., Turner-Maffei, C., Blair, A., Brimdyr, K., & McInerney, Z. M. (2004). Pain reduction and treatment of sore nipples in nursing mothers. *The Journal of Perinatal Education: An ASPO/Lamaze Publication, 13*(1), 29–35. doi:10.1624/105812404X109375

➤ HYPERADENIA

DEFINITION   Breast tissue with no nipples.

NOTES

Women can have breast or nipple tissue anywhere along the milk line, which extends from the axilla over the front of the chest and abdomen and into the groin region.

➤ HYPERBILIRUBINEMIA

DEFINITION   Presence of an excessive amount of bilirubin (a breakdown product of red blood cells). It is normal for newborn babies to break down the red blood cells they used in fetal life and replace them with adult type red blood cells.

When bilirubin accumulates, a yellow discoloration of the skin and the whites of the eyes called **jaundice** can occur. It is the most common condition requiring medical treatment in the newborn period.

Although the condition of jaundice may be benign, it can be a symptom of other serious conditions, including **kernicterus**.

ASK ABOUT

Age of the baby.
Feeding behavior.
Stooling pattern and color.
Urination pattern.

ASSESSMENT

PROMPT CARE NEEDED?

Are any of the following present?

Severe lethargy (sleepiness).

Poor feeding.

No interest in feeding for more than 6 hours.

Fever.

Meconium bowel movements after 5 days of life.

No yellow stool by day 5.

Fewer than three bowel movements daily in breastfed newborn after the first 2 days of life.

No urine in 6 hours.

Brick dust urine (uric acid crystals) after 2 days of life.

Dark-colored urine.

Fewer than four urinations daily in the breastfed newborn after day 5 of life.

Noticeably sunken fontanelles (soft spot on the top of the head).

Decreased activity.

A baby below birthweight at 10–14 days of life.

Cessation of weight gain.

Any fever in a baby younger than 3 months of age.

Fever higher than 100°F (37.7°C) in a baby older than 3 months of age.

> **IF YES,**   *Seek pediatric care now.*

ROUTINE CARE NEEDED?

Are any of the following present?

Baby sleepy during breastfeedings.

> **IF YES,**   *Call lactation care provider now.*

SELF-CARE INFORMATION

Breastfeed as soon as possible after birth.

Encourage the baby to nurse 10–12 times per 24 hours.

Colostrum has laxative properties. Stooling helps to rid the baby's body of bilirubin.

IMPORTANT CONDITIONS TO REPORT

No stool in 24 hours.

Severe lethargy (sleepiness).

Poor feeding.

Fever.

> **NOTES**

All jaundiced babies are at risk for kernicterus and should be closely monitored.

See also Bilirubin; Jaundice; Kernicterus; Late onset jaundice

➤ HYPERGALACTIA

DEFINITION   Production of excessive amounts of milk.

> **NOTES**

Excess milk production can create problems such as gas and discomfort in the baby, and recurrent plugged ducts, mastitis, and sore nipples in the mother. Lactation evaluation is indicated by these symptoms.

➤ HYPERMASTIA

DEFINITION   Refers to two conditions: excessive growth of the breasts, and existence of more than two breasts. Both of these conditions are compatible with breastfeeding.

See also Accessory breast tissue; Gigantomastia

➤ HYPERTHELIA

DEFINITION   Presence of more than one nipple per breast, or nipples with no breast tissue. These conditions are compatible with breastfeeding.

See also Accessory breast tissue

➤ HYPERTHYROIDISM

DEFINITION   An overabundance of thyroid hormone.

> **ASK ABOUT**

Age of the baby.
Weight gain pattern of the baby.

ASSESSMENT

EMERGENT CARE NEEDED?

Are any of the following present?

Meconium bowel movements after 5 days of life.

No yellow stool by day 5.

Fewer than three bowel movements daily in breastfed newborn after the first 2 days of life.

No urine in 6 hours.

Brick dust urine (uric acid crystals) after 2 days of life.

Dark-colored urine.

Fewer than four urinations daily in the breastfed newborn after day 5 of life.

Noticeably sunken fontanelles (soft spot on the top of the head).

Decreased activity (lethargy).

Baby below birthweight at 10–14 days of life.

Cessation of weight gain.

Hard to latch on.

Subtle feeding cues.

Weak suck.

A sleepy baby who is difficult to wake.

IF YES, *Seek pediatric care now.*

PROMPT CARE NEEDED?

Are any of the following present?

Inadequate weight gain.

Concern about possible inadequate weight gain.

IF YES, *Call pediatric care provider today.*

ROUTINE CARE NEEDED?

Are any of the following present?

Building up milk supply after medication adjustment.

IF YES, *Call lactation care provider today.*

SELF-CARE INFORMATION

Postpartum thyroid problems can initially present as postpartum depression or anxiety. Mothers who struggle with milk supply should have a thorough medical evaluation if the supply does not improve with increased breastfeeding frequency and milk expression.

IMPORTANT CONDITIONS TO REPORT

Increasing sleepiness in the baby.

Increasing fatigue and inability to cope in the mother.

Feelings of hopelessness or depression.

Symptoms of thyroid disease.

NOTES

Breastfeeding is not contraindicated for women who have hyperthyroidism.

A woman whose hyperthyroid problem (thyroiditis) is identified during pregnancy or lactation presents a special problem in the diagnosis and treatment. The mother should tell all healthcare providers that she is breastfeeding.

Many of the signs and symptoms of thyroid disease can seem normal to a postpartum woman. The symptom that is unique to hyperthyroidism is difficulty with initiating and maintaining an adequate milk supply.

Signs and symptoms of hyperthyroidism include:

Palpitations.

Heat intolerance.

Nervousness.

Insomnia.

Breathlessness.

Increased bowel movements.

Light or absent menstrual periods.

Fatigue.

Weight loss.

Fast heart rate.

Trembling hands.

Muscle weakness.

Warm, moist skin.

Hair loss.

Both high and low levels of thyroid hormones can affect the mother's milk supply.

See also Hyperthyroidism; Maternal fatigue

➤ HYPERTONIA

DEFINITION   Referring to tight, tense muscle response or stiffness. Hypertonia can be a symptom of illness and other problems. Hypertonic babies may arch their bodies away from the breast. Some of the problems that may be seen with breastfeeding include difficulty latching on, biting when swallowing (tonic bite reflex), and difficulty sustaining rhythmic suck.

ASK ABOUT

Age of the baby.
Onset of hypertonia.
Change in feeding behavior.
Change in urination or stooling patterns.

ASSESSMENT

EMERGENT CARE NEEDED?

Are any of the following present?

Sudden onset of change in muscle tone.

Sudden change in feeding behavior.

IF YES,   *Call pediatric care provider now.*

PROMPT CARE NEEDED?

Are any of the following present?

Feeding problems.

Weight loss or failure to initially gain weight in newborn period.

Constipation.

Decline in milk supply.

IF YES,   *Call pediatric care provider today.*

ROUTINE CARE NEEDED?

Are any of the following present?

Feeding problems.

Slow weight gain.

Problems positioning baby at breast.

Nipple discomfort.

Decline in milk supply.

> **IF YES,** *Call pediatric care provider and lactation care provider today.*

SELF-CARE INFORMATION

Breastfeeding and breastmilk are valuable for babies with high muscle tone.
Pumping may be necessary in order to maintain an adequate milk supply.
"Wearing" the baby in a safe sling or cloth baby carrier can be very helpful to
encourage flexion in a hyperextending infant.

IMPORTANT CONDITIONS TO REPORT

Change in feeding behaviors.
Change in urination or stooling patterns.
Declining breastmilk volume.

See also Attachment; Latch-on

➤ HYPOGLYCEMIA

DEFINITION A condition in which an individual's blood glucose (sugar) levels have
fallen below a predetermined amount.

> **ASK ABOUT**

Age of the baby.
Gestational age of the baby.
History of diabetes in the mother.
History of labor, especially stress.

ASSESSMENT

EMERGENT CARE NEEDED?

Are any of the following present?

Seizure activity.

Convulsions.

Coma.

Respiratory distress.

Apnea (cessation of breathing).

Cyanosis (blue color).

Thermoregulatory problems.

Jitteriness.

Hypotonia (lack of muscle tone).

Lethargy.

Listlessness.

Poor feeding.

IF YES, *Seek emergency care now.*

PROMPT CARE NEEDED?

Are any of the following present?

Feeding problems after treatment for hypoglycemia.

IF YES, *Call lactation care provider today.*

SELF-CARE INFORMATION

Establish early and frequent breastfeeding.

Keep the baby warm and dry.

Seek help with breastfeeding if the baby feeds poorly.

IMPORTANT CONDITIONS TO REPORT
Seizure activity.
Convulsions.
Coma.
Respiratory distress.
Apnea (cessation of breathing).
Cyanosis (blue color).
Thermoregulatory problems.
Jitteriness.
Hypotonia (lack of muscle tone).
Lethargy.
Listlessness.
Poor feeding.

➤ HYPOTHYROIDISM

DEFINITION   Abnormally low levels of thyroid hormone.

ASK ABOUT

Age of the baby.
Weight gain pattern of the baby.

ASSESSMENT

EMERGENT CARE NEEDED?

Are any of the following present?

About the baby:
The baby is sleepy and difficult to wake.
Meconium bowel movements after 5 days of life.
No yellow stool by day 5.
Fewer than three bowel movements daily in a breastfed newborn after the first 2 days of life.
No urine in 6 hours.

Brick dust urine (uric acid crystals) after 2 days of life.

Dark-colored urine.

Fewer than four urinations daily in the breastfed newborn after day 5 of life.

Noticeably sunken fontanelles (soft spot on the top of the head).

Decreased activity.

The baby is below birthweight at 10–14 days of life.

Cessation of weight gain.

Hard to latch on.

Subtle feeding cues.

Weak suck.

IF YES,   *Seek pediatric care now.*

PROMPT CARE NEEDED?

Are any of the following present?

About the mother:

Fatigue (may seem to be a normal postpartum condition).

Weakness.

Weight gain or difficulty losing weight (difficult to ascertain in postpartum).

Coarse, dry hair.

Dry, rough skin.

Hair loss (difficult to notice in pregnant and postpartum women unless it is severe).

Inability to tolerate cold as easily as others in the same environment.

Muscle cramps and aches.

Constipation.

Depression (may be assumed to be baby blues).

Irritability.

Memory loss.

Abnormal menstrual periods (normal to not menstruate in the early time postpartum).

Decreased sexual desire (normal in postpartum women).

IF YES,   *Seek medical care today.*

PROMPT CARE NEEDED?

Are any of the following present?

About the baby:

Inadequate weight gain.

Concern about inadequate weight gain in a breastfed baby.

> **IF YES,** *Seek pediatric care today.*

ROUTINE CARE NEEDED?

Are any of the following present?

Building up milk supply after medication adjustment.

> **IF YES,** *Call lactation care provider today.*

SELF-CARE INFORMATION

Postpartum thyroid problems can initially present as postpartum depression or simply normal tiredness or fatigue. Mothers who struggle with milk supply should have a thorough lactation and healthcare provider evaluation if the supply does not improve with increased breastfeeding frequency and milk expression.

IMPORTANT CONDITIONS TO REPORT

Increasing sleepiness in the baby.

Increasing fatigue and inability to cope in the mother.

Feelings of hopelessness or depression.

Symptoms of thyroid disease.

> **NOTES**
>
> Breastfeeding is not contraindicated for women who have hypothyroidism.
>
> Women with hypothyroidism are prescribed thyroid replacement therapy. These medications are typically compatible with breastfeeding.
>
> Many of the signs and symptoms of thyroid disease can seem normal in a postpartum woman. The symptom that is unique to hypothyroidism is difficulty with initiating and maintaining an adequate milk supply.

Hypothyroidism can occur in infants. There are indications that breastfeeding may mask the symptoms of the illness, as breastmilk contains thyroid hormones. There are no contraindications to breastfeeding with thyroid imbalance in the mother or baby.

See also Hyperthyroidism; Maternal fatigue; Milk supply, inadequate

➤ HYPOTONIA

DEFINITION Referring to loose or floppy muscle response. Babies with low muscle tone (also referred to as hypotonia) have relaxed arm and leg joints, like a rag doll. Hypotonia can be a symptom of prematurity and of physical problems or illness. Babies with low muscle tone may have breastfeeding problems such as nonrhythmic suck and weak sucking, and they may tire more easily.

ASK ABOUT

Age of the baby.
Onset of hypotonia.
Change in feeding behavior.
Change in urination or stooling patterns.
Any identified medical problems for the mother or the baby.
Any medication use.

ASSESSMENT

EMERGENT CARE NEEDED?

Are any of the following present in the infant?

Sudden change in muscle tone.
Sudden change in feeding behavior.
Sudden lethargy.

IF YES,   *Seek emergency care now.*

PROMPT CARE NEEDED?

Are any of the following present?

> Weight loss in the newborn of more than 7% from birth or continuance of weight loss by day 5 of life[181]
>
> Meconium bowel movements after 5 days of life.
>
> No yellow stool by day 5.
>
> Fewer than three bowel movements daily in a breastfed newborn after the first 2 days of life.
>
> No urine in 6 hours.
>
> Brick dust urine (uric acid crystals) after 2 days of life.
>
> Dark-colored urine.
>
> Fewer than four urinations daily in the breastfed newborn after day 5 of life.
>
> Noticeably sunken fontanelles (soft spot on the top of the head).
>
> Decreased activity.
>
> Baby below birthweight at 10–14 days of life.
>
> Cessation of weight gain or weight loss.

IF YES, *Seek pediatric care now.*

ROUTINE CARE NEEDED?

Are any of the following present?

> A breastfeeding baby with diagnosed hypotonia or a condition that includes hypotonia (such as Down syndrome).
>
> Feeding problems.
>
> Slow weight gain.
>
> Problems positioning the baby at the breast.
>
> Decline in milk supply.

IF YES, *Call lactation care provider today.*

SELF-CARE INFORMATION

Breastfeeding and breastmilk are valuable for babies with low muscle tone.

Pumping with additional hand expression may be necessary in order to maintain an adequate milk supply.

Holding the baby skin to skin in between feedings is helpful.

IMPORTANT CONDITIONS TO REPORT

Change in feeding behaviors.

Change in urination or stooling patterns.

Declining breastmilk volume.

See also Down syndrome (DS); Slow weight gain, baby

Footnote

[181]AAP Section on Breastfeeding. (2012). Breastfeeding and the use of human milk. *Pediatrics*, *129*(3), e827–e841. doi:10.1542/peds.2011-3552., p.e828

➤ HYSTERECTOMY

DEFINITION   A surgical procedure in which the uterus is removed. Women may breastfeed after this surgery.

ASK ABOUT

Date of the surgery.

Age of the baby.

ASSESSMENT

PROMPT CARE NEEDED?

Are any of the following present?

A breastfeeding mother undergoing a hysterectomy.

Breastfeeding problems in a woman who has experienced hysterectomy.

IF YES,   *Call lactation care provider today.*

SELF-CARE INFORMATION

For a woman undergoing postpartum hysterectomy:

- Express milk as much as possible to relieve pressure and maintain milk supply; aim to express milk as often as the baby would normally feed (at least eight times daily).
- Store milk as appropriate.
- Ask about the safety of any medications prescribed (make sure all care providers know you are breastfeeding).
- Arrange for transport and feeding of expressed milk to the baby.
- Ask when skin-to-skin contact and breastfeeding can resume.

IMPORTANT CONDITIONS TO REPORT

Discomfort.

Declining milk production.

Emergency hysterectomy sometimes occurs immediately after childbirth. Breastfeeding is not contraindicated in these mothers. If mothers hemorrhage severely, milk supply may be impacted because of injury to the pituitary gland (Sheehan's syndrome).

See also Abrupt weaning; Breast pump; Hand expression of breastmilk; Sheehan's syndrome

➤ IBCLC

See International Board Certified Lactation Consultant

➤ IBFAN

See International Baby Food Action Network (IBFAN)

➤ IBLCE

See International Board of Lactation Consultant Examiners (IBLCE)

➤ IDDM

See Insulin-Dependent Diabetes Mellitus (IDDM)

➤ IGA

DEFINITION   Immunoglobulin A. An immunoglobulin that protects the mucous membranes of the respiratory and digestive tracts from invasion by pathogens.

SELF-CARE INFORMATION

Nursing in the first hours after birth transfers IgA from the mother to the baby. The IgA coats the baby's intestines, lung surfaces, and other mucous membranes. This begins to protect the baby from bacteria and viruses as soon as possible.

NOTES

Human babies are born without IgA. Babies do not produce their own IgA for several months.

Human milk is a rich source of IgA, providing the first level of immune defense until babies develop their own IgA.

See also Skin-to-skin (STS) care

➤ IGA DEFICIENCY AND HUMAN MILK

DEFINITION   Selective deficiency of immunoglobulin A occurs in some adults. Often people with this disorder are asymptomatic, or they have recurrent infections, allergies, or autoimmune disorders.

NOTES

Breastfeeding is still recommended when the mother has IgA deficiency.

➤ IGE

DEFINITION   Immunoglobulin E. An immunoglobulin that combines with antigens in the gut and releases chemicals that cause changes to the permeability of the gut wall.

NOTES

Human milk contains IgE in lower concentration than IgA.

➤ IGF-I

DEFINITION   Insulin-like growth factor. A beneficial agent found in human milk that triggers growth.

NOTES

Research suggests that preterm, exclusively breastfed infants have higher serum levels of this growth-promoting factor.

➤ IHS

See DHHS/Indian Health Service

➤ ILCA

See International Lactation Consultant Association (ILCA)

➤ ILLEGAL DRUGS

DEFINITION   Street drugs, including intoxicants and hallucinogens such as amphetamines, cocaine, heroin, and marijuana.

NOTES

Breastfeeding is contraindicated in women who habitually use illegal drugs.
See Medication resources (inside back cover) for a review of specific effects of these drugs.

See also Medication resources (inside back cover)

➤ ILLICIT DRUGS

See Illegal drugs

➤ ILLNESS, ACUTE

DEFINITION   Sickness in the mother and baby are compatible with breastfeeding, except in rare contraindicated infections in the mother (e.g., HIV, HTLV-I, untreated tuberculosis, and active herpes lesions on the breast).

NOTES

An up-to-date list of contraindications to breastfeeding (such as the CDC's[182]) should be consulted to determine the safety and possible side effects of individual drugs taken during acute illness.
Newborn and premature babies are at greater risk of side effects due to limited ability to clear drugs from their systems.

See also Acute infection; Contraindicated conditions; Medication resources (inside back cover)

Footnote

[182]Centers for Disease Control & Prevention. (2009). *Breastfeeding: Diseases and Conditions*. Retrieved from http://www.cdc.gov/breastfeeding/disease/index.htm

➤ ILLNESS, CHRONIC

DEFINITION   Diseases or disorders that last for a long time or reoccur.

NOTES

Breastfeeding is known to reduce the severity or risk of developing several chronic illnesses including eczema, asthma, diabetes, multiple sclerosis, and celiac disease.

According to the Centers for Disease Control and Prevention, breastfeeding is *not* advisable if one or more of the following conditions is true:

1. An infant diagnosed with galactosemia, a rare genetic metabolic disorder
2. The infant whose mother:
   - Has been infected with the human immunodeficiency virus (HIV)
   - Is taking antiretroviral medications
   - Has untreated, active tuberculosis
   - Is infected with human T-cell lymphotropic virus type I or type II
   - Is using or is dependent upon an illicit drug
   - Is taking prescribed cancer chemotherapy agents, such as antimetabolites that interfere with DNA replication and cell division
   - Is undergoing radiation therapies; however, such nuclear medicine therapies require only a temporary interruption in breastfeeding.[183(p1)]

The AAP also recommends a temporary cessation of breastfeeding if the mother is diagnosed with untreated brucellosis.[184(p.e832)]

See also Contraindicated conditions

Footnotes

[183]Centers for Disease Control and Prevention. (2009). Breastfeeding—Diseases and conditions: When should a mother avoid breastfeeding? Retrieved from http://www.cdc.gov/breastfeeding/disease/index.htm

[184]AAP Section on Breastfeeding. (2012). Breastfeeding and the use of human milk. *Pediatrics, 129*(3), e827–e841. doi:10.1542/peds.2011-3552

➤ IMMUNE SYSTEM

DEFINITION   The complex, intricate mechanism through which the body protects itself from invasion by pathogens.

NOTES

Human milk is a rich source of bioactive factors, including antibodies, antiviral agents, white blood cells, enzymes, immune-active proteins, fats, sugars, and numerous growth and immune factors.

Breastfeeding children receive several different types of immunoglobulins as well as live immune cells and factors from their mother's milk.

See also Bioactive components of breastmilk; Bronchus-associated lymphoid tissue (BALT); Gut-associated lymphoid tissue (GALT); Lymphocytes; Macrophages; Mucosa-associated lymphoid tissue (MALT)

➤ IMMUNIZATION

DEFINITION   The process of becoming protected against a pathogen or disease. This may be naturally acquired through pathogen exposure or intentionally given by injecting dead or altered pathogens into the body.

NOTES

Immunizations taken by the mother are generally compatible with breastfeeding, with the exception of the smallpox vaccine and possibly rubella.

Contact the Centers for Disease Control and Prevention for updates regarding immunizations in the mother, as knowledge about vaccination is constantly updated.

Breastfeeding offers natural immunity to many common pathogens in the family environment.

Breastfeeding during and immediately after infant immunization is recommended to provide pain relief for the baby.

See also Vaccinations and immunizations

➤ IMMUNOGLOBULIN

DEFINITION   Proteins manufactured by the body to fight infection.

All classes of immunoglobulins—Ig, IgG, IgD, IgM, and IgE (Ig is an abbreviation for immunoglobulin)—are found in human milk. They are found in higher amounts in colostrum but continue throughout lactation.

➤ IMMUNOGLOBULIN A (IGA)

DEFINITION   An immunoglobulin that protects the mucous membranes of the respiratory and digestive tracts from invasion by pathogens.

SELF-CARE INFORMATION

Nursing in the first hours after birth transfers IgA from the mother to the baby.
    The IgA coats the baby's intestines, lung surfaces, and other mucous membranes. This begins to protect the baby from bacteria and viruses as soon as possible.

Human babies are born without IgA. Babies do not produce their own IgA for several months.
    Human milk is a rich source of IgA, providing the first level of immune defense until babies develop their own IgA.

See also Skin-to-skin (STS) care

➤ IMMUNOGLOBULIN E (IGE)

DEFINITION   An immunoglobulin that combines with antigens in the gut and releases chemicals that cause changes to the permeability of the gut wall.

Human milk contains IgE in lower concentration than IgA.

➤ IMPAIRED MOBILITY, MOTHERS WITH

DEFINITION Referring to mothers living with restrictions to physical motion. Breastfeeding is often an ideal feeding choice for mothers with impaired mobility, as it requires little preparation for feeding.

ASK ABOUT

Type of impairment.
Age of the baby.

ASSESSMENT

PROMPT CARE NEEDED?
Are any of the following present?
Mother with impaired mobility learning to breastfeed.
Ongoing breastfeeding support needed.

IF YES, *Call lactation care provider today.*

SELF-CARE INFORMATION
Set up a feeding station in the home where nonperishable snacks, drinks of water, baby changing equipment, hand wipes, and a telephone can be at the ready.

IMPORTANT CONDITIONS TO REPORT
Concern about feeding adequacy or comfort.

➤ IMPERFORATE ANUS

DEFINITION A defect in the formation of the end of the digestive system where stool exits the body. There may be a total lack of opening of the anus, narrowing of the anus, or misplacement of the opening of the anus.

Breastfeeding is compatible with this condition.

Children born with this condition require surgery and may have difficulty with stool control. Children with this problem may have associated anomalies such as esophageal atresia and cardiac defects.

➤ IMPLANTS, BREAST

DEFINITION   Devices made of saline or gel surgically inserted into the breast to increase its size or to reconstruct the breast after mastectomy or trauma.

ASK ABOUT

Onset.

Age of the baby.

Location of surgical incision.

Reason for implant.

ASSESSMENT

PROMPT MEDICAL CARE NEEDED?

Are any of the following present?

Meconium bowel movements after 5 days of life.

No yellow stool by 5 days.

Fewer than three bowel movements daily in breastfed newborn after the first 2 days of life.

No urine in 6 hours.

Brick dust urine (uric acid crystals) after 2 days of life.

Dark-colored urine.

Fewer than four urinations daily in the breastfed newborn after day 5 of life.

Noticeably sunken fontanelles (soft spot on the top of the head).

Decreased activity.

Baby below birthweight at 10–14 days.

Cessation of weight gain.

IF YES,   *Seek medical care within 4 hours.*

PROMPT LACTATION CARE NEEDED?

Are any of the following present?

Concerns about milk supply.

Slow weight gain in breastfed baby.

| IF YES, | *Call lactation care provider today.* |

SELF-CARE INFORMATION

Practice skin-to-skin contact in the first hour and frequently thereafter.

Feed the baby at the first sign of hunger cues (signs that say "feed me" include hand-to-face or hand-to-mouth movements, lip smacking, seeking with lips, rooting, and head bobbing).

Feed the baby at least 10 times per 24 hours.

Listen for signs of the baby swallowing.

Allow the baby to end feedings.

Expect at least three infant stools per 24 hours after the first 4 days of life.

Good positioning and attachment are crucial to prevent or reduce nipple pain.

If feedings are missed, hand express or pump milk to maintain supply.

IMPORTANT CONDITIONS TO REPORT

Fewer than four bowel movements daily in newborn time period.

Ongoing concerns or problems with milk supply.

NOTES

The location and extent of the incision may impact the sensation of the nerves in the nipple area. Loss of or decreased sensation may decrease milk-making potential. Trauma to the nerves may hinder the stimulation of the brain to release prolactin (the milk-making hormone) in response to suckling. Periareolar incisions suggest more potential nerve and/or injury than do incisions underneath the breast.

Babies of women who have had breast augmentation surgery should be followed closely to ensure proper growth.

If the mother reports that she had an implant in one breast only, inquire about the reason for this surgery. If augmentation corrected breast asymmetry, there may be increased concern regarding the mother's ability to make a full milk supply. Marked asymmetry may indicate insufficient glandular tissue in both breasts. The baby and the mother should be closely followed.

See Asymmetric breasts; Breast augmentation; Breast surgery

➤ INADEQUATE MILK SUPPLY

See Insufficient milk supply

➤ INADEQUATE WEIGHT GAIN

See Insufficient weight gain

➤ INCREASING MILK SUPPLY

DEFINITION Raising the amount of milk produced by the breast. This is accomplished by increasing stimulation and removal of milk from the breast.

ASK ABOUT

Reason for desire to increase milk supply.
Age of the baby.

ASSESSMENT

EMERGENT CARE NEEDED?

Are any of the following present?

Meconium bowel movements after 5 days of life.

No yellow stool by 5 days.

Fewer than three bowel movements daily in a breastfed newborn after the first 2 days of life.

No urine in 6 hours.

Brick dust urine (uric acid crystals) after 2 days of life.

Dark-colored urine.

Fewer than four urinations daily in the breastfed newborn after day 5 of life.

Noticeably sunken fontanelles (soft spot on the top of the head).

Decreased activity.

Baby below birthweight at 10–14 days of life.

Cessation of weight gain or weight loss.

IF YES, *Seek pediatric care now.*

PROMPT CARE NEEDED?

Are any of the following present?

Identified milk supply problem.

Concern about possible milk supply problems.

IF YES,   *Call lactation care provider today.*

SELF-CARE INFORMATION

Ensure baby is feeding 10–12 times per 24 hours.

Express milk after feeding.

IMPORTANT CONDITIONS TO REPORT

Persistent problems.

Recurrent problems.

See also Decrease in milk supply; Milk supply, inadequate; Relactation

➤ INDIAN HEALTH SERVICE

See DHHS/Indian Health Service

➤ INDUCED LACTATION

DEFINITION   The process of establishing a milk supply in a woman who has not given birth.

ASK ABOUT

Age of the baby.

ASSESSMENT

ROUTINE CARE NEEDED?

Are any of the following present?

Mother wishes to induce lactation for an adopted infant.

IF YES,   *Call lactation care provider.*

SELF-CARE INFORMATION

Frequent stimulation may increase milk supply.

Practice skin-to-skin contact in the first hour and frequently thereafter.

Feed the baby at the first sign of hunger cues (signs that say "feed me" include hand-to-face or hand-to-mouth movements, lip smacking, seeking with lips, rooting, and head bobbing).

Feed the baby at least 10 times per 24 hours.

Listen for signs of the baby swallowing.

Supplement as needed with milk from an HMBANA milk bank or formula.

Allow the baby to end feedings.

Expect at least three infant stools per 24 hours after the first 4 days of life.

Good positioning and attachment are crucial to prevent or reduce nipple pain.

If feedings are missed, hand express or pump milk to maintain supply.

Frequent weight checks to assure adequate nutrition and growth.

IMPORTANT CONDITIONS TO REPORT

Arrival of the baby.

First visible milk produced.

Lack of milk production after weeks of attempt.

NOTES

Feeding adopted babies at the breast can be a wonderful bonding experience for mothers and babies. Adoptive mothers can produce milk with frequent breast stimulation (from a baby or a pump). It may take weeks of stimulation for a partial supply to develop. It is essential to monitor the baby's weight gain and output closely. There is a wide range of success in terms of the volume of milk produced. Women need much practical guidance and support during this time and should consult with a lactation care provider early and often while awaiting the arrival of their adopted child.

Adopted babies may take right to the breast or may take longer to learn to feed. Devices may be used to deliver supplements to the baby at the breast in the event that the mother does not have a full milk supply.

Focus on the experience and closeness of the baby at the breast rather than the goal of producing a full milk supply.

See also At-breast supplementation

➤ INFANT

DEFINITION   A child under 12 months of age.

➤ INFANT BEHAVIOR

DEFINITION   Referring to the interplay of reflexes, levels of awareness, and response of babies to their environment.

SELF-CARE INFORMATION

Practice skin-to-skin contact in the first hour and frequently thereafter.

Infants have a predictable sequence of states in the hour after birth and their levels of awareness including deep sleep, light sleep (with rapid eye movements), quiet alert, awake, active alert, and crying.

Light sleep, quiet alert, and awake states are the best times to initiate feeding. Crying is a late feeding cue.

Signs that say "feed me" include hand-to-face or hand-to-mouth movements, lip smacking, seeking with lips, rooting, and head bobbing.

Signs of fullness include removing the mouth from the nipple with a relaxed body tone, falling asleep during feeding, and general bodily relaxation.

NOTES

Although babies are not able to speak until they are close to the end of the first year, they communicate with their caregivers and their environment through a complex set of behaviors.

Adults can learn to read feeding cues to aid in breastfeeding and the overall development of the parent–child relationship.

➤ INFANTRISK CENTER

DESCRIPTION   A call center at Texas Tech University Health Sciences Center that is "based solely on evidence-based medicine and research. We are dedicated to providing current and accurate information to pregnant and breastfeeding mothers and healthcare professionals. We are a training center for medical and pharmacy students and medical residents in the use of drugs in pregnant and breastfeeding mothers. We have underway an extensive program in clinical research."[185(p1)]

InfantRisk Center
Telephone: (806) 352-2519 (Monday–Friday, 8 a.m.–5 p.m. Central Time)
Web: www.infantrisk.com

Footnote

[185]Texas Tech University Health Services Center. (2009). InfantRisk Center—About us. Retrieved from http://www.infantrisk.com/content/about-us

➤ INFECTIONS, ACUTE

DEFINITION   Invasion and reproduction of microorganisms in the cells or tissues of the body. Infectious microorganisms include bacteria, viruses, fungi, and others. Symptoms of infection may include fever and malaise. Lack of desire to feed can be an additional symptom of infection in the baby.

ASK ABOUT

Onset.
Age of the baby.
Medications taken.
Known drug allergies.

ASSESSMENT

EMERGENT CARE NEEDED?

Are any of the following present?

About the baby:

Extreme **lethargy** in the baby.

Sudden change in the baby's muscle tone—extremely floppy (hypotonic) or extremely stiff (hypertonic).

The baby shows sudden disinterest in feeding.

Inability to wake the baby.

IF YES,   *Seek emergency care now.*

PROMPT CARE NEEDED?

Are any of the following present?

About the mother:

Fever higher than 100°F (37.7°C).

Extreme breast discomfort.

Flu-like aching throughout the body.

Extreme exhaustion.

Visible or palpable breast **abscess**.

About the baby:

Extreme discomfort.

Fever higher than 100°F (37.7°C) in a baby younger than 3 months of age.

Vomiting and diarrhea that last for more than a few hours in a child of any age.

Rash accompanied by a fever.

A cold that gets worse and includes a fever.

Ear pain or drainage from an ear.

Sore throat or problems swallowing.

Sharp or persistent pains in the abdomen or stomach.

Fever and vomiting at the same time.

Not eating for more than a day in the older baby who is eating solid foods.

IF YES,   *Seek medical or pediatric care now.*

SELF-CARE INFORMATION

Feed the baby at least 10 times per 24 hours.

Soften breasts between feedings with gentle hand expression.

Finish full course of antibiotics prescribed (unless told to stop by a physician).

Continue nonprescription pain relief as recommended.

Continue to monitor for symptoms of recurring breast infection (redness, heat, fever, chills, pain).

IMPORTANT CONDITIONS TO REPORT

Symptoms worsen or persist.

Signs of infection.

Rarely, babies experience life-threatening infections or events that cause extreme lethargy and disinterest in feeding. They may be suddenly floppy or hypertense. These symptoms indicate a medical emergency, as they may reflect botulism or other life-threatening infection.

Many mothers experiencing **mastitis** mistake symptoms of mastitis for flu.

When a mother calls to ask for recommendations of safe flu medications, remember to ask her if she has any red, painful, hot spots on her breasts. See **Mastitis** for more information.

Few infections are incompatible with breastfeeding. Infections in the breastfeeding mother that are not compatible with breastfeeding include **HIV**, **HTLV-I**, active **herpes** lesion on the nipple and/or other area that will be in contact with the baby's mouth.[186]

Mothers with certain infections may breastfeed once a period of treatment is initiated. These infections include tuberculosis, hepatitis, brucellosis, and Lyme disease. The Centers for Disease Control and Prevention and state health departments can provide further information.

See also Botulism, infantile; Breast infection; Fever

Footnote

[186]AAP Section on Breastfeeding. (2012). Breastfeeding and the use of human milk. *Pediatrics, 129* (3), e827–e841. doi: 10.1542/peds.2011-3552

➤ INFLAMMATION, BREAST

DEFINITION   The body's response to injury, infection, or foreign matter that results in pain, redness, swelling, and sometimes impaired function of the affected area. In this context, inflammation of the breast is assumed.

ASK ABOUT

Onset.
Extent of redness and involvement.

ASSESSMENT

EMERGENT CARE NEEDED?

Are any of the following present?

Sudden bilateral red streaks on the breasts with fever, aching, or chills.

IF YES, *Seek emergency care now.*

PROMPT CARE NEEDED?

Are any of the following present?

Unilateral red streaks on the breast.

Symptoms of infection.

IF YES, *Call maternal care provider today.*

SELF-CARE INFORMATION

Feed the baby at least 10 times per 24 hours.

Soften breasts between feedings with gentle hand expression.

Finish full course of treatment prescribed (unless told to stop by a provider).

Continue nonprescription pain relief as recommended.

Continue to monitor for symptoms of recurring breast infection (redness, heat, fever, chills, pain).

IMPORTANT CONDITIONS TO REPORT

Worsening symptoms.

Persistent symptoms.

Recurrent symptoms.

NOTES

An up-to-date drug reference should be consulted to determine the safety and possible side effects of medications recommended to treat inflammation.

Newborn and premature babies are at greater risk of drug side effects due to limited ability to clear drugs from their systems.

The symptoms listed above may also indicate infection.

Mothers with inflammation should continue to breastfeed. There is no reason to cease breastfeeding.

See also Acute infection; Breast infection; Mastitis; Medication resources (inside back cover)

➤ INNOCENTI DECLARATION

DEFINITION A statement made by a group of participants at a World Health Organization (WHO)/United Nations Children's Fund (UNICEF) policy makers' meeting called "Breastfeeding in the 1990s: A Global Initiative," held in Florence, Italy in 1990, and reaffirmed in 2005.

The declaration sets forth four targets to advance breastfeeding throughout the world, asking each government represented to:

1. Appoint a national breastfeeding coordinator and establish a multisectoral national breastfeeding committee.
2. Ensure that every facility providing maternity services fully practices all of the Ten Steps to Successful Breastfeeding.
3. Take action to give effect to the principles and aim of all Articles of the International Code of Marketing of Breast-Milk Substitutes.
4. Enact imaginative legislation protecting the breastfeeding rights of working women.[187]

Footnote

[187]United Nations Children's Fund. (n.d.). Innocenti Declaration. Retrieved from http://www.unicef.org/programme/breastfeeding/innocenti.htm

➤ INSUFFICIENT MILK SUPPLY

DEFINITION Inadequate production of milk in the breast. Maternal, infant, and environmental factors all have been found to contribute to milk supply problems. Milk supply can most often be increased. This is accomplished by increasing stimulation and removal of milk from the breast.

ASK ABOUT

Onset.
Age of the baby.

ASSESSMENT

EMERGENT CARE NEEDED?

Are any of the following present?

Meconium bowel movements after 5 days of life.

No yellow stool 5 days.

Fewer than three bowel movements daily in breastfed newborn after the first 2 days of life.

No urine in 6 hours.

Brick dust urine (uric acid crystals) after 2 days of life.

Dark-colored urine.

Fewer than four urinations daily in the breastfed newborn after day 5 of life.

Noticeably sunken fontanelles (soft spot on the top of the head).

Decreased activity.

Baby below birthweight at 10–14 days of life.

Cessation of weight gain.

IF YES, *Seek pediatric care now.*

PROMPT CARE NEEDED?

Are any of the following present?

Identified milk supply problem.

Concern about possible milk supply problem.

IF YES, *Call lactation care provider today.*

SELF-CARE INFORMATION

Ensure baby is feeding 10–12 times per 24 hours.

Express milk after feeding.

IMPORTANT CONDITIONS TO REPORT

Persistent problems.

Recurrent problems.

See also Milk supply, inadequate

➤ INSUFFICIENT WEIGHT GAIN

DEFINITION   Breastfed newborns should gain a minimum of 0.5 oz to 1 oz a day on average after initial weight loss. According to the AAP Section on Breastfeeding, the breastfed newborn should lose "no more than 7% from birth and no further wt loss by day 5"[188(p.e835)] New studies indicate that breastfed babies gain even faster than was previously believed, probably because breastfeeding used to be done on a schedule and not as frequently as we now know is ideal.

ASK ABOUT

Age of the baby.
Weight gain pattern.

ASSESSMENT

PROMPT CARE NEEDED?

Are any of the following present?

Lethargy.

Hard-to-rouse infant.

Sleeping at the breast without nursing first.

Meconium bowel movements after 5 days of life.

No yellow stool by day 5.

Fewer than three bowel movements daily in breastfed newborn after the first 2 days of life.

No urine in 6 hours.

Brick dust urine (uric acid crystals) after 2 days of life.

Dark-colored urine.

Fewer than four urinations daily in the breastfed newborn after day 5 of life.

Noticeably sunken fontanelles (soft spot on the top of the head).

Decreased activity.

Baby below birthweight at 10–14 days of life.

Cessation of weight gain.

IF YES,   *Seek pediatric care now.*

ROUTINE CARE NEEDED?

Are any of the following present?

Infant who sleeps at the breast after a few sucks.

Infant who is hard to latch on.

No audible swallows.

Breastfeeding problem.

Milk supply problem.

Concern about possible milk supply problem.

IF YES,   *Call lactation care provider today.*

IMPORTANT CONDITIONS TO REPORT

Decrease in frequency of urination or stools.

Increased sleepiness, hours spent sleeping.

Baby is harder to rouse.

See also Growth chart; Hypotonia; Jaundice

Footnote

[188]AAP Section on Breastfeeding. (2012). Breastfeeding and the use of human milk. *Pediatrics, 129*(3), e827–e841. doi:10.1542/peds.2011-3552

➤ INSULIN-DEPENDENT DIABETES MELLITUS (IDDM)

DEFINITION   A chronic disease causing high levels of glucose (sugar) in the blood. In this form of diabetes, the pancreas makes little or no insulin, requiring daily injections of this hormone that regulates glucose metabolism. Women with IDDM can breastfeed their babies.

ASK ABOUT

Onset.

Type of diabetes.

ASSESSMENT

EMERGENT CARE NEEDED?

Are any of the following present?

Insulin shock in the breastfeeding woman (symptoms of insulin shock include blurred vision, fast heartbeat, acting spacey, cranky, or aggressive, headache, hunger, shaking or trembling, trouble sleeping, excessive sweating, tingling, weakness, and unclear thinking).

IF YES, *Seek emergency care now.*

PROMPT CARE NEEDED?

Are any of the following present?

Difficulty maintaining blood glucose levels during breastfeeding.

IF YES, *Call medical care provider now.*

ROUTINE CARE NEEDED?

Are any of the following present?

Ongoing breastfeeding problems in the diabetic woman.

IF YES, *Call lactation care provider today.*

SELF-CARE INFORMATION

Women with diabetes are more prone to infection. Monitor breasts and nipples daily for any red, infected, or painful areas.

If insulin dependent, be aware that less insulin may be required during breastfeeding—watch for signs of low blood sugar.

IMPORTANT CONDITIONS TO REPORT

Any symptoms of infection.

Difficulty regulating blood sugar.

Women with diabetes should be encouraged to breastfeed. Breastfeeding is known to reduce the risk of developing diabetes in susceptible individuals (e.g., children of diabetic mothers).

Research suggests that women who have experienced gestational diabetes are less likely to develop diabetes if they breastfeed their babies.

See also Autoimmune diseases

➤ INSULIN-LIKE GROWTH FACTOR (IGF-I)

DEFINITION A beneficial agent found in human milk that triggers growth.

NOTES

Research suggests that preterm, exclusively breastfed infants have higher serum levels of this growth-promoting factor.

➤ INTERCOURSE

DEFINITION Resumption of sexual activity after childbirth.

ASK ABOUT

Age of the baby.

ASSESSMENT

ROUTINE MEDICAL CARE NEEDED?

Are any of the following present?

Difficult penetration.

Pain during intercourse.

IF YES, *Call obstetric care provider today.*

ROUTINE CARE NEEDED?

Are any of the following present?

Concern about sexuality in breastfeeding woman.

Concerns about the normalcy of sensual feelings during breastfeeding.

IF YES,   *Call lactation care provider today.*

SELF-CARE INFORMATION

Life changes after the birth of a baby, and it is sometimes hard for mothers to know if what they are experiencing is normal. Many breastfeeding women and their partners may worry about leaking milk, spraying milk, or the appropriateness of breast involvement in sexual activities. Talking about feelings and physical concerns can help couples adjust.

IMPORTANT CONDITIONS TO REPORT

Feelings of extreme worry or anxiety.

Difficult or painful penetration.

Pain during intercourse.

NOTES

Intercourse and sexual activity are compatible with breastfeeding, although the low estrogen level of the breastfeeding mother may contribute to vaginal dryness. There may also be residual discomfort or pain from the birth.

Women may feel differently about sexual relations after the birth of a baby. Many women feel less desire although some women feel more. No one can predict how a woman will feel.

Breastfeeding is an intimate activity that may make the rest of the family feel left out.

In addition, mothers may feel tired when they have a new baby whether or not they are breastfeeding and might not have the energy for sexual activities.

See also Fertility; Menstrual cycle

➤ INTERNATIONAL BABY FOOD ACTION NETWORK (IBFAN)

DESCRIPTION   The International Baby Food Action Network, **IBFAN**, consists of public interest groups working around the world to reduce infant and young child morbidity and mortality. IBFAN aims to improve the health and well-being of babies and young children, their mothers and their families through the protection, promotion and support of breastfeeding and optimal infant feeding practices. IBFAN works for universal and full implementation of the International Code and Resolutions 189(p1)

NOTES

International Baby Food Action Network
North American Office
Email: info@infactcanada.ca
Web: www.infactcanada.ca

Footnote

[189] International Baby Food Action Network. (2012). Retrieved from http://ibfan.org/issue-international_code.html

➤ INTERNATIONAL BOARD CERTIFIED LACTATION CONSULTANT (IBCLC)

DEFINITION   An individual who has qualified for and passed the examination administered by the International Board of Lactation Consultant Examiners. The designations International Board Certified Lactation Consultant (IBCLC) and Registered Lactation Consultant (RLC) are used to denote international board certified lactation care providers.

➤ INTERNATIONAL BOARD OF LACTATION CONSULTANT EXAMINERS (IBLCE)

DESCRIPTION   The International Board of Lactation Consultant Examiners (IBLCE) is a non-profit organization governed by a Board of Directors. It was established to develop and administer a certification examination for lactation consultants. Founded in 1985, IBLCE administers annual examinations, in multiple languages and at numerous sites around the world.[190](p1)

NOTES

International Board of Lactation Consultant Examiners (IBLCE)
Email: iblce@iblce.org
Web: www.iblce.org
   The International Board of Lactation Consultant Examiners is the independent international certification body conferring the International Board Certified Lactation Consultant (IBCLC) credential.

Footnote

[190]International Board of Lactation Consultant Examiners. (2012). About us. Retrieved from http://americas.iblce.org/about-us

➤ INTERNATIONAL CHILDBIRTH EDUCATION ASSOCIATION (ICEA)

DESCRIPTION   The International Childbirth Education Association (ICEA) as a professional organization supports educators and other healthcare providers who believe in freedom to make decisions based on knowledge of alternatives in family-centered maternity and newborn care.[191](p1)

NOTES

Email: info@icea.org
Web: www.icea.org
    ICEA provides training and continuing education programs, educational resources, and professional certification programs.

Footnote

[191]International Childbirth Education Association. (n.d.). About ICEA. Retrieved from http://icea.org/content/mission

➤ ## INTERNATIONAL CODE OF MARKETING OF BREAST-MILK SUBSTITUTES

DEFINITION A document adopted by the World Health Assembly[192] in 1981 and amended by several subsequent resolutions as a minimum requirement to protect infant health. The International Code of Marketing of Breast-milk Substitutes sets forth a series of expectations about the behavior of the infant formula industry, healthcare systems, healthcare providers, governments, and other parties regarding the protection of breastfeeding and ethical marketing of breastmilk substitutes.

NOTES

The full text of the International Code of Marketing of Breast-milk Substitutes and subsequent resolutions can be accessed through the World Health Organization's website at http://www.who.int/en/.

See also International Baby Food Action Network (IBFAN); World Health Organization (WHO)

Footnote

[192]World Health Organization. (1981). *International code of marketing of breast-milk substitutes.* Geneva, Switzerland: World Health Organization. Retrieved from http://whqlibdoc.who.int /publications/9241541601.pdf

➤ INTERNATIONAL LACTATION CONSULTANT ASSOCIATION (ILCA)

DESCRIPTION   The International Lactation Consultant Association (ILCA) is the professional association for International Board Certified Lactation Consultants (IBCLCs) and other healthcare professionals who care for breastfeeding families. Our vision is a worldwide network of lactation professionals. Our mission is to advance the profession of lactation consulting worldwide through leadership, advocacy, professional development, and research.[193(p1)]

NOTES

International Lactation Consultant Association (ILCA)
Email: info@ilca.org
Web: www.ilca.org
   ILCA provides numerous professional resources for breastfeeding, including journals, other publications, and conferences.

See also United States Lactation Consultant Association

Footnote

[193]International Lactation Consultant Association. (2012). About ILCA. Retrieved from http://www.ilca.org/i4a/pages/index.cfm?pageid=3281

➤ INTERNATIONAL SOCIETY FOR RESEARCH IN HUMAN MILK AND LACTATION (ISRHML)

DESCRIPTION   A nonprofit organization that is "dedicated to the promotion of excellence in research and the dissemination of research findings in the field of human milk and lactation."[194(p1)]

NOTES

ISRHML
Email: smcguire@wsu.edu
Web: www.isrhml.org
    ISRHML provides meetings and symposia focused on breastfeeding as well as communication among experts in the field and governmental agencies, public health authorities and others interested in human lactation.

Footnote

[194]International Society for Research in Human Milk and Lactation. (2012). Welcome! Retrieved from http://www.isrhml.org/

➤ INTRADUCTAL PAPILLOMA

DEFINITION   A small, benign (noncancerous) tumor that grows within the milk ducts. It is found within a single milk duct.

ASK ABOUT

Age of the baby.
Onset of nipple discharge.
Description of nipple discharge.

ASSESSMENT

PROMPT CARE NEEDED?

Are any of the following present?

Appearance of rust-colored milk.

Bloody discharge from the nipple.

Any other unusual nipple discharge without nipple pain or abrasion from suboptimal latch.

IF YES,   *Call obstetric care provider today.*

SELF-CARE INFORMATION

Seek prompt medical evaluation of any unusual discharge from the nipple during breastfeeding and at any other time.

See also Bleeding, breast; Blood in milk; Breast cancer

➤ INTRAUTERINE DEVICE (IUD)

DEFINITION   A contraceptive device that is placed within the uterus and left there to prevent fertilization. IUDs are compatible with breastfeeding.

See also Birth control; Contraception

➤ INVERTED NIPPLES

See Nipple, inverted

DEFINITION   Nipples that do not protrude or that retreat into the breast when the nipple is stimulated. With inverted nipples, the nipple may be hidden in a slit or a fold and may retreat further into the breast when stimulated. Some apparently inverted nipples stand out (evert) upon stimulation by hand, pump, or baby's mouth. Others do not.

ASK ABOUT

Appearance of the nipple.
Action of the nipple when the nipple or areola is stimulated.
Nipple changes during pregnancy and lactation.
Diagnosis of inverted nipple.

ASSESSMENT

PROMPT MEDICAL CARE NEEDED?

Are any of the following present?

Meconium bowel movements after 5 days of life.

No yellow stool by 5 days.

Fewer than three bowel movements daily in breastfed newborn after the first 2 days of life.

No urine in 6 hours.

Brick dust urine (uric acid crystals) after 2 days of life.

Dark-colored urine.

Fewer than four urinations daily in the breastfed newborn after day 5 of life.

Noticeably sunken fontanelles (soft spot on the top of the head).

Decreased activity.

Baby below birthweight at 10–14 days of life.

Cessation of/inadequate weight gain.

Problems with latch-on.

IF YES, *Seek pediatric care now and call lactation care provider today.*

SELF-CARE INFORMATION

Practice skin-to-skin contact in the first hour and frequently thereafter. Skin-to-skin contact immediately after birth with the baby's initial self-attachment at breast contributes to effective latch. Trying to train inverted nipples to stand out during pregnancy is ineffective.

Mothers with inverted nipples should be encouraged to express milk early and frequently until the baby is able to facilitate stretching the nipple deeply into the mouth. Close postpartum follow-up is necessary to assure adequate nutrition and weight gain of the baby.

IMPORTANT CONDITIONS TO REPORT

Poor feeding.

Poor milk transfer.

Inadequate weight gain.

Problems with latch-on.

See also Insufficient milk supply; Milk transfer, estimating; Weight gain, baby—low

➤ IRON

DEFINITION   A metal that is vital to the process of absorbing oxygen into the blood. Iron deficiency is the most common cause of anemia.

NOTES

Breastmilk contains iron in a form that is easy for the baby to absorb. Breastmilk also contains lactoferrin, a protein that keeps iron away from microorganisms in the gut that require iron to grow.

Iron supplements may be indicated for premature infants or babies with low blood iron.[195]

Taking iron supplements is compatible with breastfeeding.

Women taking high doses of iron may have suffered postpartum hemorrhage and may be experiencing **Sheehan's syndrome**.

There is a difference of opinion among AAP's experts on whether there is mandatory need for iron among breastfed infants. AAP's Committee on Nutrition (2010) states: "at 4 months of age, breastfed infants should be supplemented with 1 mg/kg per day of oral iron beginning at 4 months of age until appropriate iron-containing complementary foods (including iron-fortified cereals) are introduced in the diet."[196(p1047)]

However, AAP's Section on Breastfeeding (2012) states: "Complementary food rich in iron and zinc should be introduced at about 6 months of age. Supplementation of oral iron drops before 6 months may be needed to support iron stores."[197(p.e835)]

See also Anemia; Sheehan's syndrome

Footnotes

[195]Baker, R. D., Greer, F. R., & the Committee on Nutrition. (2010). Diagnosis and prevention of iron deficiency and iron-deficiency anemia in infants and young children (0–3 years of age). *Pediatrics, 126*(5), 1040–1050. doi:10.1542/peds.2010-2576

[196]Baker, Greer, & the Committee on Nutrition. ibid.

[197]AAP Section on Breastfeeding. (2012). Breastfeeding and the use of human milk. *Pediatrics, 129*(3), e827–e841. doi:10.1542/peds.2011-3552

➤ **ISRHML**

See International Society for Research in Human Milk and Lactation (ISRHML)

➤ **IUD**

DEFINITION   Intrauterine device. A contraceptive device that is placed within the uterus and left there to prevent fertilization. IUDs are compatible with breastfeeding.

See also Birth control; Contraception

➤ **JAUNDICE**

DEFINITION   A condition caused by excess bilirubin. It is the most common condition requiring medical treatment during the newborn period.

ASK ABOUT

Age of the baby.
Feeding behavior.
Stooling pattern and color.
Urination pattern.

ASSESSMENT

PROMPT CARE NEEDED?

Are any of the following present?

Severe lethargy (sleepiness).

Poor feeding.

No interest in feeding for more than 6 hours.

Fever.

Meconium bowel movements after 5 days of life.

No yellow stool by 5 days.

Fewer than three bowel movements daily in breastfed newborn after the first
2 days of life

No urine in 6 hours.

Brick dust urine (uric acid crystals) after 2 days of life.

Dark-colored urine.

Fewer than four urinations daily in the breastfed newborn after day 5 of life.

Noticeably sunken fontanelles (soft spot on the top of the head).

Decreased activity.

Baby below birthweight at 10–14 days of life.

Cessation of weight gain.

Any fever in a baby younger than 3 months of age.

| IF YES, | *Seek pediatric care now.* |

ROUTINE CARE NEEDED?

Are any of the following present?

Breastfeeding in a jaundiced baby.

Baby sleepy during breastfeedings.

Milk supply problem.

Concern about possible milk supply problem.

| IF YES, | *Call lactation care provider now.* |

SELF-CARE INFORMATION

Breastfeed as soon as possible after birth.

Encourage the baby to nurse 10–12 times per 24 hours.

Colostrum has laxative properties. Stooling helps to rid the baby's body of bilirubin.

IMPORTANT CONDITIONS TO REPORT

No stool in 24 hours.

Severe lethargy (sleepiness).

Poor feeding.

Fever.

NOTES

Newborns produce bilirubin as they break down the extra red blood cells required to absorb oxygen over the placenta. The baby with high bilirubin levels will develop a yellow (or tan or light orange) tone to the skin and the sclera (whites) of the eyes.

Although the condition of jaundice may be benign, it can be a symptom of other serious conditions, including **kernicterus**.

All jaundiced infants are at risk for kernicterus and should be closely monitored.

See also Hyperbilirubinemia; Kernicterus; Late onset jaundice

➤ KANGAROO CARE (KC)

DEFINITION   A form of skin contact encouraged between parents and premature babies, also referred to as "Kangaroo Mother Care (KMC)." The baby is usually placed between the mother's breasts. Kangaroo care can be continuous or intermittent. Skin contact is beneficial to all parents and babies, but is particularly helpful in establishing breastfeeding and bonding, and in helping the premature baby to regulate body temperature, respiratory rate, and oxygenation.

See also Skin-to-skin (STS) care

➤ KC

See Kangaroo care

➤ KERNICTERUS

DEFINITION Damage to the brain, spinal cord, and nerve cells caused by buildup of bilirubin in these tissues. Any jaundiced baby is at risk for kernicterus. Babies with **jaundice** should be closely monitored.

See also Bilirubin; Hyperbilirubinemia; Jaundice

➤ KMC

See Kangaroo care (KC)

➤ KWASHIORKOR

DEFINITION A form of malnutrition caused by inadequate protein intake.

> **NOTES**
>
> Breastmilk is an excellent source of protein. Kwashiorkor is not associated with breast-feeding.
>
> This disorder is rare in the United States but may occur after weaning in locations where protein-rich food is scarce.

➤ LACTATIONAL AMENORRHEA METHOD (LAM)

DEFINITION A form of natural family planning that is thought to be effective in the first 6 months following the birth of a baby, so long as the mother's menses have not returned, her baby is exclusively breastfed, and there are no long periods of time between feedings, day and night.[198] Once the baby is older than 6 months, or any of the aforementioned criteria is no longer true, LAM is no longer effective, and mothers should utilize other forms of birth control.

NOTES

Refer mothers with questions about this contraceptive method to a lactation care provider, medical care provider, or family planning counselor.

Footnote

[198]Kennedy, K. I. (2002). Efficacy and effectiveness of LAM. *Advances in Experimental Medicine and Biology, 503*, 207–216.

➤ LACTATION CARE PROVIDERS

DEFINITION   Individuals who have education and skill in assisting breastfeeding mothers.

NOTES

Lactation care providers have different professional backgrounds and different levels of training.

To find a local lactation care provider, contact the International Board of Lactation Consultant Examiners (IBLCE), the Academy of Lactation Policy and Practice, the International Lactation Consultant Association (ILCA) [in the United States, through the United States Lactation Consultant Association], Nursing Mothers' Council, state breastfeeding coalitions, breastfeeding task forces, WIC Program, or local hospitals and birth centers.

➤ LACTATION STUDY CENTER

DESCRIPTION   A center at the University of Rochester Medical Center that "encourages and promotes human lactation and breastfeeding through physician education and support. The goal is to provide the information that will help the practitioner encourage and support breastfeeding for all patients."[199(p943)]

NOTES

Lactation Study Center
Telephone: 585-275-0088, 8 a.m. to 5 p.m. Eastern Time
   The Study Center has an extensive data bank on drugs, medical conditions, and research articles. Dr. Ruth A. Lawrence, MD, professor of pediatrics and of obstetrics/gynecology, leads the study center.

Footnote

[199]Lawrence, R. A., & Lawrence, R. M. (2011). *Breastfeeding: A guide for the medical profession* (7th ed.). St. Louis, MO: Elsevier/Mosby.

➤ LACTIFEROUS DUCT

DEFINITION   The tube-shaped structures in the breast that carry milk from the alveoli to the nipple. There are thought to be fewer than nine major ducts in the breast, corresponding with pores in the surface of the nipple. Ducts divide into smaller ductules in a branching fashion beginning close to the base of the nipple.

➤ LACTIFEROUS SINUS

DEFINITION   A concept suggesting a pooling area behind the areola where milk is stored. This concept has been challenged by ultrasound evidence[200] that showed no presence of a permanent sinus, but rather a temporary widening of the diameter of the ducts.

Footnote

[200]Ramsay, D. T., Kent, J. C., Owens, R. A., & Hartmann, P. E. (2004). Ultrasound imaging of milk ejection in the breast of lactating women. *Pediatrics, 113,* 361–367.

➤ LACTMED

DESCRIPTION   "LactMed, a free online database with information on drugs and lactation, is one of the newest additions to the National Library of Medicine's TOXNET system, a Web-based collection of resources covering toxicology, chemical safety, and environmental health."[201(p1)]

NOTES

LactMed
Web: http://toxnet.nlm.nih.gov/cgi-bin/sis/htmlgen?LACT
   Geared to the healthcare practitioner and nursing mother, LactMed contains over 450 drug records. It includes information such as maternal levels in breastmilk, infant levels in blood, potential effects in breastfeeding infants and on lactation itself, the American Academy of Pediatrics category indicating the level of compatibility of the drugs with breastfeeding, and alternate drugs to consider. References are included, as is nomenclature information, such as each drug's Chemical Abstract Service's (CAS) registry number and its broad drug class.

Footnote

[201]U.S. National Library of Medicine. (2006). LactMed: A new NLM database on drugs and lactation. Announcements, news. Retrieved from http://www.nlm.nih.gov/news/lactmed_announce_06 .html

➤ LACTOENGINEERING

DEFINITION   Laboratory techniques used to increase the nutrient content of expressed milk especially intended to be fed to premature infants.

NOTES

May include concentrating expressed mothers' milk, adding minerals, fat, and protein to expressed milk, or adding cow's milk products to expressed milk.

See also Human milk fortification; Premature infant

➤ LACTOFERRIN

DEFINITION A milk protein that binds to iron, making it easier for the baby to absorb.

NOTES

Lactoferrin also serves the purpose of keeping iron away from the many microorganisms that require iron for growth.

➤ LACTOSE

DEFINITION A double sugar (disaccharide) made up of the simple sugars glucose and galactose. It is found only in the milk of mammals.

➤ LACTOSE INTOLERANCE

DEFINITION An inability to digest lactose into the simple sugars glucose and galactose.

NOTES

Lactose intolerance is a common condition in adults. However, lactose intolerance is rarely seen in children prior to 3 years of age.

Lactose intolerance in the mother is compatible with breastfeeding.

Concerns about lactose intolerance in infants should be referred to the healthcare provider.

Lactose intolerance arises from lack of adequate production of lactase, an enzyme made in the cells that line the intestinal wall. The role of lactase is to break lactose into the simpler sugars that can be absorbed into the bloodstream. Lack of lactase results in an overload of lactose in the intestine, creating abdominal cramps, gas, diarrhea, and discomfort. Shiny, green, mucous stools may be noted.

The prevalence of lactose intolerance in many adult populations worldwide is thought to be related to the fact that historically, few populations consumed dairy foods past childhood. Typically, lactase is made by the cells of the gut in response to the amount of lactose in the diet. Thus, when milk is not consumed regularly, the body may lose its ability to digest lactose well.

See also Diarrhea

➤ LA LECHE LEAGUE, INTERNATIONAL

DESCRIPTION   Organization whose mission is "to help mothers worldwide to breast-feed through mother-to-mother support, education, information, and encouragement and to promote a better understanding of breastfeeding as an important element in the healthy development of the baby and mother."[202(p1)]

NOTES

La Leche League International
Web: www.lalecheleague.org
   La Leche League has numerous documents about breastfeeding on its website, as well as research reviews in the newsletter, *Breastfeeding Abstracts*.

Footnote

[202]La Leche League International. (2012). All about La Leche League. Retrieved from http://www.llli.org/ab.html?m=1

➤ LAM

See Lactational amenorrhea method (LAM)

➤ LAMAZE INTERNATIONAL

DESCRIPTION   Organization whose mission is "to promote, support and protect normal birth through education and advocacy through the dedicated efforts of professional childbirth educators, providers and parents."[203(p1)]

NOTES

Lamaze International
Web: www.lamaze.org
   Among its other activities promoting childbirth education, Lamaze convenes the Lamaze Institute for Normal Birth.

Footnote

[203]Lamaze International. (2012). About Lamaze International. Retrieved from http://www.lamaze.org/AboutLamaze

➤ LANOLIN

DEFINITION   A cream containing fatty acids and cholesterol extracted from sheep's wool. Lanolin has been suggested as a topical treatment for maintaining or healing nipple integrity.

ASK ABOUT

Nipple pain.

ASSESSMENT

PROMPT CARE NEEDED?

Are any of the following present?

Extreme nipple pain.

Bleeding from nipples.

Unable to breastfeed due to pain.

IF YES,   *Call lactation care provider now.*

ROUTINE CARE NEEDED?

Are any of the following present?

Feeding discomfort.

Trauma to nipple or breasts.

Misshapen nipple after feedings.

Visible fissures on nipples.

IF YES,   *Call lactation care provider today.*

SELF-CARE INFORMATION

Any substance that is applied to the nipple area will be consumed by the nursing baby. Check out the safety of any substance you put on your nipples.

Creams do not cure the causes of nipple pain.

Report nipple pain to your lactation care provider.

Most nipple pain/trauma occurs due to ineffective latch or inappropriately fitting pump parts.

IMPORTANT CONDITIONS TO REPORT

Symptoms worsen or persist.

Signs of infection.

Feeding or stooling expectations are not met.

NOTES

Questions about lanolin and other nipple creams suggest that a mother may be experiencing nipple pain. Research does not support effectiveness without optimizing the latch.[204]

Breast milk and Montgomery gland secretions provide natural antimicrobial lubrication of the nipple and areola.

Women experiencing **nipple pain** may self-treat with this and other substances, some of which may be inappropriate for the baby to consume (which is what happens when creams are applied to the nipple).

Women experiencing nipple pain should have a breastfeeding evaluation. There is no magic fix. Face-to-face counseling with a breastfeeding assessment and corrective intervention is effective in assessing and resolving nipple pain.

See also Breastfeeding assessment tools; Nipple pain; Sore nipples

Footnote

[204]Cadwell, K., Turner-Maffei, C., Blair, A., Brimdyr, K., & McInerney, Z. M. (2004). Pain reduction and treatment of sore nipples in nursing mothers. *The Journal of Perinatal Education: An ASPO/Lamaze Publication*, *13*(1), 29–35. doi:10.1624/105812404X109375

➤ LARGE FOR GESTATIONAL AGE (LGA)

DEFINITION   Babies whose birth weight is greater than the 90th percentile or greater than two standard deviations from the mean for babies of the same age.

➤ LATCH-ON

DEFINITION   The way in which the nursing baby attaches to the breast.

ASK ABOUT

Nipple pain.
Weight gain pattern.

ASSESSMENT

PROMPT CARE NEEDED?

Are any of the following present?

Inadequate stooling pattern (less than three stools daily) after the first 2 days of life.

No yellow stool by day 5.

Weight loss of more than 7% from birth or further weight loss by day 5.

Inadequate weight gain.

IF YES,   *Call pediatric care provider today.*

Are any of the following present?

Extreme nipple pain.

Bleeding from nipples.

Unable to breastfeed due to pain.

IF YES,   *Call lactation care provider now.*

Are any of the following present?

Breastfeeding lasting longer than 20 minutes.

Weight gain of less than 0.5 oz per day on average.

No change in suckling rhythm to a suck–swallow ratio of 2:1 or 1:1.

Feeding discomfort.

Trauma to nipple or breasts.

Misshapen nipple after feedings.

Visible fissures (cracks) on nipples.

IF YES,   *Call lactation care provider today.*

SELF-CARE INFORMATION

Any substance that is applied to the nipple area will be consumed by the nursing baby. Check out the safety of any substance you put on your nipples.

Creams do not cure the causes of nipple pain.

Report nipple pain to your lactation care provider.

IMPORTANT CONDITIONS TO REPORT

Increased infant lethargy.

Decrease in number of stools and wet diapers.

Weight loss, failure to gain weight after initial weight loss, or slow weight gain in the breastfed baby.

NOTES

Correct attachment of the baby to the breast is crucial to comfortable breastfeeding, to adequate milk manufacture and transfer, and ultimately to infant growth. When a baby is attached well, the mother should feel no pain or discomfort and should hear sounds of swallowing by the baby.

Since concerns about pain and inadequate milk are major reasons mothers stop breastfeeding, mothers should be seen for a feeding evaluation within 48 hours of stated breastfeeding concerns.

Women experiencing nipple pain or infants with slow weight gain should have a breastfeeding evaluation. Face-to-face counseling is effective in assessing and resolving these problems.

See also Asymmetric latch; Nipple pain; Slow weight gain, baby; Sore nipples

➤ LATE ONSET JAUNDICE

DEFINITION   A form of jaundice that occurs after the first week of life in breastfed infants. This type of jaundice is unusual and not well understood. It is also called "breastmilk jaundice."

IMPORTANT CONDITIONS TO REPORT

Jaundice that begins after 5 days after birth.

Jaundice that does not subside with treatment.

No stool in 24 hours.

Pale or gray stool.

Severe lethargy (sleepiness).

Poor feeding.

Fever higher than 100°F (37.7°C) in a baby younger than 3 months of age.

NOTES

Medical evaluation is indicated to rule out other metabolic reasons for jaundice, including urinary tract infection, glucose-6-phosphate dehydrogenase deficiency (G6PD), Gilbert Syndrome, galactosemia, etc.

All jaundiced infants are at risk for **kernicterus** and should be closely monitored.

See also Jaundice; Kernicterus

➤ LAXATIVES

DEFINITION   Drugs taken to relieve constipation.

NOTES

Occasional laxative use in the breastfeeding mother is not thought to affect the breastfeeding baby.

Questions about giving laxatives to the breastfed infant should be directed to the pediatric care provider. Constipation is not normal in the breastfed infant.

An up-to-date drug reference should be consulted to determine the safety and possible side effects of individual drugs.

Newborn and premature babies are at greater risk of drug side effects due to limited ability to clear drugs from their systems.

See also Constipation; Medication resources (inside back cover)

➤ LCPUFAS

DEFINITION   Long chain polyunsaturated fatty acids. These fatty acids are present in human milk and known to assist in the development of nerve and brain tissue.

See also Arachidonic acid (AA, also ARA); Docosahexaenoic acid (DHA) in breastmilk; Fat in breastmilk

➤ LEAD IN BREASTMILK

DEFINITION   A heavy metal that can damage the nervous system and kidneys. Overdose of lead is known as lead poisoning. Lead poisoning is of particular concern in babies and children due to the rapid growth of their brains and other organs.

ASSESSMENT

PROMPT CARE NEEDED?

Are any of the following present?

Breastfeeding woman diagnosed with lead poisoning.

Breastfed infant diagnosed with lead poisoning.

IF YES,   *Seek medical care within 4 hours.*

NOTES

Regarding the mother's blood levels, Lawrence states, "A lead level of 40 mg/dL is considered below the level of transfer through the breast milk."[205(p397)]

Footnote

[205]Lawrence, R. A., & Lawrence, R. M. (2011). *Breastfeeding: A guide for the medical profession* (7th ed.). St. Louis, MO: Elsevier/Mosby.

➤ LEAKING BREASTMILK

DEFINITION   Phenomenon of milk dripping from the breast between feedings or from the opposite breast during feedings. Leaking is a nuisance for many women but is not associated with breastfeeding problems.

SELF-CARE INFORMATION

Choose soft, absorbent breast pads.

Replace damp pads with fresh ones frequently to avoid irritation of the nipple.

Avoid waterproof or plastic-lined pads, which can cause irritation.

Breast pads are easily made by cutting appropriately sized circles out of new cloth diapers (edge stitching is recommended to hold the pad together in the wash).

Press the forearms against the nipples to cause temporary cessation of milk flow.

Wearing shirts or dresses with multicolored patterns may make leakage less visible.

➤ LET-DOWN REFLEX

DEFINITION   The neurohormonal response that compresses the myoepithelial cells that surround the alveoli, forcing milk to be squeezed down through the ducts and out the nipple. Also called "milk ejection reflex."

SELF-CARE INFORMATION

The breastfed newborn should gain well (0.5–1 oz per day on average). If the baby is gaining less than this, have a face-to-face breastfeeding evaluation.

At the breast, the baby should have sucking pattern that includes slow, deep sucks. After the first few days, the baby's swallows can be heard, and the newborn baby should have at least six wet diapers and at least four yellow stools each day.

IMPORTANT CONDITIONS TO REPORT

Inadequate weight gain.

Inadequate number of urinations and stools.

NOTES

This reflex is caused by a spike in the hormone oxytocin, one of the two major hormones of lactation (the other is prolactin). Oxytocin is released from the posterior lobe of the pituitary gland and stimulates the contraction of the smooth muscle of the uterus during labor. This hormone is also responsible for the ejection of milk from the breast.

Researchers have found that oxytocin is released in the first hours postpartum by the baby's hand massage of the breast.

Oxytocin is also released by the baby stretching the nipple sufficiently in the mouth. This is why a good latch is so important to milk transfer.

Oxytocin is also released through a conditioned response over time.

The mother's oxytocin response in the first days may be muted by the administration of Pitocin (oxytocin) during labor.[206]

See also Milk-ejection reflex; Oxytocin; Overactive let-down reflex

Footnote

[206]Jonas, K., Johansson, L. M., Nissen, E., Ejdebäck, M., Ransjö-Arvidson, A. B., & Uvnäs-Moberg, K. (2009). Effects of intrapartum oxytocin administration and epidural analgesia on the concentration of plasma oxytocin and prolactin, in response to suckling during the second day postpartum. *Breastfeeding Medicine: The Official Journal of the Academy of Breastfeeding Medicine, 4*(2), 71–82. doi:10.1089/bfm.2008.0002

➤ LETHARGY

DEFINITION   A state of sleepiness, sluggishness, or lack of desire to move about and interact.

NOTES

Lethargy can be a symptom of several diseases and disorders including anemia, botulism, sepsis, infection, meningitis, or other acute illness, dehydration, depression, and thyroid conditions.

In the infant, lethargy is a symptom requiring immediate medical evaluation.

➤ LGA

DEFINITION   Large for gestational age. This term is used to describe babies whose birth weight is greater than the 90th percentile or greater than two standard deviations from the mean for babies of the same age.

➤ LOBES

DEFINITION   Sections of milk-making tissue in the breast. There are many lobes of milk-making tissue, articulating with the ductal system, which carries milk to the nipple pores. Lobes branch into lobules that contain hundreds of alveolar units.

➤ LOCHIA

DEFINITION   Discharge of blood from the vagina after delivery. Three types of lochia are recognized, including lochia rubra (red), lochia serosa (pink), and lochia alba (white). Lochia rubra, a red discharge, begins after delivery and continues for 2–3 days. Lochia serosa, a paler, pinkish discharge, continues for the next week or so. Lochia alba, a whitish discharge, starts around the 10th day postpartum and should be resolved within a month.[207(p1043)]

ASK ABOUT

Onset.
Date of delivery.

ASSESSMENT

EMERGENT CARE NEEDED?

Are any of the following present?

Soaking a sanitary napkin with bright red blood at a rate of one napkin or more per hour.

Clots in the bloody discharge.

Foul odor to the discharge (even if occasional).

Dizziness.

Fever.

Abdominal pain.

IF YES,   *Call obstetric care provider now or seek emergency care now.*

PROMPT CARE NEEDED?

Are any of the following present?

Soaking a sanitary napkin with bright red blood at a rate of one napkin every 2–3 hours.

Abdominal tenderness.

Lightheadedness.

Sudden resumption of lochia rubra (bright red blood flow).

Continuation of lochia rubra after 4 days postpartum.

Continuation of lochia serosa after 2 weeks postpartum.

Signs of infection (fever, chills, pain, malaise, and overall aching).

Milk supply problems coupled with ongoing lochia rubra or serosa.

IF YES,   *Call obstetric care provider now.*

SELF-CARE INFORMATION

Monitor blood flow.

IMPORTANT CONDITIONS TO REPORT

Continuation of symptoms.

Sudden gushing of blood.

Multiple blood clots passed.

Concerns about milk supply.

NOTES

As time progresses, the volume of lochia should also decrease. Sudden return of bright red bleeding is of concern and should be evaluated by the healthcare provider. Retained placental fragments can be indicated by ongoing lochia rubra. In this event, mature milk production may not occur until placental fragments are expelled or removed.

See also Placental fragments, retained

Footnote

[207]Varney, H., Kriebs, J. M., & Gegor, C. L. (Eds.). (2004). *Varney's midwifery* (4th ed.). Sudbury, MA: Jones and Bartlett.

➤ LONG CHAIN POLYUNSATURATED FATTY ACIDS (LCPUFAS)

DEFINITION   Fatty acids present in human milk known to assist in the development of nerve and brain tissue.

See also Arachidonic acid (AA, also ARA); Docosahexaenoic acid (DHA) in breastmilk; Fat in breastmilk

➤ LOW MUSCLE TONE (HYPOTONIA)

DEFINITION   Loose or floppy muscle response. Babies with low muscle tone (also referred to as hypotonia) have relaxed arm and leg joints and weak neck muscles, like a rag doll.

Hypotonia can be a symptom of prematurity and of physical problems or illness.

Babies with low muscle tone may have breastfeeding problems such as non-rhythmic suck and weak sucking, and they may tire more easily.

ASK ABOUT

Age of the baby.
Onset of hypotonia.
Change in feeding behavior.
Change in urination or stooling patterns.

ASSESSMENT

EMERGENT CARE NEEDED?

Are any of the following present?

Sudden change in muscle tone.
Sudden change in feeding behavior.
Sudden lethargy.

IF YES,   *Seek emergency care now.*

PROMPT CARE NEEDED?

Are any of the following present?

Meconium bowel movements after 5 days of life.

No yellow stool by 5 days.

Fewer than three bowel movements daily in a breastfed newborn after the first 2 days of life.

No urine in 6 hours.

Brick dust urine (uric acid crystals) after 2 days of life.

Dark-colored urine.

Fewer than four urinations daily in the breastfed newborn after day 5 of life.

Noticeably sunken fontanelles (soft spot on the top of the head).

Decreased activity.

Weight loss of more than 7% from birth or further weight loss by day 5.

Cessation of weight gain.

IF YES,   *Seek pediatric care now.*

ROUTINE CARE NEEDED?

Are any of the following present?

Feeding problems.

Slow weight gain.

Problems positioning baby at breast.

Decline in milk supply.

Inadequate milk supply.

Concerns about adequate milk supply.

IF YES,   *Call lactation care provider today.*

SELF-CARE INFORMATION

Breastfeeding and breastmilk are valuable for babies with low muscle tone. Pumping may be necessary in order to maintain an adequate milk supply.

IMPORTANT CONDITIONS TO REPORT

Change in feeding behaviors.

Change in urination or stooling patterns.

Declining breastmilk volume.

See also Slow weight gain, baby

➤ LYME DISEASE

DEFINITION An inflammatory response to the bacterium *Borrelia burgdorferi*, received from a deer tick bite. Symptoms of Lyme disease include a circular rash at the site of the bite, fever, headache, muscle pain, inflammation of the joints, and malaise.

SELF-CARE INFORMATION

Make sure that all medical personnel caring for you know that you are breastfeeding. Some drugs used to treat this condition are not recommended while breastfeeding. Ask your healthcare provider about safe alternatives to these drugs.

NOTES

Breastfeeding is compatible with Lyme disease as soon as treatment has been initiated.[208]
Antibiotics and anti-inflammatory drugs may be prescribed for Lyme disease. An up-to-date drug reference should be consulted to determine the safety and possible side effects of individual drugs.

See also Acute infection; Medication resources (inside back cover)

Footnote

[208]Lawrence, R. A., & Lawrence, R. M. (2011). *Breastfeeding: A guide for the medical profession* (7th ed.). St. Louis, MO: Elsevier/Mosby.

➤ LYMPHOCYTES

DEFINITION White blood cells that are active in defending the body against infection.

NOTES

Some of the lymphocytes in milk are B-cells, so named because they are specialized in the bone marrow. B-cells respond to the presence of antigens by causing the production of the specific antibody to destroy the antigen recognized.

Other lymphocytes are T-cells, named for the thymus where they are specialized. T-cells are sometimes called "helper T-cells" because they either kill infected cells or send out messages to mobilize macrophages and other immune cells.

➤ LYSOZYME

DEFINITION An enzyme that breaks down the cell wall of bacteria. Lysozyme is found in human milk and serves as part of the army of immunologic agents working to benefit the baby's health.

➤ MACROBIOTIC DIET OF THE MOTHER

DEFINITION A particular type of vegetarian diet. A mother on a macrobiotic diet may be eating a diet consisting mostly of grains. Although many vegetarian diets are compatible with breastfeeding, some vegetarian diets (macrobiotic and vegan, for example) may not be nutritionally adequate and can put the breastfed infant at risk of malnutrition. The major concerns are deficiencies of vitamins B_{12}, B_2, and D.

ASK ABOUT

Type of diet.
Age of the baby.
Nutritional supplements taken.

ASSESSMENT

EMERGENT CARE NEEDED?

Are any of the following present?

Infant tetany (a condition characterized by painful muscle spasms and tremors).
Infant seizures.

IF YES,   *Seek emergency care now.*

PROMPT CARE NEEDED?

Are any of the following present?

Infant lethargy.
Change in infant feeding behavior.
Infant weight loss after the first week of life.
Slow growth in the breastfed infant of a macrobiotic mother.

IF YES,   *Seek pediatric care within 4 hours.*

ROUTINE CARE NEEDED?

Are any of the following present?

Macrobiotic diet of the breastfeeding mother.

Vegan diet of the breastfeeding mother.

Ovo-lacto vegetarian diet of the breastfeeding mother.

| IF YES, | *Seek dietary consultation.* |

SELF-CARE INFORMATION

Nutritional risks of vegetarian diets are especially associated with protein, vitamins B_{12}, B_2, and D, and zinc deficiencies.

IMPORTANT CONDITIONS TO REPORT

Lethargy, fussiness, and poor feeding behavior can be early signs of nutritional inadequacies.

NOTES

Many people who are vegetarians are knowledgeable about including foods and supplements that balance their diets.

See also Maternal diet; Maternal diet, vegetarian

➤ MACRONUTRIENTS IN HUMAN MILK

DEFINITION   The three macronutrients in human milk are carbohydrate, fat, and protein. Human milk also contains micronutrients and water as well as immunologic properties, cellular components, and other substances.

➤ MACROPHAGES

DEFINITION   Components of both colostrum and mature milk. They are large-complex cells whose functions include phagocytosis (engulfing and destroying) of fungi and bacteria, killing bacteria, and production of other human milk components such as lysozyme and lactoferrin.

➤ MADONNA POSTURE

DEFINITION   The Madonna posture is also called the cradle position or cradle posture. The baby is positioned across the mother's lap and turned toward the mother. In this position, the weight of the baby is often carried on the arm of the mother on the same side as the breast that is being nursed.

See also **Cradle posture**

➤ MALABSORPTION SYNDROME

DEFINITION   Any alteration in the ability of the intestine to absorb nutrients adequately. It is often characterized by 2 or more weeks of diarrhea that continues even after treatment, as well as bloating, gas, cramping, and weight loss.

➤ MALAISE, MATERNAL

DEFINITION   A generalized feeling of discomfort, illness, or lack of well-being. Malaise is a nonspecific symptom that can occur along with other specific symptoms of significant disease or illness.

In breastfeeding mothers, malaise may be an early sign of mastitis or abscess. Malaise may also be a sign of any infection or illness.

ASK ABOUT

Onset.
Age of the baby.
Medications taken.
Other symptoms.

ASSESSMENT

EMERGENT CARE NEEDED?

Are any of the following present?

Suicidal thoughts.

Thoughts of harming the baby.

IF YES, *Seek emergency care now.*

Are any of the following present?

Visible red areas on breast.

Fever higher than 101°F (38.5°C).

Extreme breast discomfort.

Flu-like aching throughout body.

Extreme anxiety.

IF YES, *Seek medical care now.*

PROMPT CARE NEEDED?

Are any of the following present?

Persistent sadness.

Inability to function.

Fatigue.

Difficulty eating or sleeping.

IF YES, *Call healthcare provider today.*

ROUTINE CARE NEEDED?

Are any of the following present?

Feeling of malaise lasting for more than 2 days without any other symptoms developing.

IF YES, *Call medical care provider.*

SELF-CARE INFORMATION

Report new symptoms to your healthcare provider.

IMPORTANT CONDITIONS TO REPORT

Watch for any of the following symptoms:

Visible red areas on breast.

Fever higher than 101°F (38.5°C).

Extreme breast discomfort.

Flu-like aching throughout body.

Persistent fatigue, anxiety, or sadness.

NOTES

Physical feelings of malaise can be also associated with depression and other postpartum mood disorders.

See also Abscess, breast; Hypothyroidism; Mastitis; Postpartum depression

➤ MALARIA

DEFINITION   Malaria is a parasitic disease characterized by fever, chills, headache, and anemia. It is transmitted from one human to another by the bite of an infected mosquito. It is a major health problem in many of the world's tropic and subtropic locations. Malaria can also be transmitted congenitally and by blood transfusions.

SELF-CARE INFORMATION

Make sure that all medical personnel caring for you know that you are breastfeeding. Some drugs used to treat this condition are not recommended while breastfeeding. Ask your healthcare provider about safe alternatives to these drugs.

NOTES

Breastfeeding does not transmit malaria. Breastfeeding is not contraindicated for mothers who are being treated for malaria. Many of the drugs used to prevent and treat malaria are compatible with breastfeeding.

More information is available from the Centers for Disease Control and Prevention. Visit www.cdc.gov for the latest information.

➤ MALNOURISHED MOTHER

DEFINITION Poor nourishment in a mother due to inadequate diet or presence of disease or other disorder decreasing absorption and digestion.

NOTES

Exercise, hard work, and weight loss do not change the volume of milk produced by nursing mothers. Extremely malnourished women or severely dehydrated women may have a decreased volume of milk.

Improving the poorly nourished mother's diet may prolong breastfeeding duration as well as the duration of exclusive breastfeeding. Malnourished mothers whose diets are improved have more energy and are more interactive with their baby.

See also Macrobiotic diet of the mother; Maternal diet; Maternal diet, vegetarian; Milk production

➤ MALT

See Mucosa-associated lymphoid tissue (MALT)

➤ MAMMAPLASTY

DEFINITION Breast reduction or augmentation surgery.

See also Breast augmentation; Breast reduction; Breast surgery

➤ MAMMOGENESIS

DEFINITION Mammogenesis is the development of the mammary gland. This development begins early in fetal life and continues through lactation. The mammary gland is one of the few tissues in mammals that can repeatedly undergo growth, functional differentiation, and regression or involution.

➤ MANUAL EXPRESSION OF BREASTMILK

DEFINITION   A method of removing milk from the lactating breast that does not require any device with the exception of a hand and a bowl or jar to collect milk. Hand expression is a simple skill that should be taught to all breastfeeding mothers.

ASK ABOUT

Reason mother plans to express milk.

ASSESSMENT

PROMPT CARE NEEDED?

Are any of the following present?

Imminent separation of mother and baby.

IF YES,   *Call lactation care provider today.*

ROUTINE CARE NEEDED?

Are any of the following present?

Desire to learn hand expression.

Desire to pump.

Questions about storage and handling of breastmilk.

Questions about donating milk to a milk bank.

IF YES,   *Call lactation care provider.*

SELF-CARE INFORMATION

Wash hands before beginning.

When baby is latched onto one breast, practice hand expression on the other breast.

Gently massage and then compress the breast with thumb and pointer finger opposite each other on the areola. Repeat.

Your skill will improve with practice.

Store expressed milk in the refrigerator, a cooler with ice packs, or the freezer if it will not be used within 48 hours.

Follow safe milk storage guidelines.

IMPORTANT CONDITIONS TO REPORT
Questions or problems with hand expression.
Concerns about volume of milk expressed.

See also Breast pump; Collection and storage of breastmilk

➤ MANUAL PUMP

DEFINITION   A device designed to remove milk from the breast. Manual pumps work by hand pressure, squeezing a lever or contracting levers, or pulling out a cylinder to generate pressure to operate the pump.

➤ MANUFACTURED INFANT MILKS

DEFINITION   May also be called artificial baby milks, manufactured baby milk, infant formula, artificial milks, formulated baby milks, or breastmilk substitutes.

See also Formula, infant

➤ MARIJUANA

DEFINITION   Marijuana, although illegal for recreational use in many parts of the United States, is commonly used. Portions of the plant *Cannabis sativa* are dried and, most commonly, smoked. Marijuana has been placed in the category of drugs that are contraindicated for breastfeeding mothers by the American Academy of Pediatrics Committee on Drugs. Hale rates cannabis as an L5 (contraindicated) drug during lactation.[209(pp180-181)]

See also Contraindicated medications; Illegal drugs

Footnote
[209]Hale, T. (2012). *Medications and mothers' milk* (15th ed.). Amarillo, TX: Hale Pub.

➤ MASSAGE, BREAST

DEFINITION A technique used to encourage milk to flow from the breast. When the suckling baby pauses, the mother gently but firmly massages and compresses the breast to which the baby is attached, thereby increasing the transfer of milk and encouraging the suckling again.

NOTES

This technique is used with sleepy or inefficient feeders, especially those who are premature, have low muscle tone, or cleft lip/palate.

See also Alternate breast massage; Premature infant; Slow weight gain, baby

➤ MASTALGIA

DEFINITION Breast pain with no certain cause. There can be many reasons for pain in the breast including breast infection or inflammation, clogs, or cysts.

NOTES

Breastfeeding should not be painful. Advise mothers to seek medical or lactation care for breast pain.

See also Mastitis; Painful breastfeeding; Plugged ducts; Sore nipples

➤ MASTITIS

DEFINITION Breast inflammation. It can be infective or noninfective.

ASK ABOUT

Onset.
Prior breast inflammation.
Sore nipples.
Known drug allergies.

ASSESSMENT

EMERGENT CARE NEEDED?

Are any of the following present?

Visible red areas on the breast(s).

Fever higher than 101°F (38.5°C).

Extreme breast discomfort.

Flu-like aching throughout the body.

Continuing fever after treatment.

Reaction to antibiotic prescribed.

IF YES, *Seek emergency care urgently if red streaks or red areas are found on both breasts and other symptoms are also present. Seek medical care within 4 hours with other symptoms if red area is on one breast only.*

PROMPT MEDICAL CARE NEEDED?

Are any of the following present?

Continuing symptoms after treatment.

IF YES, *Call obstetric care provider now.*

PROMPT LACTATION CARE NEEDED?

Are any of the following present?

Difficulty breastfeeding during mastitis.

IF YES, *Call lactation care provider now.*

SELF-CARE INFORMATION

Breastfeed on both breasts, keeping them as soft as possible.

Start on the unaffected breast.

Take care of yourself as though you have the flu (bed rest, plenty of fluids, help for other children and household chores).

Antibiotics and anti-inflammatory drugs that are used to treat mastitis are generally compatible with breastfeeding. Use an up-to-date drug reference to be sure.

Take medications as they have been prescribed, even after you feel better.

IMPORTANT CONDITIONS TO REPORT
Symptoms that worsen or do not resolve.

NOTES

Simultaneous bilateral mastitis may indicate more severe infection. *Immediate emergency care is indicated.*

See also Acute infection; Bilateral mastitis; Breast inflammation; Mastitis; Medication resources (inside back cover)

➤ MATERNAL CHILD HEALTH BUREAU

See DHHS/Health Resources Services Administration (HRSA), Maternal Child Health Bureau

➤ MATERNAL DIET

DEFINITION   Foods and beverages consumed by a woman who is breastfeeding. Mothers can produce enough milk and milk of good quality, even when the mothers' supply of nutrients is limited.[210] Rules about eating or not eating certain foods during lactation are not warranted, may be hard to follow, and may decrease the mother's enjoyment of breastfeeding. However, there may be individual cases where certain foods affect the baby. Most commonly, the mother's drinking of liquid cow's milk has been associated with colic symptoms in some babies. If this is the case, improvement may be seen after the mother eliminates cow's milk from her diet for at least a week. Mothers should seek further information about diet and breastfeeding on an individual basis.

With the exception of cow's milk and possibly a few other allergens such as soy, corn, egg, wheat, and tree nuts, there is little evidence that anything that mothers consume negatively affect their babies. Gas and flatulence are normal occurrences in the newborn, as in all humans.

Adults associate eating cabbage and other cruciferous vegetables with gas, due to difficulty digesting complex sugars in these foods. These sugars do not pass into the nursing baby's gastrointestinal tract in the same form (at least until the baby eats solid foods), so there is unlikely to be any effect for the baby.

Many mothers will put themselves on increasingly restrictive diets without seeking help for their baby's symptoms.

Clinicians should carefully evaluate a mother's concerns and her baby's symptoms to distinguish normal gas from colic or other digestive difficulty.

See also **Macrobiotic diet of the mother; Maternal diet, vegetarian**

Footnotes

[210]Subcommittee on Nutrition, National Academy of Sciences. (1991). *Nutrition during lactation.* Washington, DC: National Academy Press.

➤ MATERNAL DIET, VEGETARIAN

DEFINITION Although many vegetarian diets are compatible with breastfeeding, some vegetarian diets (macrobiotic and vegan for example) may not be nutritionally adequate and can put the breastfed infant at risk of malnutrition. The major concerns are deficiencies of vitamins B_{12}, B_2, and D.

ASK ABOUT

Type of diet.
Age of the baby.
Nutritional supplements taken.

ASSESSMENT

EMERGENT CARE NEEDED?

Are any of the following present?

Infant tetany (a condition characterized by painful muscle spasms and tremors).

Infant seizures.

IF YES,   *Seek emergency care now.*

PROMPT CARE NEEDED?

Are any of the following present?

Infant lethargy.

Change in infant feeding behavior.

Infant weight loss after the first week of life.

Slow growth in the breastfed infant of a macrobiotic or vegan mother.

IF YES,   *Seek pediatric care now.*

ROUTINE CARE NEEDED?

Are any of the following present?

Macrobiotic diet of the mother.

Vegan diet of the mother.

Ovo-lacto vegetarian diet of the mother.

IF YES,   *Seek dietary consultation.*

SELF-CARE INFORMATION

Dietary risks of vegetarian diets are especially associated with protein, vitamins B_{12}, B_2, and D, and zinc deficiencies.

IMPORTANT CONDITIONS TO REPORT

Fussiness, lethargy, and poor feeding behavior can be early signs of nutritional inadequacies.

NOTES

Many people who are vegetarians are knowledgeable about including foods and supplements that balance their diets.

See also Macrobiotic diet of the mother; Maternal diet

➤ MATERNAL DIET AND WEIGHT LOSS

DEFINITION   Weight loss of up to 5 lb a month in the first months postpartum has not been associated with poorer growth of the nursing baby. Nursing mothers are likely to be closer to their prepregnancy weight at 6 months than formula feeding mothers. A pattern of short, frequent feedings has been associated with greater weight loss than a pattern of longer, less frequent feedings.

See also Maternal exercise; Weight loss, mother

➤ MATERNAL EMPLOYMENT

DEFINITION   Mothers who work for pay may do so away from home or in the home. Employed mothers may be separated from their baby or have the baby nearby. In the United States, more than half of the mothers with babies under the age of 1 year are employed.[211]

ASK ABOUT

Amount of separation—hours per day, days per week.
Start date of work.
Age of the baby.
Mother's plans to continue breastfeeding.
Mother's plans to express milk.
Accommodations at work for expressing and saving milk.
How the baby will be fed away from the mother.

ASSESSMENT

ROUTINE CARE NEEDED?
   Are any of the following present?
      Information about managing work and breastfeeding.

   IF YES,   *Call lactation care provider.*

SELF-CARE INFORMATION

Stress does not seem to affect milk supply but frequent milk removal is needed to maintain or improve the milk supply.

Milk can be collected and frozen in the early weeks to supplement milk collected after the mother's return to work.

Milk supply is best maintained by hand expression or combining hand expression with pumping using a pump that is intended for that purpose along with breastfeeding.

Select child care facilities carefully.

Expressed milk is a raw food and should be refrigerated immediately if possible. Get information about storage, use, and feeding expressed milk from your lactation care provider.

The timing of return to work and the number of hours spent away from the baby affect the duration of breastfeeding more than the type of work a woman does.

IMPORTANT CONDITIONS TO REPORT

Problems with expressing milk (check that the equipment is working properly).

Breast problems.

Problems with the infant accepting expressed milk.

NOTES

The Patient Protection and Affordable Care Act, passed by Congress in 2010, specifies that employers are required to provide "reasonable break time for an employee to express breast milk for her nursing child for 1 year after the child's birth each time such employee has need to express the milk." Employers are also required to provide "a place, other than a bathroom, that is shielded from view and free from intrusion from coworkers and the public, which may be used by an employee to express breast milk."212(p1)

Ongoing support and help with problem solving may be needed after returning to work.

See also Breast pump; Collection and storage of breastmilk; Day care; Decrease in milk supply; Storage of breastmilk; Working mothers

Footnotes

[211]U.S. Department of Labor, Bureau of Labor Statistics. (2012, April 26). Employment characteristics of families summary. Retrieved from http://www.bls.gov/news.release/famee.nr0.htm

[212]U.S. Department of Labor. (2010, December). Wage and Hour Division (WHD)—fact sheet. Retrieved from http://www.dol.gov/whd/regs/compliance/whdfs73.htm

➤ MATERNAL EXERCISE

DEFINITION   Physical exertion is a normal part of the life of lactating women around the globe. There is no reason for lactating women not to exercise in moderation during lactation, even women who have previously been sedentary. For comfort, mothers may want to select a well-fitting supportive bra that does not compress their breasts.

ASK ABOUT

Age of the baby.
Type and amount of exercise.
Prior cautions against exercise.

SELF-CARE INFORMATION

Moderate exercise does not decrease milk production.
Mothers may be more comfortable with a supportive (but not too constricting bra).
Mothers may be more comfortable exercising after nursing, when the breasts are the most soft.
Mothers should be advised to discuss new physical activities with their health-care providers.

➤ MATERNAL FATIGUE

DEFINITION   Exhaustion, weariness, or lack of energy. May be the result of lack of sleep. May also be associated with anemia, postpartum mood disorder, infection, underactive or overactive thyroid, pain, and the use of some drugs (including prescription drugs).

ASK ABOUT

Onset of symptom of fatigue.
Age of the baby.
Weight gain of baby.
Medication and/or drugs used.

ASSESSMENT

EMERGENT CARE NEEDED?

Are any of the following present?

Fever.

Confusion.

Dizziness.

Blurred vision.

Swelling, weight gain, and little or no urine.

IF YES, *Seek emergency care now.*

PROMPT CARE NEEDED?

Are any of the following present?

Ongoing fatigue.

Sadness or depression.

Intolerance to cold.

Dry skin.

Headache.

Insomnia.

Constipation.

IF YES, *Seek medical care today.*

ROUTINE CARE NEEDED?

Are any of the following present?

Concern about frequency of nighttime and daytime nursing.

Concern about weight gain pattern of the breastfed baby.

Questions about fatigue and breastfeeding.

IF YES, *Call lactation care provider.*

SELF-CARE INFORMATION

Although tiredness is common postpartum, fatigue should be investigated since it can be a nonspecific symptom of other problems.

IMPORTANT CONDITIONS TO REPORT

Fatigue that is not relieved by sleep.

See also Anemia; Postpartum depression; Thyroid disease; Hypothyroidism

➤ MATERNAL HOSPITALIZATION

DEFINITION Hospitalization of breastfeeding mothers in an emergency, because of chronic health problems, for psychiatric reasons, for tests, or for elective surgery.

ASK ABOUT

Age of the baby.
Dependence of baby on mother's milk/exclusivity of breastfeeding.
Drugs the mother may be given.
Ability of the mother to express milk in the hospital.
Practicality of breastfeeding the baby in the hospital.

ASSESSMENT

PROMPT CARE NEEDED?

Are any of the following present?

Imminent hospitalization of breastfeeding woman.

IF YES, *Call lactation care provider now.*

ROUTINE CARE NEEDED?

Are any of the following present?

Possible hospitalization of a breastfeeding woman.

IF YES, *Call lactation care provider.*

SELF-CARE INFORMATION

Tell all of the healthcare providers that you are nursing and that you want to continue (assuming this is the case).

Make a plan for expressing milk in order to maintain the milk supply and provide milk for the baby.

Ask if it is possible for the baby to visit or stay in the hospital room with you.

See also Abrupt weaning; Breast pump; Hand expression of breastmilk

➤ MATERNAL MEDICATIONS

DEFINITION   Many factors influence whether a drug the mother takes will be found in her milk, the amount of the drug that is found in the milk, and the effect of the drug on the baby. Some drugs can also affect the milk supply.

ASK ABOUT

Age of the baby.

Weight of the baby.

History of taking medication (e.g., was the drug taken during pregnancy?).

How long the medication will be taken.

ASSESSMENT

PROMPT CARE NEEDED?

Are any of the following present?

Questions regarding drug compatibility with lactation.

IF YES, *Consult up-to-date drug references and seek advice from the healthcare provider within 4 hours regarding safety of medications or possible drug substitutions and call lactation care provider for assistance with managing milk supply.*

SELF-CARE INFORMATION

Do not self-medicate while breastfeeding without discussing the drug with your healthcare provider.

Tell every healthcare provider that you are breastfeeding.

If you are prescribed a drug that is incompatible with breastfeeding, ask your healthcare provider about alternative drugs that are compatible.

IMPORTANT CONDITIONS TO REPORT

Any changes in the baby's behavior or appearance.

Any changes in your milk supply.

See also Contraindicated medications; Medication resources (inside back cover); Over-the-counter (OTC) drugs

➤ MATURE MILK

DEFINITION   Milk that is produced after delivery of the placenta until the time of weaning.

➤ MCHB

See DHHS/Health Resources Services Administration (HRSA), Maternal Child Health Bureau

➤ MECONIUM

DEFINITION   Thick, sticky, and greenish-black in color, meconium is the first stool (feces) of the newborn. The passage of meconium indicates that the intestines are working properly.

SELF-CARE INFORMATION

Passage of meconium is facilitated by frequent nursing in the first days so that the baby receives many colostrum feedings.

Because it is so sticky, meconium may be hard to clean off of the baby's bottom. Putting on a light coating of cream or oil when the diaper is changed can help.

Over the first days, the dark, early stool becomes greener (transitional stool) and then, for the breastfed infant, yellow.

If baby is still passing dark green meconium stools on day 5 or later, call pediatric care provider immediately.

See also Bowel movements, infant

➤ MEDICATIONS

DEFINITION   Prescription, over-the-counter drugs, herbal remedies, and other substances thought to have curative effects that may be taken by an individual. Many factors influence whether a drug the mother takes will be found in her milk, the amount of the drug that is found in the milk, and the effect of the drug on the baby. Some drugs can also affect the milk supply.

ASK ABOUT

Age of the baby.

Weight of the baby.

History of taking medication (e.g., was the drug taken during pregnancy?).

How long the medication will be taken.

ASSESSMENT

PROMPT CARE NEEDED?

Are any of the following present?

Questions regarding drug compatibility with lactation.

IF YES,   *Consult up-to-date drug references and seek advice from the health-care provider within 4 hours regarding safety of medications or possible drug substitutions and call lactation care provider for assistance with managing milk supply.*

SELF-CARE INFORMATION

Do not self-medicate while breastfeeding without discussing the drug with your healthcare provider.

Tell every healthcare provider that you are breastfeeding.

If you are prescribed a drug that is incompatible with breastfeeding, ask your healthcare provider about alternative drugs that are compatible.

IMPORTANT CONDITIONS TO REPORT

Any changes in the baby's behavior or appearance.

Any changes in your milk supply.

See also Contraindicated medications; Medication resources (inside back cover); Over-the-counter (OTC) drugs

➤ MEDICINAL HERBS

DEFINITION Plants or plant parts that can be valued for their medicinal qualities.

SELF-CARE INFORMATION

Tell all healthcare providers about any herbs and natural supplements you are taking.

Some herbs, such as fenugreek, may interfere with the absorption of any medication used concurrently,[213(p261)] and have other potentially dangerous side effects. Investigate medicinal herbs with the same care you would with prescribed and over-the-counter medications.

IMPORTANT CONDITIONS TO REPORT

Any change in the baby's physical condition or behavior such as problems sleeping, vomiting, rash, or irritability.

NOTES

Herbs can have powerful effects. As with some drugs taken by breastfeeding mothers, troubling effects have also been reported in breastfed babies whose mothers have taken certain medicinal herbs.

See also Fenugreek; Medication resources (inside back cover); Over-the-counter (OTC) drugs

Footnote

[213]Skidmore-Roth, L. (2010). *Mosby's handbook of herbs & natural supplements*. St. Louis, MO: Elsevier Mosby.

➤ MENINGITIS

DEFINITION   Inflammation of the outer membrane of the brain and spinal cord, typically caused by viral or bacterial infection.

NOTES

Symptoms of meningitis in an infant include fever, vomiting, stiffness of the neck, lethargy, and irritability that is not calmed by cuddling. If the baby has symptoms of meningitis, seek emergency care immediately.

See also Lethargy

➤ MENSTRUAL CYCLE

DEFINITION   The recurring pattern of physical changes in the ovaries and uterus under control of hormones that regulate a woman's fertility. Research continues in order to better understand the relationship between menstruation, fertility, and breastfeeding. The time after childbirth and before menstruation resumes in nursing mothers is called lactational amenorrhea.

SELF-CARE INFORMATION

It is impossible to predict when any woman will get her first period after her baby is born if she is breastfeeding.

Periods can be irregular, or lighter or heavier than when not breastfeeding.

Fertility may return before the first period after childbirth.

The return of menstruation does not mean the end of breastfeeding.

Some mothers report that their nursing babies are less interested in breastfeeding during their periods.

Some mothers experience nipple soreness during menstruation.

IMPORTANT CONDITIONS TO REPORT

Menstruation before 4 weeks postpartum if breastfeeding.

See also Amenorrhea; Birth interval; Fertility; Lactational amenorrhea method (LAM); Placental fragments, retained

➤ METABOLIC DISORDER, GALACTOSEMIA

DEFINITION   A rare genetic metabolic disorder diagnosed through newborn screening in which the infant must be placed on a galactose-free diet because the liver enzyme needed to break down galactose is missing.

ASK ABOUT

Age of the baby.

ASSESSMENT

EMERGENT CARE NEEDED?

Are any of the following present?

Jaundice (yellow appearance).

Vomiting.

Diarrhea.

Weight loss.

IF YES,   *Seek pediatric care now.*

PROMPT CARE NEEDED?

Are any of the following present?

If the mother has been breastfeeding prior to diagnosis, she may need assistance with finding comfort until milk production ceases.

> **IF YES,**   *Call lactation care provider today.*

SELF-CARE INFORMATION

Suddenly stopping breastfeeding or expressing after the baby is diagnosed with galactosemia can lead to breast problems such as mastitis and abscess development.

Milk expression can help to keep the breasts comfortable until milk production slows and ceases. Consider donating expressed milk to a milk bank.

IMPORTANT CONDITIONS TO REPORT

Breast inflammation (redness) and painful areas on the breast.

Fever higher than 101°F (38.5°C).

Extreme breast discomfort.

Flu-like aching throughout body.

> **NOTES**

Galactosemia is usually diagnosed in the first week via heel stick screening or the appearance of symptoms including prolonged jaundice, vomiting, and diarrhea.

Classic galactosemia is an absolute contraindication to breastfeeding. A rarer variant of galactosemia, Duarte's galactosemia, may allow partial breastfeeding of the affected baby. For this reason, along with many false positives on newborn screening, it may be beneficial to help mothers maintain their milk production until testing is conclusive.

See also Abrupt weaning; Contraindicated conditions; Weaning

➤ METABOLIC DISORDER, PHENYLKETONURIA

DEFINITION   A rare genetic inborn error of metabolism that is detectable during the first days of life through newborn screening. **Phenylketonuria (PKU)** is characterized by the absence or deficiency of the enzyme that is necessary to process the essential amino acid phenylalanine. Babies with PKU may be partially breastfed together with consumption of a phenylalanine-free formula, per physician's order. These babies must be monitored carefully to protect the central nervous system from damage caused by high levels of phenylalanine.

PROMPT CARE NEEDED?

Are any of the following present?

Management of breastfeeding, breasts, and milk.

IF YES,   *Call lactation care provider today.*

SELF-CARE INFORMATION

The healthcare provider will prescribe a phenylalanine-free formula and determine how often the baby's blood levels will be tested for phenylalanine.

Even babies with PKU require some of the amino acid phenylalanine that is found in formula and breastmilk.

Human milk is lower in phenylalanine than standard formulas.

Research indicates that children who had received their mother's milk in addition to the special phenylalanine-free formula during infancy had more than a 10-point IQ advantage compared to children who had received the special formula alone or compared to a standard formula.[214]

IMPORTANT CONDITIONS TO REPORT

Any breastfeeding or formula feeding problems.

Footnote

[214]Riva, E., Agostoni, C., Biasucci, G., Trojan, S., Luotti, D., Fiori, L., & Giovanni, M.. (1996). Early breastfeeding is linked to higher intelligence quotient scores in dietary treated phenylketonuric children. *Acta Paediatrica, 85,* 56.

➤ METABOLISM

DEFINITION   The processing of a substance by the body, breaking it down into usable fragments.

➤ MFCI

DESCRIPTION Mother-Friendly Childbirth Initiative. A set of 10 steps for hospitals, birth centers, and other birth services for provision of mother-friendly care during childbirth. This initiative is a project of the Coalition for Improving Maternity Services.

See also Coalition for Improving Maternity Services (CIMS)

➤ MILK BANKS

DEFINITION Donor human milk banks have been in operation since the early 1900s. They collect milk from mothers who have extra milk, beyond what they need for their thriving babies. Mothers are screened by history, and their blood and milk are tested for exposure to bacteria and viruses of concern. In addition, milk is heat treated, or pasteurized. In the United States, milk is distributed only by prescription.

ASK ABOUT

Age of the baby.
Does the mother wish to donate?
Does the baby need donor milk?

NOTES

Mothers who wish to donate milk should be encouraged to contact the Human Milk Banking Association to find a location that is accepting donations. Informal donation of milk from one mother to another cannot be condoned, as it is possible to pass illnesses through unscreened and untreated milk.

Donor milk from a recognized human milk bank will have gone through several different screening processes (history and serology of the donor, bacteriology of the milk before and after heat treatment, etc.) and will be heat-treated to remove most pathogens.

The uses of donor milk are many, including providing nourishment to preterm or chronically ill infants, such as those with feeding intolerance, malabsorption, cardiac problems, metabolic problems, and diarrhea.

Use of donor milk in preterm infants is thought to be preventive of necrotizing enterocolitis.

A prescription is necessary for donor milk to be dispensed from the milk bank.

There is a processing cost associated with obtaining donor milk; this fee may be covered by insurance, waived, or reduced if cost prohibitive.

Milk banks can be located by contacting the following organization:

Human Milk Banking Association of North America (HMBANA)
Web: www.hmbana.org

See also Human Milk Banking Association of North American (HMBANA)

➤ MILK BLISTER, BLEB

DEFINITION   A tiny, white, milky blockage of a single duct opening on the surface of the nipple. Mothers often describe excruciating, pinpoint pain at the site of the blockage radiating toward the spine. Blebs may need to be lanced by a medical care provider.

ASK ABOUT

Onset.

Age of the baby.

History of herpes lesions or other skin conditions on breast or nipple.

ASSESSMENT

EMERGENT CARE NEEDED?

Are any of the following present?

History of herpes lesions on the nipple.

History of herpes elsewhere on the mother or partner's body with current bleb or lesion on the nipple or breast.

IF YES,   *Seek medical care now.*

PROMPT CARE NEEDED?

Are any of the following present?

Painful, protuberant bleb on the nipple.

IF YES,   *Seek medical care today.*
Call lactation care provider today.

SELF-CARE INFORMATION

Some mothers find manual massage of the area helps the bleb to dislodge and move out of the breast. Others prefer warmth, such as a warm, wet towel.

If lanced, follow directions for postlancing care. Breastfeeding can usually resume right away.

IMPORTANT CONDITIONS TO REPORT

Symptoms of infection (fever, aching, chills, or redness at site).

NOTES

Blisters may appear on the nipple and breast for several reasons, including poor latch, trauma, damage from nipple shields, abscess, and blebs.

Emergency differential diagnosis is crucial in women with history of herpes lesions on the nipple or elsewhere on the mother's or partner's body. As herpes can be fatal to the newborn, breastfeeding should be discontinued on the affected nipple until differential diagnosis is obtained. Active herpes or chicken pox lesions on the nipple and breast are potentially life threatening for the baby. Herpes lesions elsewhere on the body do not contraindicate breastfeeding. However, parents should practice very careful hand-washing techniques to avoid touching lesions and then touching the baby.

Other conditions to consider include poison ivy, allergic response to surface antigens (contact dermatitis), and eczema.

A bleb is a tiny white, milky blockage of a single duct opening on the surface of the nipple. Mothers often describe excruciating, pinpoint pain at the site of the blockage. Counseling and visual inspection may be required to assure correct diagnosis. A bleb "may be 'cured' or disappear when the health professional opens it with a sterile needle or lances it. It may reappear and have to be opened again."[215(p267)]

Because of the serious nature of some infectious conditions, including herpes, women reporting rashes or lesions on the breast and nipple should be seen immediately by a qualified healthcare provider to rule out contraindicated infections.

See also Blisters on nipple or breast; Nipple pain

Footnote

[215]Lawrence, R. A., & Lawrence, R. M. (2011). *Breastfeeding: A guide for the medical profession* (7th ed.). St. Louis, MO: Elsevier/Mosby.

➤ MILK COLLECTION AND STORAGE

DEFINITION   Procedure by which milk is safely expressed and stored.

SELF-CARE INFORMATION

Milk collection may be done by hand or pump expression or a combination.

Begin all milk collection by washing hands, pump, and collection device carefully.

Massage breasts prior to expressing.

Label each container with date of expression and name of the infant (if it will be used in a multichild setting).

Glass and hard plastic containers with tight lids are recommended. All containers should be food grade. Plastic bags designed for milk storage may be used, but prevent spillage and puncture of these bags.

Milk can be safely stored:[216]

   Up to 4 hours at room temperature (66°–72° F), but should be refrigerated immediately if possible (with a frozen gel pack in an insulated lunch bag or cooler if a refrigerator is not available).

   Three to five days in the refrigerator (32°–50°F).

   Up to 3 months in the built-in freezer section (0°–32°F) of a refrigerator.

   Up to 6 months in a deep freezer (-20°F or less).

Milk that will not be used fresh within 5 days should be frozen as soon as possible.

Thaw milk in its container.

Milk can be safely thawed by:

   Placing frozen containers in the refrigerator overnight.

   Holding frozen containers under lukewarm running tap water.

   Placing frozen containers in lukewarm water.

Hot water is not recommended due to potential nutrient loss.

Milk should never be boiled or microwaved.

Milk does not need to be overly warm before being fed to infant.

See also Containers for milk storage; Storage of breastmilk; Thawing and warming frozen breastmilk

Footnote

[216]Cadwell, K., & Turner-Maffei, C. (2014). *Pocket guide for lactation management* (2nd ed.). Burlington, MA: Jones & Bartlett Learning.

➤ MILK-EJECTION REFLEX

DEFINITION   The neurohormonal response that compresses the myoepithelial cells that surround the alveoli, forcing milk to be squeezed down through the ducts and out the nipple. Also called "let-down reflex."

SELF-CARE INFORMATION

The breastfed newborn should gain well (0.5–1 oz per day on average). If the baby is gaining less than this, have a face-to-face breastfeeding evaluation.

At the breast, the baby should have sucking pattern that includes slow, deep sucks. After the first few days, the baby's swallows can be heard, and the baby should have at least six wet diapers at least four yellow stools each day.

IMPORTANT CONDITIONS TO REPORT

Inadequate weight gain.

Inadequate number of urinations and stools.

NOTES

This reflex is caused by a spike in the hormone oxytocin, one of the two major hormones of lactation (the other is prolactin). Oxytocin is released from the posterior lobe of the pituitary gland and stimulates the contraction of the smooth muscle of the uterus during labor. This hormone is also responsible for ejection of milk from the breast.

Researchers have found that oxytocin is released in the first hours postpartum by the baby's hand massage of the breast.

Oxytocin is also released by the baby stretching the nipple sufficiently in the mouth. This is why a good latch is so important to milk transfer.

Oxytocin is also released through a conditioned response over time.

The mother's oxytocin response in the first days may be muted by administration of Pitocin (oxytocin) during labor.[217]

See also Oxytocin; Overactive let-down reflex

Footnote

[217]Jonas, K., Johansson, L. M., Nissen, E., Ejdebäck, M., Ransjö-Arvidson, A. B., & Uvnäs-Moberg, K. (2009). Effects of intrapartum oxytocin administration and epidural analgesia on the concentration of plasma oxytocin and prolactin, in response to suckling during the second day postpartum. *Breastfeeding Medicine: The Official Journal of the Academy of Breastfeeding Medicine, 4*(2), 71–82. doi:10.1089/bfm.2008.0002

➤ MILK FED TO WRONG BABY

DEFINITION Accidental feeding of one mother's expressed breastmilk to another baby. This may happen in the hospital or daycare setting. Concern has been raised about the possibility of disease transmission from the milk to the infant.

NOTES

The Centers for Disease Control and Prevention states that this accident should be treated as any other accidental exposure to bodily fluids.
   According to the Centers for Disease Control and Prevention:

> HIV and other serious infectious diseases can be transmitted through breast milk. However, the risk of infection from a single bottle of breast milk, even if the mother is HIV positive, is extremely small. For women who do not have HIV or other serious infectious diseases, there is little risk to the child who receives her breast milk. See Diseases and Conditions[218] for more information.[219]("What can happen" section)

Footnotes

[218]CDC. (2010, April 19). Breastfeeding: Frequently asked questions (FAQs); What can happen if someone else's breast milk is given to another child? Retrieved May from http://www.cdc.gov/breastfeeding/faq/index.htm

[219]CDC. (2009, October 20). Breastfeeding: Diseases and conditions; Hepatitis B and C infections. Retrieved from http://www.cdc.gov/breastfeeding/disease/hepatitis.htm

➤ MILK FLOW, TOO FAST

DEFINITION Rapid milk flow that may overwhelm the baby's ability to suck, swallow, and breathe comfortably. This may be due to the oversupply of milk, a forceful let-down reflex, or both.

ASK ABOUT

Age of the baby.
Weight gain of the baby.

ASSESSMENT

ROUTINE CARE NEEDED?

Are any of the following present?

Gagging, choking, or coughing at the breast as if the milk is coming too fast.

Baby spits up and is gassy.

Baby pulls off the breast while nursing and milk sprays.

The nipple is compressed at the end of the nursing.

IF YES,   *Call lactation care provider today.*

PROMPT CARE NEEDED?

Are any of the following present?

Perception of overabundant milk supply.

Excessively large or frequent stools in a breastfed baby.

Recurrent engorgement or mastitis.

Baby has difficulty managing excessive milk flow including pulling away from the breast.

Baby is unsettled after feeding.

IF YES,   *Call lactation care provider today.*

SELF-CARE INFORMATION

Frequency of feeding and amount of milk removal drives milk supply. The rapid milk flow is often accompanied by an abundant milk supply. Many women with oversupply may need to gradually decrease breast stimulation.

Positioning the baby in an upright position, with no pressure on the back of the head, may give the baby an opportunity to find the best nursing position.

Try nursing the baby on only one breast at each feeding to decrease the supply. Decrease milk expression, if practiced.

Some mothers successfully manage the flow by nursing while lying on their backs with the baby lying on the mother's abdomen. This technique is known as the "reclining posture," "the Australian posture," and "nursing down under." The baby has complete head control in this position, and the milk is spraying against gravity. In these postures, the weight of the baby is on the mother's chest and abdomen and the baby is clearly upright.

IMPORTANT CONDITIONS TO REPORT

Worsening of symptoms

Continuation of symptoms

Ongoing concerns

Any symptoms of mastitis, including:

    Plugged ducts.

    Visible red areas on the breast(s).

    Fever higher than 101°F (38.5°C).

    Extreme breast discomfort.

    Flu-like aching throughout the body.

NOTES

Because production of milk relies on many different body systems in both mother and baby, any milk supply problem requires consideration of maternal and infant factors.

Occasionally, medical factors such as endocrine imbalance and the use of medications require evaluation.

See also Australian posture; Block nursing; Clenching or clamping onto the nipple/areola; Mastitis; Plugged ducts; Milk flow, too fast; Overactive let-down reflex; Oversupply

➤ MILK FLOW, TOO SLOW

DEFINITION   Delayed or slow milk flow may be due to a low milk supply, poor let-down, or both. The nipple may be stretched inadequately due to faulty latch. Rarely, flow may be impeded temporarily by sudden high levels of adrenalin due to acute stress or crisis.

ASK ABOUT

Age of the baby.

Weight gain pattern of baby.

History of breast surgery.

ASSESSMENT

PROMPT MEDICAL CARE NEEDED?

Are any of the following present?

Meconium bowel movements after 5 days of life.

No yellow stool by day 5.

Fewer than three bowel movements daily in breastfed newborn after the first 2 days of life.

No urine in 6 hours.

Brick dust urine (uric acid crystals) after 2 days of life.

Dark-colored urine.

Fewer than four urinations daily in the breastfed newborn after day 5 of life.

Noticeably sunken fontanelles (soft spot on the top of the head).

Decreased activity.

Weight loss of more than 7% from birth or further weight loss by day 5.

Cessation of weight gain.

IF YES,   *Seek pediatric care now and call lactation care provider today.*

PROMPT LACTATION CARE NEEDED?

Are any of the following present?

Breastfeeding lasting longer than 20 minutes.

Newborn weight gain of less than 0.5 oz per day on average.

No change in suckling rhythm to a suck-to-swallow ratio of 2:1 or 1:1 in bursts.

Concern about adequacy of milk supply.

IF YES,   *Seek lactation care today.*

SELF-CARE INFORMATION

Some mothers never feel the sensation of let-down or any of the signs of let-down such as thirst and uterine contractions.

Collecting milk by using a breast pump or hand expression is not the same as breastfeeding; you cannot determine how much a baby is transferring by how much milk is collected.

Milk flow can be enhanced with alternate breast massage and compression.

IMPORTANT CONDITIONS TO REPORT
Increased infant lethargy.
Decrease in number of stools and wet diapers.
Decrease in infant weight gain.

NOTES

Babies with a history of long feedings (more than 20 minutes per breast) should be evaluated by a lactation care provider.

See also Alternate breast massage; Insufficient milk supply; Latch-on; Let-down reflex; Milk-ejection reflex; Slow weight gain, baby

➤ MILK PRODUCTION

DEFINITION The synthesis of a nutritive fluid by mammary cells in the breast. There is a wide variance in the volume of milk intake among healthy breastfed infants, but during the first 4 months, women produce about 750 ml per day.[220] But women can make much more; some women can make more than 4,000 ml per day.[221]

See also Increasing milk supply; Milk production; Test weighing

Footnotes

[220]Butte, N. F., Wong, W. W., Garza, C., Stuff, J. E., Smith, E. O., Klein, P. D., & Nichols, B. L. (1991). Energy requirements of breast-fed infants. *Journal of the American College of Nutrition, 10*, 190–195.

[221]Saint, L., Maggiore, P., & Hartmann, P. E. (1986). Yield and nutrient content of milk in eight women breast-feeding twins and one woman breast-feeding triplets. *British Journal of Nutrition, 56*, 49–58.

➤ MILK STORAGE BAGS

DEFINITION   Soft waterproof bags specifically designed to store milk. Some are suitable for collecting milk into directly, refrigerating or freezing the milk, and fitting into a rigid holder for feeding.

SELF-CARE INFORMATION

Be sure to read and follow the manufacturer's instructions carefully.

If you are freezing the milk, leave room for expansion (liquids expand when they are frozen).

Prevent spillage and puncture.

See also Collection and storage of breastmilk

➤ MILK SUPPLY, INADEQUATE

DEFINITION   Insufficient amount of milk produced by the breast. Maternal, infant, and environmental factors all contribute to milk supply problems.

Milk supply can usually be increased by increasing stimulation and removal of milk from the breast.

ASK ABOUT

Onset.

Age of the baby.

ASSESSMENT

EMERGENT CARE NEEDED?

Are any of the following present?

Exclusively breastfed newborn baby with less than one stool per day.

Meconium bowel movements after 5 days of life.

No yellow stool by day 5.

Fewer than three bowel movements daily in breastfed newborn after the first 2 days of life.

No urine in 6 hours.

Brick dust urine (uric acid crystals) after 2 days of life.

Dark-colored urine.

Fewer than four urinations daily in the breastfed newborn after day 5 of life.

Noticeably sunken fontanelles (soft spot on the top of the head).

Decreased activity.

Weight loss of more than 7% from birth or further weight loss by day 5.

Cessation of weight gain.

IF YES,   *Seek pediatric care now.*

PROMPT LACTATION CARE NEEDED?

Are any of the following present?

Identified milk supply problem.

Concern about possible milk supply problem.

IF YES,   *Call lactation care provider today.*

SELF-CARE INFORMATION

Ensure baby is feeding 10–12 times per 24 hours.

Express milk after feeding.

IMPORTANT CONDITIONS TO REPORT
Persistent problems.
Recurrent problems.

See also Increasing milk supply

➤ MILK TRANSFER, ESTIMATING

DEFINITION   Estimate of milk transfer by weighing the baby before and after nursing with an accurate (to 2 grams) digital scale. It is important to realize that the same volume of milk is probably not transferred at each nursing.

NOTES

The amount of milk a woman pumps or collects via hand expression may not be related to the amount the baby can transfer.

See also Electronic scales; Increasing milk supply; Milk production

➤ MIXED FEEDS

DEFINITION   Combining formula or solid foods with breastfeeding.

ASK ABOUT

Age of the baby.
Diet of the baby.
Weight gain of the baby.

ASSESSMENT

EMERGENT CARE NEEDED?

Are any of the following present?

Difficulty breathing

Meconium bowel movements after 5 days of life.

No yellow stool by day 5.

Fewer than three bowel movements daily in breastfed newborn after the first 2 days of life.

No urine in 6 hours.

Brick dust urine (uric acid crystals) after 2 days of life.

Dark-colored urine.

Fewer than four urinations daily in the breastfed newborn after day 5 of life.

Noticeably sunken fontanelles (soft spot on the top of the head).

Decreased activity.

Irritability and excessive crying.

IF YES,   *Seek pediatric care now.*

PROMPT MEDICAL CARE NEEDED?

Are any of the following present?

Eczema.

Hives.

Vomiting.

Diarrhea.

Blood in the stools.

IF YES,   *Seek medical care today.*

PROMPT LACTATION CARE NEEDED?

Are any of the following present?

Identified milk supply problem.

Desire to increase milk supply.

Education needed about combining breast and formula feeding or adding family foods.

IF YES,   *Call lactation care provider today.*

SELF-CARE INFORMATION

Solid foods do not help babies sleep through the night.

IMPORTANT CONDITIONS TO REPORT

Signs of dehydration (scanty, dark urine).

Difficulty breathing.

Eczema.

Hives.

Vomiting.

Diarrhea.

Blood in the stools.

Irritability and excessive crying.

NOTES

Full (exclusive) breastfeeding for about the first 6 months of life is recommended by the American Academy of Pediatrics Committee on Breastfeeding, the World Health Organization, the U.S. Breastfeeding Committee, and other policy groups.

See also Allergy in the breastfed infant; Formula, infant; Supplemental feeding devices

➤ MOMSRISING

DESCRIPTION MomsRising describes itself as a "transformative online and on-the-ground multicultural organization of more than million members and over a hundred aligned organizations working to increase family economic security, to end discrimination against women and mothers, and to build a nation where both businesses and families can thrive."[222(p1)]

Footnote

[222]MomsRising. (2011). About MomsRising. Retrieved from http://www.momsrising.org/page /moms/aboutmomsrising

➤ MONTGOMERY GLANDS (MONTGOMERY'S TUBERCLES)

DEFINITION   A group of 12–20 tubercles scattered around the areola of the breast that enlarge during pregnancy and lactation. These tubercles are connected to a combination of lactiferous glands and sebaceous glands. The substance secreted is both lubricating and antimicrobial.

SELF-CARE INFORMATION

Excessive cleaning of the breast and areola is not necessary and is not recommended.

IMPORTANT CONDITIONS TO REPORT

Blocked or infected Montgomery glands.

NOTES

Blocked or infected Montgomery glands look very similar to herpes lesions. Herpes can be deadly to newborns. Because of this, appearance of blocked or infected Montgomery glands must always be referred immediately to a healthcare provider.

See also Breast structure

➤ MONTGOMERY'S TUBERCLES

See Montgomery glands (Montgomery's tubercles)

➤ MOTHER-FRIENDLY CHILDBIRTH INITIATIVE (MFCI)

DEFINITION   A set of 10 steps for hospitals, birth centers, and other birth services for provision of mother-friendly care during childbirth. This initiative is a project of the Coalition for Improving Maternity Services.

See also Coalition for Improving Maternity Services (CIMS)

➤ MOTHER OF PRETERM INFANT

DEFINITION   Mothers of babies who are born before completion of the 37 weeks from the onset of the last menstrual period.

ASK ABOUT

Gestational age of the baby.
Drugs prescribed for the mother.

ASSESSMENT

ROUTINE CARE NEEDED?

Are any of the following present?

Declining milk supply.
Difficulty transitioning the baby to breastfeeding.
Questions about breast pumps or expressing milk.

IF YES,   *Call lactation care provider today.*

SELF-CARE INFORMATION

Begin hand expression as soon as possible after the baby is born. Add pumping with a breast pump when milk volume warrants. Continue to hand express after each pumping.

Begin skin-to-skin contact and kangaroo care with the baby as soon as permitted.

Express milk at least eight times a day for best milk supply.

Use a pump designed for pump-dependent mothers (an automatic cycling pump that can remove milk from both breasts at the same time).

IMPORTANT CONDITIONS TO REPORT

Concern about milk supply.

See also Breast pump; Decrease in milk supply; Increasing milk supply; Kangaroo care; Preterm milk; Transition to breastfeeding

➤ MOTHER-TO-MOTHER COUNSELING

DEFINITION   Delivery of breastfeeding support via trained, knowledgeable women who have breastfed a child of their own.

See also La Leche League, International; Peer counseling

➤ MS

See Multiple sclerosis (MS)

➤ MUCOSA-ASSOCIATED LYMPHOID TISSUE (MALT)

DEFINITION   Lymphoid tissue in the human body is associated with the mucosal system. Mucosa-associated lymphoid tissue (MALT) is scattered along the body's mucosal linings and serves to protect the body from antigens that could potentially enter along mucosal surfaces. The direct secretion of secretory immunoglobulin A (IgA) onto mucosal epithelia represents the major mechanism of MALT.

➤ MULTIPLE INFANTS (TWINS, TRIPLETS, AND HIGHER ORDER MULTIPLES)

DEFINITION   Refers to the birth of more than one infant from the same pregnancy. Mothers can nurse more than one baby. Increased suckling, especially nursing two babies simultaneously, stimulates an increased supply of milk.

Multiples may be born prematurely, spend weeks or months in the hospital before discharge, and may not be discharged on the same day.

Mothers may express milk to be fed to hospitalized babies. Hand expression should start as soon after the babies are born as possible with pumping using an electric pump added as soon as volume warrants. Continue hand expression after pumping. Mothers should express eight or more times per day.

ASK ABOUT

Age of the babies.

ASSESSMENT

PROMPT CARE NEEDED?

Are any of the following present?

Imminent birth of multiple infants in a woman planning to breastfeed.

Initiation of breastfeeding in a woman with multiple hospitalized babies.

Problems with breastfeeding multiples.

IF YES,   *Call lactation care provider now.*

ROUTINE CARE NEEDED?

Are any of the following present?

Need for strategies for managing the nursing of multiples.

Strategies for managing milk supply for multiples.

IF YES,   *Call lactation care provider today.*

SELF-CARE INFORMATION

Nursing babies simultaneously is helpful for building a milk supply, but may be difficult to manage at first. Ask for help with positioning.

At first, switch the babies from one breast to another. As the babies get older, they may prefer nursing on a particular breast.

Many mothers have found it helpful at first to write down who nursed when to ensure that each baby gets enough.

IMPORTANT CONDITIONS TO REPORT

Lethargy.

Decrease in urine and stools.

Change in breastfeeding behavior.

Problems with feeding.

NOTES

Mothers carrying multiple infants are more likely to deliver prematurely, especially when carrying higher order multiples. Additional time is needed for mothers to recover from multiple pregnancy and birth. Focus on the mother's needs as well as those of the babies.

See also Breast pump; Higher order multiples (HOM); Premature infant; Triplets; Twins

➤ MULTIPLE SCLEROSIS (MS)

DEFINITION   An autoimmune disease of the central nervous system (CNS). In general, people with MS can experience partial or complete loss of any function that is controlled by or passes through the brain or spinal cord.

SELF-CARE INFORMATION

Being breastfed and breastfeeding may be related to a decreased chance of MS in later life.[223]

NOTES

Breastfeeding is not contraindicated for a woman with MS.

See also Autoimmune diseases

Footnote

[223]Pisacane, A., Impagliazzo, N., Russo, M., Valiani, R., Mandarini, A., Florio, C., & Vivo, P. (1994). Breast feeding and multiple sclerosis. *British Medical Journal, 308*, 1411–1412.

➤ MUSCLE TONE OF INFANT

DEFINITION   Tone refers to the ability of the muscles to be firm and to tense, allowing motion in the body. Infant muscle tone can be normal, low, or overreactive. Infants with normal tone have flexed elbows and knees. Low muscle tone is called hypotonia. Overreactive tone is called hypertonia. Hypotonic babies seem floppy. Their elbows and knees are loosely extended. Hypertonic babies may arch their bodies away from the breast. Babies who have these symptoms can be more difficult to breastfeed.

Hypotonia and hypertonia can sometimes be symptoms of other problems. Some of the problems that may be seen with breastfeeding include a nonrhythmic suck, biting when swallowing (tonic bite reflex), weak reflexes for sucking, swallowing, and gagging. Babies also may tire more easily.

Malnourished babies have decreased muscle tone.

ASK ABOUT

Age of the baby.
Onset of hypotonia or hypertonia.
Change in feeding behavior.
Change in urination or stooling patterns.

ASSESSMENT

EMERGENT CARE NEEDED?

Are any of the following present?

Sudden change in muscle tone.

Sudden change in feeding behavior.

IF YES,   *Seek emergency care now and contact pediatric care provider immediately.*

PROMPT CARE NEEDED?

Are any of the following present?

Feeding problems.

Weight loss or slow/inadequate weight gain.

Constipation or decrease in stool output.

IF YES,   *Seek pediatric care today.*

ROUTINE CARE NEEDED?

Are any of the following present?

Problems positioning baby at breast.

Concerns about milk supply.

IF YES,   *Call lactation care provider today.*

SELF-CARE INFORMATION

Breastfeeding and breastmilk are valuable for babies with low or overreactive muscle tone.

Hand expression and pumping may be necessary to maintain an adequate milk supply.

"Wearing" the baby in a safe sling or baby carrier can be very helpful to encourage flexion in a hyperextending infant.

IMPORTANT CONDITIONS TO REPORT

Change in feeding behaviors.

Change in urination or stooling patterns.

Declining breastmilk volume.

NOTES

Because low muscle tone can be a sign of malnutrition, floppy babies should always be evaluated promptly. Similarly, stiffness can be a marker of infection and should be evaluated promptly as well.

See also Milk production; Premature infant; Test weighing

➤ MYOEPITHELIAL CELLS

DEFINITION   Specialized, smooth muscle-like cells that surround the milk-making cells. The hormone oxytocin causes these cells to contract. This moves the milk toward the nipple and out of the breast. The action of the myoepithelial cells is called the "let-down" or "milk-ejection" reflex.

See also Let-down reflex; Milk-ejection reflex; Oxytocin

➤ NABA

See National Alliance for Breastfeeding Advocacy: Research, Education, and Legal (NABA-REAL)

➤ NAPNAP

See National Association of Pediatric Nurse Practitioners (NAPNAP)

➤ NATIONAL ALLIANCE FOR BREASTFEEDING ADVOCACY: RESEARCH, EDUCATION, AND LEGAL (NABA REAL)

DESCRIPTION Organization that "functions to educate the public, state and federal legislators, policymakers, government agencies, and the health care system about breastfeeding and the hazards of not breastfeeding. It does this through numerous activities, including Code monitoring."[224(p1)]

NOTES

NABA REAL
Email: Barbara@naba-breastfeeding.org
Web: www.naba-breastfeeding.org
   NABA REAL monitors the WHO International Code of Marketing of Breast-milk Substitutes in the United States through a variety of activities.

Footnote

[224]National Alliance for Breastfeeding Advocacy. (n.d.). NABA REAL. Retrieved from http://www.naba-breastfeeding.org/nabareal.htm

➤ NATIONAL ASSOCIATION OF PEDIATRIC NURSE PRACTITIONERS (NAPNAP)

DEFINITION NAPNAP is the professional association for PNPs and other advanced practice nurses who care for children. Established in 1973, NAPNAP has been actively advocating for children's health by: providing funding, education, and research opportunities to PNPs; influencing legislation that affects maternal/child health care; and producing and distributing educational materials to parents and families.[225(p1)]

National Association of Pediatric Nurse Practitioners (NAPNAP)
Email: info@napnap.org
Web: www.napnap.org
   NAPNAP includes information and articles about breastfeeding in its publications, website, and educational offerings.

Footnote

[225]National Association of Pediatric Nurse Practitioners. (2010). About NAPNAP. Retrieved from http://www.napnap.org/aboutUs.aspx

➤ NATIONAL BLACK NURSES ASSOCIATION

DESCRIPTION   "The National Black Nurses Association (NBNA) was organized in 1971 under the leadership of Dr. Lauranne Sams, former Dean and Professor of Nursing, School of Nursing, Tuskegee University, Tuskegee, Alabama. NBNA is a non-profit organization incorporated on September 2, 1972 in the state of Ohio . . . The NBNA mission is 'to provide a forum for collective action by African American nurses to investigate, define and determine what the health care needs of African Americans are and to implement change to make available to African Americans and other minorities health care commensurate with that of the larger society.'"[226(p1)]

National Black Nurses Association (NBNA)
Email: contact@nbna.org
Web: www.nbna.org/
   NBNA offers education and information about breastfeeding through its educational offerings and publications.

Footnote

[226]National Black Nurses Association. (2012). Who we are. Retrieved from http://www.nbna.org/index.php?option=com_content&view=article&id=44&Itemid=60

➤ NATIONAL COMMISSION ON DONOR MILK BANKING

See American Breastfeeding Institute (ABI)

➤ NATIONAL HEALTHY MOTHERS, HEALTHY BABIES COALITION (HMHB)

DESCRIPTION "The National Healthy Mothers, Healthy Babies Coalition (HMHB) is a recognized leader and resource in maternal and child health, reaching an estimated 10 million health care professionals, parents, and policymakers through its membership of over 100 local, state and national organizations. HMHB's mission is to improve the health and safety of mothers, babies and families through educational materials and collaborative partnerships."[227](p1)

NOTES

National Healthy Mothers, Healthy Babies Coalition (HMHB)
Email: info@hmhb.org
Web: www.hmhb.org
   National and local HMHB coalitions often engage in breastfeeding promotion activities.

Footnote

[227]National Healthy Mothers, Healthy Babies Coalition. (2011). About us. Retrieved from http://www.hmhb.org/aboutus.html

➤ NATIONAL PERINATAL ASSOCIATION (NPA)

DESCRIPTION An organization that "promotes the health and well being of mothers and infants enriching families, communities and our world. NPA will engage the broadest possible coalition to improve social, cultural and economic environments for the optimal health and well being of mothers, infants and families."[228](Mission & Vision)

NOTES

Email: npa@nationalperinatal.org
Web: www.nationalperinatal.org/

Footnote

[230]National Perinatal Association. (2012). History. Retrieved from http://www.nationalperinatal .org/history.php

➤ NATIONAL WIC ASSOCIATION (NWA)

DESCRIPTION   "The National WIC Association (NWA) is the non-profit education arm and advocacy voice of the Special Supplemental Nutrition Program for Women, Infants and Children Program (WIC), the over 9 million mothers and young children served by WIC and the 12,000 service provider Agencies who are the front lines of WIC's public health nutrition services for the nation's nutritionally at-risk mothers and young children."[229(p1)]

NOTES

Web: www.nwica.org
   NWA advocates and educates about breastfeeding through workshops, position papers, and other activities.

See also United States Department of Agriculture (USDA), Special Supplemental Food Program for Women, Infants, and Children (WIC)

Footnote

[229]National WIC Association. (2011). About NWA. Retrieved from http://www.nwica.org/?q=nwa/1

➤ NATURAL FAMILY PLANNING

DEFINITION   Refers to child spacing methods that do not require use of medications or devices. Natural family planning is focused on planning or preventing pregnancy based on when a woman is fertile. Women may want to use natural family planning methods for religious, medical, or personal reasons. The **lactational amenorrhea method (LAM)** is a type of natural family planning that can be used during the first 6 months of breastfeeding.

See also Bellagio Consensus; Child spacing; Fertility; Lactational amenorrhea method (LAM)

➤ NEC

See Necrotizing enterocolitis (NEC); Premature infant; Preterm milk

➤ NECROTIZING ENTEROCOLITIS (NEC)

DEFINITION   The most common surgical emergency in newborns, especially premature babies. The intestine reacts with an inflammatory response to feedings, leading to intestinal necrosis (tissue death). There is no single explanation for why NEC happens, but formula feeding is one factor that has been associated with its incidence.

See also Premature infant; Preterm milk

➤ NEONATAL HYPOGLYCEMIA

DEFINITION   Low blood sugar in an infant. It happens because the infant's blood glucose (sugar) levels have fallen below a recommended or acceptable level.

ASK ABOUT

Age of the baby.
Gestational age of the baby.
History of diabetes in the mother.
History of labor, especially stress.

ASSESSMENT

EMERGENT CARE NEEDED?

Are any of the following present?

Seizure activity.

Convulsions.

Coma.

Respiratory distress.

Apnea (cessation of breathing).

Cyanosis (blue color of the skin).

Thermoregulatory problems.

Jitteriness.

Hypotonia (floppy or low muscle tone).

Lethargy.

Listlessness.

Poor feeding.

IF YES,   *Seek emergency care and call pediatrician immediately.*

PROMPT CARE NEEDED?

Are any of the following present?

Breastfed infant with identified hypoglycemia.

Breastfeeding problems or questions.

Concern about milk supply.

IF YES,   *Call lactation care provider now.*

SELF-CARE INFORMATION

Establish early and frequent breastfeeding.

Keep the baby warm and dry.

Practice frequent skin-to-skin contact at the breast (babies can stay very warm in your arms). To do this, strip the baby down to a diaper, remove your bra, and place the baby against your skin, inside your shirt. Put a hat on the baby's head and cover yourself and the baby with a blanket if the room air is cold.

Seek help with breastfeeding if the baby feeds poorly.

IMPORTANT CONDITIONS TO REPORT

Seizure activity.

Convulsions.

Coma.

Respiratory distress.

Apnea (cessation of breathing).

Cyanosis (blue color).

Thermoregulatory problems.

Jitteriness.

Hypotonia (floppy muscle tone).

Lethargy.

Listlessness.

Poor feeding.

See also Colostrum; Muscle tone of infant

➤ NEONATAL INTENSIVE CARE UNIT (NICU)

DEFINITION   A special hospital unit providing care for premature and ill infants.

➤ NEONATAL JAUNDICE

DEFINITION   Neonatal jaundice is a condition caused by an excessive amount of bilirubin. It is the most common condition requiring medical treatment in the newborn period. Because bilirubin is yellow, the color accumulates in the baby's skin and the sclera (whites) of the eyes. The baby may appear tan, yellow, or light orange in color. Bilirubin is removed from the blood by the liver. Although the condition of jaundice may be benign, it may be associated with serious conditions such as **kernicterus**, hemolysis, and liver disease.

ASK ABOUT

Age of the baby.
Feeding behavior.
Stooling pattern and color.
Urination pattern.

ASSESSMENT

EMERGENT CARE NEEDED?

Are any of the following present?

No stool in 24 hours.
Severe lethargy (sleepiness) or irritability.
Poor feeding.
Fever.
Yellow skin.
Gray or white stool.

IF YES,   *Seek emergency care now and call pediatric care provider immediately.*

PROMPT CARE NEEDED?

Are any of the following present?

Breastfed baby with jaundice diagnosis.

IF YES,   *Call lactation care provider today.*

SELF-CARE INFORMATION

Breastfeed as soon as possible after birth.

Encourage the baby to nurse 10–12 times per 24 hours.

Colostrum has laxative properties. Stooling helps to rid the baby's body of bilirubin.

IMPORTANT CONDITIONS TO REPORT

No stool in 24 hours.

Severe lethargy (sleepiness).

Poor feeding.

Fever.

Yellow skin.

Gray or white stool.

NOTES

All jaundiced babies are at risk for kernicterus and should be closely monitored. Gray or white stool may indicate biliary atresia, a serious congenital problem with the bile ducts of the liver.

See also Bilirubin; Colostrum; Jaundice; Kernicterus; Late-onset jaundice

➤ NEONATE

DEFINITION   A newborn infant. The World Health Organization defines the neonatal period as that time which "commences at birth and ends 28 completed days after birth."[230]

Footnote

[230]World Health Organization. (2012). Health Status Statistics: Mortality. *WHO*. Retrieved from http://www.who.int/healthinfo/statistics/indneonatalmortality/en/

➤ NEURAL TUBE DEFECTS

DEFINITION   Congenital problems involving the covering of the nervous system. As the baby develops in utero, the neural tube is the part of the baby that will grow into the spinal cord and brain. Normally, bones grow around the brain and spinal cord, and then skin covers the bones. A neural tube defect results when this has not happened. Spina bifida is the most common neural tube defect. Anencephaly is a neural tube defect in which the brain and spinal cord do not form properly. Anencephaly is always fatal.

SELF-CARE INFORMATION

A mother of a baby with spina bifida can express milk for her baby until the baby's condition allows breastfeeding.

IMPORTANT CONDITIONS TO REPORT

Problems expressing milk.
Decreased amount of expressed milk.

See also Breast pump; Hospitalization; Increasing milk supply; Milk production

➤ NEWBORN

DEFINITION   A neonate. The World Health Organization defines the neonatal period as that time which "commences at birth and ends 28 completed days after birth."[231]

Footnote

[231] World Health Organization. (2012). Health Status Statistics: Mortality. *WHO*. Retrieved from http://www.who.int/healthinfo/statistics/indneonatalmortality/en/

➤ NICOTINE

DEFINITION Chief addictive component of tobacco.

ASK ABOUT

Age of the baby.
Weight gain pattern of baby.

ASSESSMENT

ROUTINE CARE NEEDED?

Are any of the following present?

Using pacifier to delay, shorten, or eliminate breastfeeding.

More than 12 feedings daily.

Irritable baby.

Smoking in the baby's environment.

Concern about milk supply.

Poor feeding.

Desire to cut down on or stop smoking.

Upper respiratory problems in the baby (coughing, runny nose, etc.).

IF YES, *Seek pediatric care now and call lactation care provider today.*

SELF-CARE INFORMATION

Babies and children should always be protected from second- and third-hand smoke.

Research indicates that mothers who smoke may make and secrete less milk, but if they cut down or stop smoking, their milk supply may rebound.

Breastfeeding mothers who smoke should encourage frequent feedings to stimulate milk production and should also avoid excessive pacifier use, as this may decrease milk supply.

Breastfeeding may mitigate the effects to the baby of smoking during pregnancy.[232]

IMPORTANT CONDITIONS TO REPORT

Weight loss or poor weight gain pattern.

Poor feeding.

Upper respiratory problems in the baby (coughing or runny nose).

NOTES

Mothers who smoke tobacco may breastfeed, but they should cut down on smoking and be encouraged to quit if possible. Babies should always be protected from secondhand (that breathed from the smoke of cigarettes) and thirdhand (that carried on clothing, furniture, etc.) smoke.

Exposing babies and children to secondhand smoke can have serious health consequences and should be avoided.

See also Medications; Smoking

Footnote

[232]Batstra, L., Neeleman, J., & Hadders-Algra, M. (2003). Can breastfeeding modify the adverse effects of smoking during pregnancy on the child's cognitive development? *Journal of Epidemiology and Community Health, 57*(6), 403–404.

➤ NICU

DEFINITION   Neonatal intensive care unit. A special hospital unit providing care for premature and ill infants.

➤ NICU, MILK STORAGE AND HANDLING IN

DEFINITION   Special requirements for milk collection and storage for ill, hospitalized babies.

NOTES

Each neonatal care unit provides its own directions for methods and materials used to collect and store milk for ill babies.

Encourage mothers to contact the NICU for specific requirements of the unit where their babies are hospitalized.

Contact the **Human Milk Banking Association of North America (HMBANA)** for recommended milk storage guidelines for NICU settings.

See also Breast pump; Collection and storage of breastmilk; Human Milk Banking Association of North America (HMBANA)

➤ NIGHT NURSINGS

DEFINITION   Refers to at-breast feeding episodes that occur during the night. Night-time nursings are desirable in the early months to ensure that babies are getting enough to eat. Sleeping longer than 5 hours at a stretch is the operative definition of sleeping through the night.

ASK ABOUT

Age of the baby.
Weight gain pattern.

ASSESSMENT

ROUTINE CARE NEEDED?

Are any of the following present?

> Baby older than 4 months.
> Parents want fewer night feedings.

IF YES,   *Call lactation care provider.*

SELF-CARE INFORMATION

Daytime interventions work best to cut back on nighttime nursings. Babies who sleep a lot during the day and feed infrequently need to make up for the lack of nourishment by nursing frequently at night.

IMPORTANT CONDITIONS TO REPORT

Poor feedings.
Increased wakening.
Weight loss or poor weight gain.

NOTES

Many mothers find it more comforting to nurse their babies back to sleep, as compared to training the baby to go back to sleep. Baby training should never be attempted with babies younger than 4 months, babies who are poor nursers, or babies who are not gaining well.

See also Maternal fatigue

➤ NINE STAGES

DEFINITION   The normal sequence of newborn activities culminating in feeding and sleep that are seen in the first hours after birth when the infant is placed on the mother's chest and kept there in direct skin-to-skin contact continuously and uninterrupted.[233]

Footnote

[233]Widström, A.-M., Lilja, G., Aaltomaa-Michalias, P., Dahllöf, A., Lintula, M., & Nissen, E. (2011). Newborn behaviour to locate the breast when skin-to-skin: A possible method for enabling early self-regulation. *Acta Paediatrica (Oslo, Norway: 1992), 100*(1), 79–85. doi:10.1111/j.1651-2227 .2010.01983.x

➤ NIPPLE

DEFINITION   The protuberant part of the breast that contains the endings of the lactiferous ducts from which the milk flows.

➤ NIPPLE CREAMS OR OINTMENTS

DEFINITION   Topical preparations that have been made for several purposes, such as to protect the skin, to decrease itching, to clean the skin (antiseptics), and to moisturize the skin.

ASK ABOUT

Nipple discomfort.

ASSESSMENT

ROUTINE CARE NEEDED?

Are any of the following present?

Sore nipples.

Painful breastfeeding.

Skin rash, breakouts, or itching on the breast, areola, and nipple.

IF YES,   *Report symptoms to obstetric care provider today and call lactation care provider today to schedule a feeding evaluation.*

SELF-CARE INFORMATION

Most ointments and creams are not intended for ingestion. When a mother applies an ointment or cream to her areola or nipple, her baby will be exposed to the ingredients during nursing.

Only use ointments and creams on the breast that are recommended for this purpose. Never use a product that has been prescribed for another problem.

Mothers can have adverse reactions to ointments and creams. Report any changes immediately.

Breast milk and Montgomery gland secretions provide natural antimicrobial lubrication of the nipple and areola.

IMPORTANT CONDITIONS TO REPORT

Symptoms worsen or persist.

Signs of infection.

Feeding or stooling expectations are not met.

NOTES

Women experiencing **nipple pain** may self-treat with these and other inappropriate substances.

Women experiencing nipple pain should have a breastfeeding evaluation. Face-to-face counseling is effective in assessing and resolving nipple pain.

See also Breast inflammation; Breast pain; Creams and ointments; Nipple pain; Sore nipples

➤ NIPPLE EVERTER

DEFINITION   A device designed to pull out inverted nipples.

NOTES

Research does not support use of such devices.

See also Nipple, inverted

➤ NIPPLE, FLAT

DEFINITION   Nipples that appear level with surrounding tissue.

ASK ABOUT

Appearance of the nipple.
Change in nipple appearance after feeding or pumping.
Action of the nipple when exposed to the cold.
Nipple changes during pregnancy and lactation.
Diagnosis of flat nipple.

ASSESSMENT

PROMPT CARE NEEDED?

Are any of the following present?

> Poor feeding.
>
> Poor milk transfer.
>
> Inadequate weight gain.
>
> Problems with latch-on.
>
> Concern about milk supply.

IF YES, *Report symptoms to pediatric care provider and call lactation care provider today.*

SELF-CARE INFORMATION

Mothers with flat nipples should be encouraged to express milk early and frequently until the baby is able to facilitate nipple stretching well into the mouth.

IMPORTANT CONDITIONS TO REPORT

Poor feeding.
Poor milk transfer.
Inadequate weight gain.
Problems with latch-on.

NOTES

Training flat nipples to stand out during pregnancy is an ineffective technique.

See also Milk transfer, estimating; Weight gain, baby–low

➤ NIPPLE, INVERTED

DEFINITION   The nipple is the protuberant part of the breast that contains the endings of the lactiferous ducts from which the milk flows as well as the nerve endings that signal the release of prolactin and oxytocin. With inverted nipples, the nipple looks like a slit or a fold and may retreat further into the breast when stimulated. The nipple does not protrude when stimulated.

ASK ABOUT

Appearance of the nipple.
Action of the nipple when the nipple or areola is stimulated.
Nipple changes during pregnancy and lactation.
Diagnosis of inverted nipple.

ASSESSMENT

PROMPT MEDICAL CARE NEEDED?

Are any of the following present?

Meconium bowel movements after 5 days of life.
Fewer than three bowel movements daily in a breastfed newborn after the first 2 days of life.
No urine in 6 hours.
Brick dust urine (uric acid crystals) after 2 days of life.
No yellow stool by 5 days.
Dark-colored urine.
Fewer than four urinations daily in the breastfed newborn after day 5 of life.
Noticeably sunken fontanelles (soft spot on the top of the head).
Decreased activity.
Baby below birthweight at 10–14 days of life.
Cessation of/inadequate weight gain.
Problems with latch-on.

IF YES,   *Seek pediatric care now and call lactation care provider today.*

SELF-CARE INFORMATION

Practice skin-to-skin contact in the first hour and frequently thereafter. Skin-to-skin immediately after birth with the baby's initial self-attachment at the breast contributes to effective latch. Trying to train inverted nipples to stand out during pregnancy is ineffective.

Mothers with inverted nipples should be encouraged to express milk early and frequently until the baby is able to facilitate stretching the nipple deeply into the mouth. Close postpartum follow-up is necessary to assure adequate nutrition and weight gain of the baby.

IMPORTANT CONDITIONS TO REPORT

Poor feeding.

Poor milk transfer.

Inadequate weight gain.

Problems with latch-on.

See also Insufficient milk supply; Milk transfer, estimating; Weight gain, baby—low

➤ NIPPLE PAIN

DEFINITION   Uncomfortable sensation in the nipples. Pain is not an expected part of breastfeeding and indicates need for feeding evaluation. There can be many reasons for pain in the breast, including nipple trauma, bleb, milk blisters, poor latch and/or positioning and infection.

ASK ABOUT

Onset.

Location of pain.

Whether the pain is unilateral or bilateral.

ASSESSMENT

PROMPT MEDICAL CARE NEEDED?

Are any of the following present?

Open fissure of nipple with pus.

Maternal fever.

Maternal malaise.

Pain combined with color change of nipple(s).

IF YES, *Call obstetric or primary care provider now.*

PROMPT LACTATION CARE NEEDED?

Are any of the following present?

Persistent pain with feeding.

Persistent pain between feedings.

Constant pain.

Pain combined with color change of nipple(s).

Pain with visible fissure or bleeding of the nipple(s).

IF YES, *Call lactation care provider now to schedule a feeding evaluation.*

ROUTINE CARE NEEDED?

Are any of the following present?

Brief nipple pain at beginning of feeding.

Mild, recurrent nipple pain.

IF YES, *Call lactation care provider today.*

SELF-CARE INFORMATION

Practice skin-to-skin contact in the first hour and frequently thereafter.

Feed the baby at the first sign of hunger cues (signs that say "feed me" include hand-to-face or hand-to-mouth movements, lip smacking, seeking with lips, rooting, and head bobbing).

Feed the baby at least 10 times per 24 hours.

Listen for signs of the baby swallowing.

Allow the baby to end feedings.

Expect at least three infant stools per 24 hours after the first 4 days of life.

Expect yellow stools by day 5.

Good positioning and attachment are crucial to prevent or reduce nipple pain.

If feedings are missed, hand express or pump milk to maintain supply.

NOTES

Breastfeeding should not be painful. Advise mothers to seek medical or lactation care for breast pain.

See also Bleb; Blisters on nipple or breast; Latch-on; Mastitis; Nipple shields; Raynaud's phenomenon/syndrome; Sore nipples

➤ NIPPLE SHIELDS

DEFINITION   Nipple shields are devices made of silicone or rubber that are used to cover the surface of the nipple during a feeding. They come in a variety of sizes and shapes. These devices are commonly used to help with latch-on problems and nipple pain; however, a 2010 review of the literature on their use concluded that "current published research does not provide evidence for safety or effectiveness of contemporary nipple shield use."[234(p309)]

ASK ABOUT

Age of the baby.

History of weight gain.

Stooling pattern.

Urination pattern.

ASSESSMENT

PROMPT CARE NEEDED?

Are any of the following present?

Desire to obtain a nipple shield.

Desire to wean the baby off a nipple shield.

Concern about adequacy of milk supply.

IF YES,   *Call lactation care provider today.*

SELF-CARE INFORMATION

Use of nipple shields has been associated with decreased milk transfer and poor weight gain in babies.

Frequent weight checks and milk transfer assessments should be part of the baby's routine care when a mother uses a nipple shield for feedings.

IMPORTANT CONDITIONS TO REPORT

Lethargy or poor feeding.

Weight loss or slow weight gain.

Decrease in the stooling or urination pattern.

NOTES

Nipple shields have been shown to be helpful for premature babies transitioning to the breast. The mother continues to express her milk in order to maintain her milk supply.

See also Nipple pain

Footnote

[234]McKechnie, A. C., & Eglash, A. (2010). Nipple shields: A review of the literature. *Breastfeeding Medicine: The Official Journal of the Academy of Breastfeeding Medicine, 5*(6), 309–314. doi:10.1089/bfm.2010.0003

➤ NNS

See Nonnutritive suckling (NNS)

➤ NONNUTRITIVE SUCKLING (NNS)

DEFINITION   The situation in which the baby suckles but there is low milk transfer.

> **NOTES**
>
> NNS may be intentional, as with a premature infant who may be unable to manage a fast flow of milk. In this case, the mother expresses her milk prior to nursing to facilitate NNS.
>
> It is common and normal for the rate of milk flow to change during a nursing. Some of the sucks will transfer less milk than others.
>
> This term may also be used to refer to suckling on a pacifier or thumb, during which time no milk is transferred.

➤ NONPUERPERAL LACTATION

DEFINITION   Lactation in a woman who has not given birth. This condition is abnormal, except with induced lactation.

IMPORTANT CONDITIONS TO REPORT

Breast secretions in a nonpuerperal woman, except in the case of induced lactation.

See also Galactorrhea; Induced lactation

➤ NPA

See National Perinatal Association (NPA)

➤ NURSING

DEFINITION   A term used in the United States to denote feeding a child at the breast. Also used to indicate the professional care activities of nurses. In other English-speaking cultures, nursing refers to caring for a child.

➤ NURSING-BOTTLE CARIES

DEFINITION   Cavities in the teeth that occur in a distinct pattern and are usually associated with bottle feeding.

SELF-CARE INFORMATION

Cavities, though very rare, can occur in the teeth of older breastfeeding babies.

Cavities in nursing children may be associated with eating sticky, gummy, or sugary snacks, drinking sugary beverages, or administering sugary liquid medicines (such as cough medicine) at bedtime. Cavities are also associated with inadequate tooth cleaning.

As soon as a baby erupts a tooth, a tooth cleaning routine should be started. At first, the baby's teeth can be cleaned with a soft, wet facecloth. Later, brush the teeth as instructed by a dental health professional.

Begin visits to the dentist early, especially if there is a family history of caries and problems with the enamel of the teeth.

IMPORTANT CONDITIONS TO REPORT

Discolorations on the teeth.

Toothache.

Any unusual mouth discomfort.

➤ NURSING PADS, PILLOWS, AND STOOLS

DEFINITION   A variety of commonly available items that may help the mother position the baby (or babies, in the case of multiples) at the breast in a more optimal way.

Breastfeeding equipment is available from breast pump rental depots, baby product stores, and catalogues such as the one from La Leche League.

➤ NURSING STRIKE

DEFINITION   A nursing strike is the sudden refusal of the baby to nurse. This can happen with a baby of any age. It is not intended to be the end of breastfeeding, but it may be incorrectly interpreted as baby's desire to wean.

ASK ABOUT

Age of the baby.
Nursing history.

ASSESSMENT

PROMPT CARE NEEDED?

Are any of the following present?

Baby refuses to nurse along with any of the following symptoms:

Sudden onset of inconsolable crying.

Change in stooling, urination, or sleep patterns.

Lethargy.

Vomiting.

Breathing difficulties.

Refusal to eat other age-appropriate foods.

Fever.

IF YES,   *Seek emergency care now and call pediatric provider immediately.*

PROMPT LACTATION CARE NEEDED?

Are any of the following present?

The baby refuses to nurse but otherwise seems normal.

The baby feeds well on one breast and not on the other.

Concerns about adequacy of milk supply.

IF YES,   *Call lactation care provider today.*

SELF-CARE INFORMATION

Mothers whose babies go on strike need to express milk for comfort and to maintain supply.

Many babies who have gone on strike return to the breast once the problem has been resolved.

Do not starve the baby back to the breast. Babies need to be fed.

Babies go on strike when something is wrong in their lives. Some of the reasons reported for strikes include:

Teething.

Stuffy nose.

Ear infection.

Baby has bitten the mother who yelled; this frightened the baby.

Reaction to being left unattended to cry it out.

Family stress.

Recent separation of the mother and baby, such as the mother's return to work.

To end a nursing strike:

Find out and correct what started the strike.

Give the baby lots of skin-to-skin contact, such as snuggling.

Do not force the baby to the breast. Try offering the breast just before bedtime, a nap, or first thing in the morning when the baby is drowsy.

Avoid feeding the baby via a bottle. Try cup feeding.

Offer the breast to the sleeping baby.

Try peer pressure. Attend a breastfeeding support meeting with the baby, or bring the baby to visit with a nursing friend.

IMPORTANT CONDITIONS TO REPORT

Change in stooling or urination patterns.

Sleepiness, lethargy.

Breathing difficulties.

Vomiting.

Inconsolable crying.

See also Abrupt weaning; Breast refusal; Goldsmith's sign

➤ NUTRITIONAL VALUES OF BREASTMILK

DEFINITION At more than 87% water, human milk is one of the most dilute of mammal milks and is easily digested by human babies. That means that babies should nurse frequently—10–12 times per 24 hours at first.

Lactose (the primary carbohydrate in human milk) constitutes about 7% of human milk's volume. Fat constitutes about 4%, protein constitutes about 1%, and the ash (mineral) content constitutes less than 1%.

Mother's milk has approximately 22 calories per ounce (75 kcal per 100 ml).

Milk composition is dynamic, changing throughout each feeding, throughout the day, and throughout the months of breastfeeding.

SELF-CARE INFORMATION

Eat in moderation from a wide variety of healthy foods.

There are no forbidden foods.

Consult a dietitian if you are following a strict diet for any reason.

NOTES

Humans make human milk. Women on excessively restrictive diets (complete vegetarian diets such as vegan or macrobiotic, and women who avoid all dairy foods) should seek dietary counseling because certain important components (such as vitamins B_{12} and D) may be transferring into their milk in lowered amounts. These women may be advised to add nutritional supplements to their routine.

Healthcare providers should avoid telling women that they must have perfect diets to breastfeed. There is little difference in the composition of milk of well-nourished women and malnourished women. Women should be encouraged to eat well to protect their own health and energy.

See also Macrobiotic diet of the mother; Maternal diet; Maternal diet, vegetarian; Vitamin supplements

➤ NWA

See National WIC Association (NWA)

➤ OBESITY

DEFINITION Breastfeeding has been identified as one of several strategies to reduce childhood obesity by the Institute of Medicine, the Centers for Disease Control and Prevention, and the American Academy of Pediatrics. Other strategies include eating more healthful foods such as fruits and vegetables, increasing exercise, drinking fewer sugary beverages, and spending less time watching television or engaging in other sedentary activities. Mothers should be encouraged to breastfeed and be supported in their decision.

Researchers have found that a longer duration of breastfeeding may result in a lower incidence of obesity within a population of people.

Breastfed infants normally gain weight faster in the first months after birth compared to formula-fed infants. Their weight gain slows around 4–6 months.

Some studies have shown that obese mothers may encounter more problems with breastfeeding, especially during the first week. However, the likely cause of these breastfeeding problems is thought to be the underlying reason(s) for the mother's excess weight that may impact breastfeeding. Conditions such as hypo- or hyperthyroidism and polycystic ovary syndrome (PCOS), which both affect weight, may also have a direct impact on milk volume.

NOTES

Ensure that the baby's growth is compared to the normal growth pattern of breastfed infants.

Advise overweight mothers with milk supply problems to have a complete physical evaluation.

See also Growth chart; Hyperthyroidism; Hypothyroidism; Maternal diet; Polycystic ovary syndrome (PCOS); Weight loss, mother

➤ OBTURATOR, PALATAL

DEFINITION A device that is fitted individually for the baby with a cleft palate. The obturator blocks the cleft opening and allows for easier suckling.

Modern obturators are made from the same material as athletic mouth guards and take only a few minutes to fit. As the baby grows, new obturators must be made. After the palatal repair, the obturator will no longer be needed.

For babies with cleft palates, nipple shields have been used to improve breastfeeding before the obturator is fitted.

Advise the mother to follow cleaning instructions for the obturator that has been provided to her and to return for scheduled refittings.

See also Cleft lip and palate (CL/CP)

➤ OCCUPATIONAL THERAPY

DEFINITION   Skilled treatment that helps individuals achieve the skills for living that they need. An occupational therapist can help develop feeding skills in babies with physical and developmental challenges.

➤ OFFICE ON WOMEN'S HEALTH (OWH)

See DHHS/Office on Women's Health (OWH)

➤ OINTMENTS AND CREAMS

DEFINITION   Topical preparations that have been made for several purposes, such as to protect the skin, to decrease itching, to clean the skin (antiseptics), and to moisturize the skin.

ASK ABOUT

Nipple discomfort.

ASSESSMENT

ROUTINE CARE NEEDED?

Are any of the following present?

Sore nipples.

Painful breastfeeding.

Skin rash, breakouts, or itching on the breast, areola, and nipple.

IF YES,	*Call mother's healthcare provider today and call lactation care provider to schedule a feeding evaluation today.*

SELF-CARE INFORMATION

Most ointments and creams are not intended for ingestion. When a mother puts an ointment or cream on her areola or nipple, her baby will be exposed to the ingredients during nursing.

Only use ointments and creams on the breast that are recommended for this purpose. Never use a product that has been prescribed for another problem.

Mothers can have reactions to ointments and creams. Report any changes immediately.

IMPORTANT CONDITIONS TO REPORT

Symptoms worsen or persist.

Signs of infection.

Feeding or stooling expectations are not met.

NOTES

Women experiencing **nipple pain** may self-treat with this and other inappropriate substances.

Women experiencing nipple pain should have a breastfeeding evaluation. Face-to-face counseling and breastfeeding assessment with corrective intervention is effective in assessing and resolving nipple pain.

See also Breast pain; Nipple pain; Sore nipples

➤ OLIGOSACCHARIDES IN BREASTMILK

DEFINITION   Short chains of sugar molecules. Researchers have found that some of the oligosaccharides in human milk have a protective effect against pathogens, especially in the urinary tract. Oligosaccharides are unique to human milk.

See also Bioactive components of breastmilk

➤ ONE-SIDED NURSING

DEFINITION   Nursing in which the baby prefers one breast over the other. The nipples may be different from one side to the other, the flow of milk or the volume of milk may be greater or less, or the baby may be more comfortable positioned at one breast compared to the other.

ASK ABOUT

Age of the baby.

ASSESSMENT

PROMPT CARE NEEDED?

Are any of the following present?

About the mother:

Fever higher than 101°F (38.5°C).

Reddened area on the breast.

Flu-like symptoms.

About the baby:

Sudden refusal of one breast.

Inconsolable crying.

Decrease in stooling or urination.

IF YES,   *Call healthcare provider now and call lactation care provider now.*

ROUTINE CARE NEEDED?

Are any of the following present?

Gradual preference of one breast over the other.

IF YES,   *Call lactation care provider.*

SELF-CARE INFORMATION

Sudden refusal of the breast, or refusal of one breast from birth can be a symptom of a medical problem in the baby or the mother. Common reasons include mastitis in the mother or nasal stuffiness in the baby.

There can be more serious medical problems that should be investigated when a baby refuses to nurse. Breast refusal has been associated with undetected breast cancer, for example.

If the baby is nursing less because of a stuffy nose or ear infection for example, the mother should express her milk in order to maintain lactation and stay comfortable.

IMPORTANT CONDITIONS TO REPORT

Decrease in baby's stooling or urination.

Fever or flu-like feelings in mother.

Fever or inconsolable crying in baby.

See also Breast refusal; Goldsmith's sign

➤ ORAL CONTRACEPTIVES

DEFINITION   Medications used to disrupt fertility, decreasing chances of pregnancy. Oral contraceptives have been studied in relation to breastfeeding. Some oral contraceptives are a combination of estrogen and progestin. Others are progestin-only.

ASK ABOUT

Age of the baby.

Duration of oral contraceptive use.

ASSESSMENT

PROMPT CARE NEEDED?

Are any of the following present?

Inadequate weight gain.

Perception of decreased milk supply.

IF YES,   *Call lactation care provider today.*

ROUTINE CARE NEEDED?

Are any of the following present?

More information desired about oral contraception and breastfeeding.

More information desired about breastfeeding and family planning or birth control.

IF YES,   *Consult up-to-date drug references, call obstetric care provider, and call lactation care provider.*

SELF-CARE INFORMATION

Consider the **lactational amenorrhea method (LAM)**, other natural family planning methods, and barrier methods of contraception if hormonal contraceptives are not acceptable. They are all compatible with breastfeeding.

IMPORTANT CONDITIONS TO REPORT

Decreased milk supply.

Decreased stooling or urination in the baby.

NOTES

Hale states that the healthcare provider should "suggest that the mother establish a good flow (60–90 days) prior to beginning oral contraceptives. Avoid combination (estrogen-progestin) contraceptives if at all possible. Use oral progestin-only preparations initially preferably after 6 weeks postpartum. Warn mothers that even progestin-only preparations may rarely suppress milk production."[235(p779)] Hale rates oral contraceptives as L3 (moderately safe) drugs.

See also Birth control; Fertility; Hormonal contraceptive methods; Lactational amenorrhea method (LAM); Progestin-only contraceptives

Footnote

[235]Hale, T. (2012). *Medications and mothers' milk* (15th ed.). Amarillo, TX: Hale Pub.

➤ ORAL REHYDRATION THERAPY (ORT)

DEFINITION   Use of special fluids to treat dehydration. Oral rehydration therapy (ORT) is promoted by the World Health Organization (WHO) to reduce the number of infant deaths from dehydration due to diarrhea. Research confirms that rehydration solution made from inexpensive ingredients (glucose and electrolytes) is advantageous. Breastfed infants receiving ORT should continue breastfeeding.

See also Diarrhea

➤ ORT

See Oral rehydration therapy (ORT)

➤ OSTEOPOROSIS

DEFINITION   A disease in which the bones become extremely porous, often causing fracture. This is typically a problem of women after menopause.
Breastfeeding is thought to provide some protection against osteoporosis.

See also Bone loss; Bone mineral density (BMD)

➤ OTC DRUGS

See Over-the-counter (OTC) drugs

➤ OTITIS MEDIA

DEFINITION   Otitis media is an infection or inflammation of the middle ear. The inflammation may begin with an infection that causes a sore throat, cold, or other respiratory or breathing problem. Babies who are breastfed have a lower incidence of otitis media compared to babies who are not. Pacifier use increases the incidence of otitis media.

ASK ABOUT

Age of the baby.

History of sore throat, cold, or respiratory problem.

Change in breastfeeding behavior.

ASSESSMENT

PROMPT CARE NEEDED?

Are any of the following present?

Unusual irritability.

Difficulty sleeping.

Tugging or pulling at one or both ears.

Fever.

Fluid draining from one or both ears.

Difficulty breastfeeding.

Crying at the breast or pulling away and crying after a few sucks.

IF YES,   *Seek pediatric care now and call lactation care provider today.*

ROUTINE CARE NEEDED?

Are any of the following present?

Baby has been treated for ear infection but continues to fret or cry at the breast.

IF YES,   *Call lactation care provider.*

SELF-CARE INFORMATION

Even after the otitis media has resolved, the baby may be uncomfortable nursing or may remember the pain of nursing with the ear infection. Changing positions may help. If the problem persists, have the baby's ears checked again by the healthcare provider.

Keep the breasts soft and express excess milk during the time the baby is not nursing well.

IMPORTANT CONDITIONS TO REPORT

Less urination or stooling.

Continued symptoms of otitis media after treatment.

Continued problems with breastfeeding after treatment is initiated.

NOTES

Pacifier use has been associated with ear infection[236] and should be reexamined in babies with recurrent ear infection.

See also Ear infection; Nursing strike; Weaning

Footnote

[236]Niemela, M., Pihakari, O., & Pokka, T. (2000). Pacifier as a risk factor for acute otitis media: A randomized, controlled trial of parental counseling. *Pediatrics, 106*(3), 483–488.

➤ OVERACTIVE LET-DOWN REFLEX

DEFINITION   Rapid milk flow that may overwhelm the baby's ability to suck, swallow, and breathe comfortably. This may be due to the oversupply of milk, a forceful let-down reflex, or both.

ASK ABOUT

Age of the baby.

Weight gain of the baby.

ASSESSMENT

ROUTINE CARE NEEDED?

Are any of the following present?

Gagging, choking, or coughing at the breast as if the milk is coming too fast.

The baby spits up and is gassy.

The baby pulls off the breast while nursing and milk sprays.

The nipple is compressed at the end of the nursing.

IF YES,   *Call lactation care provider today.*

PROMPT CARE NEEDED?

Are any of the following present?

Perception of overabundant milk supply.

Excessively large or frequent stools in a breastfed baby.

Recurrent engorgement or mastitis.

The baby has difficulty managing excessive milk flow, including pulling away from the breast.

The baby is unsettled after feeding.

IF YES, *Call lactation care provider today.*

SELF-CARE INFORMATION

Frequency of feeding and amount of milk removal drives milk supply. The rapid milk flow is often accompanied by an abundant milk supply. Many women with oversupply may need to gradually decrease breast stimulation.

Positioning the baby in an upright position, with no pressure on the back of the head, may give the baby an opportunity to find the best nursing position.

Try nursing the baby on only one breast at each feeding to decrease the supply. Decrease milk expression, if practiced. Some mothers successfully manage the flow by nursing while lying on their backs with the baby lying on the mother's abdomen. This technique is known as "posture feeding," "the Australian posture," and "nursing down under." The baby has complete head control in this position, and the milk is spraying against gravity. Another posture is the reclining posture where the weight of the baby is on the mother's chest and abdomen and the baby is clearly upright.

IMPORTANT CONDITIONS TO REPORT

Worsening of symptoms

Continuation of symptoms

Ongoing concerns

Any symptoms of mastitis, including:

Plugged ducts.

Visible red areas on the breast(s).

Fever higher than 101°F (38.5°C).

Extreme breast discomfort.

Flu-like aching throughout body.

NOTES

Because production of milk relies on many different body systems in both the mother and the baby, any milk supply problem requires consideration of maternal and infant factors. Occasionally, medical factors such as endocrine imbalance and the use of some medications require evaluation.

See also Australian posture; Block nursing; Clenching or clamping onto the nipple/areola; Mastitis; Plugged ducts; Milk flow, too fast; Oversupply; Reclining posture

➤ OVERSUPPLY

DEFINITION An extremely abundant milk supply. Rapid milk flow that may overwhelm baby's ability to suck, swallow, and breathe comfortably. This may be due to a forceful let-down reflex.

ASK ABOUT

Age of the baby.
Weight gain of the baby.

ASSESSMENT

ROUTINE CARE NEEDED?

Are any of the following present?

Gagging, choking, or coughing at the breast as if the milk is coming too fast.
The baby spits up and is gassy.
The baby pulls off the breast while nursing, and milk sprays.
The nipple is compressed at the end of the nursing.

IF YES, *Call lactation care provider today.*

PROMPT CARE NEEDED?

Are any of the following present?

Perception of overabundant milk supply.

Excessively large or frequent stools in a breastfed baby.

Recurrent engorgement or mastitis.

The baby has difficulty managing excessive milk flow including pulling away from the breast.

The baby is unsettled after feeding.

IF YES, *Call lactation care provider today.*

SELF-CARE INFORMATION

Frequency of feeding and amount of milk removal drives milk supply. The rapid milk flow is often accompanied by an abundant milk supply. Many women with oversupply need to gradually decrease breast stimulation.

Positioning the baby in an upright position with no pressure on the back of the head may give the baby an opportunity to find the best nursing position.

Try nursing the baby on only one breast at each feeding to decrease the supply. Decrease milk expression, if practiced. Some mothers successfully manage the flow by nursing while lying on their backs with the baby lying on the mother's abdomen. This technique is known as "posture feeding," "the Australian posture," and "nursing down under." The baby has complete head control in this position, and the milk is spraying against gravity. Another posture is the reclining posture where the weight of the baby is on the mother's chest and abdomen and the baby is clearly upright.

IMPORTANT CONDITIONS TO REPORT

Worsening of symptoms

Continuation of symptoms

Ongoing concerns

Any symptoms of mastitis, including:

Plugged ducts.

Visible red areas on the breast(s).

Fever higher than 101°F (38.5°C).

Extreme breast discomfort.

Flu-like aching throughout the body.

> **NOTES**

Because production of milk relies on many different body systems in both the mother and the baby, any milk supply problem requires consideration of maternal and infant factors.
Occasionally medical factors such as endocrine imbalance and the use of medications require evaluation.

See also Australian posture; Block nursing; Clenching or clamping onto the nipple/areola; Mastitis; Plugged ducts; Milk flow, too fast; Overactive let-down reflex; Reclining posture

➤ OVER-THE-COUNTER (OTC) DRUGS

DEFINITION Medications that are available to the public without a prescription. However, their convenient availability does not guarantee they are compatible with breastfeeding.

SELF-CARE INFORMATION

Use up-to-date drug references to determine compatibility of OTC drugs with breastfeeding.

IMPORTANT CONDITIONS TO REPORT

Report any changes in the baby as soon as they are noticed.
Report any changes in milk supply as soon as they are noticed.

See also Medication resources (inside back cover); Medicinal herbs

➤ OVULATION AND LACTATION

DEFINITION Refers to changes in the production of eggs (ovum) during breastfeeding. Research continues to help healthcare providers better understand the relationship between menstruation, fertility, and breastfeeding. After childbirth, the absence of menstruation in nursing mothers is called "lactational amenorrhea." Ovulation may happen before the first menstrual period after childbirth.

SELF-CARE INFORMATION

It is impossible to predict when any woman breastfeeding woman will ovulate or get her first period after her baby is born.

Fertility may return before the first menstrual period after childbirth.

Home care products and natural methods can be used to detect ovulation.

Periods can be lighter, heavier, or more irregular than when not breastfeeding.

The return of menstruation does not mean the end of breastfeeding.

Some mothers report that their nursing babies are less interested in breastfeeding during their periods.

Some mothers experience nipple soreness during menstruation.

IMPORTANT CONDITIONS TO REPORT

Menstruation before 4 weeks postpartum if breastfeeding.

See also Amenorrhea; Fertility; Lactational amenorrhea method (LAM); Menstrual cycle

➤ OWH

See DHHS/Office on Women's Health (OWH)

➤ OXYTOCIN

DEFINITION   Oxytocin is one of the two major hormones of lactation (the other is prolactin). Oxytocin is released from the posterior lobe of the pituitary gland and stimulates the contraction of the smooth muscle of the uterus during labor. Oxytocin is responsible for the let-down (ejection) of milk.

SELF-CARE INFORMATION

The breastfed baby should gain well (0.5 oz to 1 oz per day on average). If the baby is gaining less than this, have a face-to-face breastfeeding evaluation.

At the breast, the baby should have a sucking pattern that includes slow, deep sucks. After the first few days, the baby's swallows can be heard. The baby should have at least six wet diapers and four stools each day after day 4. The baby should begin to have yellow stools by day 5.

IMPORTANT CONDITIONS TO REPORT

Meconium bowel movements after 5 days of life.

No yellow stools by day 5.

Fewer than three bowel movements daily in breastfed newborn after the first 2 days of life.

No urine in 6 hours.

Brick dust urine (uric acid crystals) after 2 days of life.

Dark-colored urine.

Fewer than four urinations daily in the breastfed newborn after day 5 of life.

Noticeably sunken fontanelles (soft spot on the top of the head).

Decreased activity.

Weight loss of more than 7% from birth or further weight loss by day 5.

Cessation of weight gain.

NOTES

Researchers have found that oxytocin is released in the first hours postpartum by the baby's hand massage of the breast, as well as by suckling.

Oxytocin is also released by the baby stretching the nipple sufficiently in the mouth. This is why a good latch is so important to milk transfer.

Oxytocin is also released through a conditioned response over time.

The amount of natural oxytocin a woman releases in response to breastfeeding in the early days may be inversely related to the amount of prolactin she received during labor.[237]

See also Hormones; Let-down reflex; Milk-ejection reflex

Footnote

[237]Jonas, K., Johansson, L. M., Nissen, E., Ejdebäck, M., Ransjö-Arvidson, A. B., & Uvnäs-Moberg, K. (2009). Effects of intrapartum oxytocin administration and epidural analgesia on the concentration of plasma oxytocin and prolactin, in response to suckling during the second day postpartum. *Breastfeeding Medicine: The Official Journal of the Academy of Breastfeeding Medicine, 4*(2), 71–82. doi:10.1089/bfm.2008.0002

➤ PACIFIER

DEFINITION   An artificial nipple, usually connected to a ring or solid backing. Pacifiers are sometimes called "dummies."

SELF-CARE INFORMATION

Pacifiers have been controversial in relation to breastfeeding. Research indicates that breastfed babies who use pacifiers spend less time nursing, are more likely to be given formula supplements, and are weaned from the breast at a younger age.[238] Babies who are given pacifiers have a higher risk of ear infection (otitis media).[239] Premature babies who cannot suck at the breast because they are being tube fed grow better if they can suck on a pacifier during the tube feeding.

NOTES

Pacifiers are used to calm babies, but their use may result in underfeeding. The American Academy of Pediatrics suggests that:

> Because pacifier use has been associated with a reduction in SIDS incidence, mothers of healthy term infants should be instructed to use pacifiers at infant nap or sleep time after breastfeeding is well established, at approximately three to four weeks of age.[240(p.e835)]

Footnotes

[238]Howard, C. R., Howard, F. M., Lanphear, B., deBlieck, E. A., Eberly, S., & Lawrence, R. A. (1999). The effects of early pacifier use on breastfeeding duration. *Pediatrics, 103*(3), E33.

[239]Jackson, J. M., & Mourino, A. P. (1999). Pacifier use and otitis media in infants twelve months of age or younger. *Pediatric Dentistry, 21*(4), 255–260.

[240]AAP Section on Breastfeeding. (2012). Breastfeeding and the use of human milk. *Pediatrics, 129*(3), e827–e841. doi: 10.1542/peds.2011-3552

➤ PAGET'S DISEASE OF THE BREAST

DEFINITION   Paget's disease of the breast is a form of breast cancer affecting the nipple and the areola. It has also been referred to as Paget's disease of the nipple.

Symptoms mimic allergic skin reaction of the nipple and areolar area, including itchy, flaky, scaly skin, sometimes with bloody nipple discharge. This typically happens only on one breast. Eventually the growth of cells will obliterate the normal contour and appearance of the nipple area.

Refer all women with reoccurring symptoms such as those described above to their healthcare provider when improved latch and breastfeeding does not alleviate symptoms.

➤ PAINFUL BREASTFEEDING

DEFINITION Uncomfortable sensations in the breast. Pain is not an expected part of breastfeeding and indicates the need for a feeding evaluation.

ASK ABOUT

Onset.

Location of pain.

Whether pain is unilateral or bilateral.

ASSESSMENT

PROMPT MEDICAL CARE NEEDED?

Are any of the following present?

Visible red areas on the breast(s).

Fever higher than 101°F (38.5°C).

Extreme breast discomfort.

Flu-like aching throughout body.

Continuing fever after treatment.

Reaction to antibiotic prescribed.

IF YES, *Seek emergency care if red streaks are found on both breasts and other symptoms are also present.*

Seek medical care within 4 hours with other symptoms in the absence of red areas on both breasts.

PROMPT LACTATION CARE NEEDED?

Are any of the following present?

Persistent pain during nursing.

Persistent pain between feedings.

Constant pain.

Pain combined with color change of nipple(s).

Pain with visible fissure or bleeding of the nipple.

IF YES,   *Call lactation care provider now.*

ROUTINE CARE NEEDED?

Are any of the following present?

Brief pain at beginning of feeding.

Mild recurrent pain.

IF YES,   *Call lactation care provider today.*

SELF-CARE INFORMATION

Practice skin-to-skin contact in the first hour and frequently thereafter.

Feed the baby at the first sign of hunger cues (signs that say "feed me" include hand-to-face or hand-to-mouth movements, lip smacking, seeking with lips, rooting, and head bobbing).

Feed the baby at least 10 times per 24 hours.

Listen for signs of the baby swallowing.

Allow the baby to end feedings.

Expect at least four infant stools per 24 hours after the first 4 days of life.

Good positioning and attachment are crucial to prevent or reduce nipple pain.

If feedings are missed, hand express or pump milk or both to maintain supply.

NOTES

There can be many reasons for pain in the breast including breast infection or inflammation, clogs, or cysts. Poor latch-on or positioning can also cause pain.

Breastfeeding should not be painful. Advise mothers to seek medical or lactation care for breast pain.

See also Latch-on; Mastitis; Plugged ducts; Sore nipples

➤ PALADAI

DEFINITION   A paladai is a South Indian feeding device shaped like a miniature gravy boat. The infant sips from the paladai when he or she is separated from the mother and is unable to breastfeed. Research comparing behavior of babies feeding from cups, bottles, and paladai shows that babies feed better and sleep longer between feedings when they are fed from the paladai.[241]

See also Cup feeding; Feeding methods, alternate; Supplemental feeding devices

Footnote

[241]Malhotra, N., Vishwambaran, L., Sundaram, K. R., & Narayanan, I. (1999). A controlled trial of alternative methods of oral feeding in neonates. *Early Human Development, 54,* 29–38.

➤ PALATAL OBTURATOR

DEFINITION   A palatal obturator is a device that is fitted individually for the baby with a cleft palate. The obturator blocks the cleft opening and allows for easier suckling. Modern obturators are made from the same material as athletic mouth guards and take only a few minutes to fit. As the baby grows, new obturators must be made. After the palatal repair, the obturator will no longer be needed.

NOTES

For babies with cleft palates, nipple shields have been used to improve breastfeeding before the obturator is fitted.

Advise the mother to follow cleaning instructions for the obturator that has been provided to her, and return to her child's pediatric dentist for scheduled refittings.

See also Cleft lip and palate (CL/CP)

➤ PALATE, ABNORMAL

DEFINITION The palate is the roof of the mouth. Both the hard and soft palate play an important role in suckling. One in 700 babies is born with a cleft of the lip or palate.

NOTES

Intact palates may have a high arch, making placement of the nipple and effective suckling difficult.

Babies with abnormal palates can breastfeed or be fed expressed breastmilk. Pediatric occupational/speech, therapists and/or speech/language pathologists should be consulted.

See also Cleft lip and palate (CL/CP); Palatal obturator

➤ PAPILLOMA, INTRADUCTAL

DEFINITION An intraductal papilloma is a small, benign (noncancerous) tumor that grows within a single milk duct.

ASK ABOUT

Age of the baby.
Onset of nipple discharge.
Description of nipple discharge.

ASSESSMENT

PROMPT CARE NEEDED?

Are any of the following present?

Appearance of rust-colored milk.

Bloody discharge from the nipple.

Any other unusual nipple discharge without nipple pain or abrasion from suboptimal latch.

IF YES, *Call obstetric care provider today.*

SELF-CARE INFORMATION
Seek prompt medical evaluation of any unusual discharge from the nipple during breastfeeding and at any other time.

See also Bleeding, breast; Blood in milk; Breast cancer

➤ PASTEURIZATION

DEFINITION The process of pasteurization was named after Louis Pasteur who discovered that organisms that could spoil wine were inactivated by heating to temperatures below the boiling point. This process was later applied to milk. Pasteurization of human milk has been studied at a variety of temperatures and times. Some of the components of human milk are lost with heat treatment along with the targeted microorganisms, but the composition of human milk remains essentially the same. The Food and Drug Administration and the Centers for Disease Control and Prevention do not recommend the use of donor milk without heat treatment. Milk from milk banks has been pasteurized.

See also Donor milk; Milk banks

➤ PATHOGEN

DEFINITION An invading microorganism or toxin.

➤ PCOS

See Polycystic ovary syndrome (PCOS)

➤ PEDICLE TECHNIQUE FOR BREAST REDUCTION

DEFINITION   With the pedicle technique for breast reduction surgery, the nipple and areola remain attached while excess breast tissue is removed.

Breastfeeding women who have had breast reduction surgery will need careful evaluation and close monitoring. Their babies need close pediatric follow-up over several weeks to assure adequate nutrition.

See also Breast reduction; Breast surgery

➤ PEER COUNSELING

DEFINITION   Delivery of breastfeeding support via trained peers.

See also La Leche League, International; United States Department of Agriculture (USDA) Special Supplemental Food Program for Women, Infants, and Children (WIC)

➤ PESTICIDES AND POLLUTANTS IN BREASTMILK

DEFINITION   Refers to environmental toxins that may be found in human milk. All foods, including breastmilk, may contain traces of chemical contaminants present in the environment. Breastmilk is one of the easiest and least painful body tissues to sample. For this reason, it is used to monitor population exposure to chemicals. Low-level exposure to contaminants should not contraindicate breastfeeding. The greatest exposure for the baby is during pregnancy.

ASK ABOUT

Known contaminant exposure.
Age of the baby.

ASSESSMENT

EMERGENT CARE NEEDED?

Are any of the following present?

Sudden exposure of mother to toxic chemical.

IF YES,   *Seek emergency care now.*

PROMPT CARE NEEDED?

Are any of the following present?

History of high-level exposure to toxic chemicals in a breastfeeding woman.

IF YES,   *Seek medical care today.*

ROUTINE CARE NEEDED?

Are any of the following present?

General questions about environmental exposure.

IF YES,   *Call lactation care provider today.*

IMPORTANT CONDITIONS TO REPORT

Known history of environmental or workplace exposure to toxic chemicals.
Any negative effects of past exposure.

NOTES

Women who know they have been exposed to specific chemicals or pollutants should consult with their physician regarding analysis of the contaminant content of their milk.

See also Chemical contaminants in breastmilk

➤ PHENYLKETONURIA (PKU)

DEFINITION   Phenylketonuria (PKU) is a rare genetic inborn error of metabolism that is detectable during the first days of life through newborn screening. PKU is characterized by the absence or deficiency of the enzyme that is necessary to process the essential amino acid phenylalanine. Babies with PKU may be partially breastfed together with consumption of a phenylalanine-free formula, per physician's order. These babies must be monitored carefully to protect the central nervous system from damage caused by high levels of phenylalanine.

ASSESSMENT

PROMPT CARE NEEDED?

Are any of the following present?

Questions about management of breastfeeding after diagnosis of PKU.

IF YES,   *Call lactation care provider today.*

SELF-CARE INFORMATION

The healthcare provider will prescribe a phenylalanine-free formula and determine how often the baby's blood levels will be tested for phenylalanine.

Even babies with PKU require some of the amino acid phenylalanine that is found in formula and breastmilk.

Human milk is lower in phenylalanine than standard formulas.

Research indicates that children who had received their mother's milk in addition to the special phenylalanine-free formula during infancy had more than a 10-point IQ advantage compared to children who had received the special formula alone or compared to a standard formula.[242]

IMPORTANT CONDITIONS TO REPORT

Any breastfeeding or formula feeding problems.

Footnote

[242]Riva, E., Agostoni, C., Biasucci, G., Trojan, S., Luotti, D., Fiori, L., & Giovannini, M. (1996). Early breastfeeding is linked to higher intelligence quotient scores in dietary treated phenylketonuric children. *Acta Paediatrica, 85,* 56.

➤ PHOTOTHERAPY

DEFINITION   Phototherapy is the process of using light to treat certain medical conditions. In infants, phototherapy is commonly used to treat jaundice (hyperbilirubinemia).

SELF-CARE INFORMATION

If the baby is too sleepy to nurse effectively, the mother should express her milk frequently to feed to jaundiced infant, and to encourage her supply.

NOTES

The baby is exposed to a fluorescent light that is absorbed by the skin. During this process, the bilirubin is changed and is more easily moved out of the baby's body.

As much of the baby's skin as possible is exposed to the light.

The baby's eyes are covered to protect them.

There is no need to stop breastfeeding, although the baby may be sleepy and need coaxing as well as shorter, more frequent feedings.

The baby's bilirubin will be monitored, and when it is low enough, the lights will no longer be required.

See also Bilirubin; Hyperbilirubinemia; Jaundice

➤ PIERRE ROBIN SEQUENCE

DEFINITION   Pierre Robin sequence is also called "Pierre Robin complex" or "syndrome." Many children with this syndrome have difficulty with feeding and/or breathing. It is a condition present at birth that is characterized by the coexistence of two or more of the following conditions:

A very small jaw with a receding chin.

A tongue that appears large (due to the small size of the jaw) and is placed unusually far back in the mouth.

High arched palate.

Cleft soft palate.

Choking on tongue.

Presence of teeth at birth.

Diagnosis of Pierre Robin sequence in the baby.

ASSESSMENT

PROMPT CARE NEEDED?

Are any of the following present?

Diagnosis of Pierre Robin sequence in a breastfed baby.

IF YES, *Call lactation care provider today.*

SELF-CARE INFORMATION

Begin expressing milk as soon as possible after birth. Breastmilk may be fed to the baby even before breastfeeding can begin.

Babies with Pierre Robin sequence often have swallowing problems. At-breast feeding devices can be helpful.

See also At-breast supplementation; Breast pump; Cleft lip and palate (CL/CP); Palate, abnormal

➤ PKU

See Phenylketonuria (PKU)

➤ PLACENTAL FRAGMENTS, RETAINED

DEFINITION Small pieces of placenta (fragments) retained in the uterus after the placenta is delivered. The fragment continues to be supported, but may subsequently break away. When this happens, the area of the uterus continues to bleed. The mother may hemorrhage and lose a considerable amount of blood.

A sign of retained placental fragments is the continued vaginal flow of red blood after the early days postpartum.

Retained placental fragments are associated in some women with failure to produce sufficient milk due to hormonal influence of progesterone, a hormone of pregnancy that is produced by the placenta.

ASK ABOUT

Age of the baby.
Current vaginal bleeding.
Breastfeeding difficulties.

ASSESSMENT

EMERGENT CARE NEEDED?

Are any of the following present?

Soaking a sanitary napkin with bright red blood at a rate of one napkin or
more per hour.

Clots in the bloody discharge.

Foul odor to the discharge (even if occasional).

Dizziness.

Fever.

Abdominal pain.

IF YES, *Call obstetric care provider now or seek emergency care now.*

PROMPT MEDICAL CARE NEEDED?

Are any of the following present?

Soaking a sanitary napkin with bright red blood at a rate of one napkin every
2 to 3 hours.

Abdominal tenderness.

Low-grade fever.

Lightheadedness.

IF YES, *Call obstetric care provider within 4 hours.*

PROMPT LACTATION CARE NEEDED?

Are any of the following present?

Problems with milk supply in a woman diagnosed with retained
placental fragments.

IF YES, *Call lactation care provider today.*

ROUTINE CARE NEEDED?

Are any of the following present?

Soaking a sanitary napkin with bright red blood at a rate of one napkin every 3 or more hours.

Abdominal tenderness.

IF YES,   *Call obstetric care provider today.*

SELF-CARE INFORMATION

Rapid soaking of a sanitary napkin with bright red blood after the early days postpartum may be associated with retained placental fragments and can be the first sign of hemorrhage.

Retained placental fragments have been associated with the failure to establish an adequate milk supply.

IMPORTANT CONDITIONS TO REPORT

Increase in bright red blood flow.

Bright red blood after 2 weeks postpartum.

See also Bleeding, postpartum vaginal; Lochia; Retained placental fragments; Slow weight gain, baby

➤ PLUGGED DUCTS

DEFINITION   Presence of clogs in the tubes that drain the breast. The milk ducts of the breast may become plugged with dried milk. The mother may experience tenderness and feel a lump at the site of the plug.

ASK ABOUT

Age of the baby.

Location of the lump.

Tenderness around the lump.

When the lump was first noted.

ASSESSMENT

PROMPT CARE NEEDED?

Are any of the following present?

Temperature higher than 101°F (38.5°C).

Reddened area on the breast.

Identified lump or lumps on the breast that persist and do not move for more than 48 hours.

IF YES, *Call obstetric care provider now and call lactation care provider now.*

ROUTINE CARE NEEDED?

Are any of the following present?

Identified lump or lumps on the breast which persist for more than 48 hours with no other symptoms.

IF YES, *Call obstetric care provider and call lactation care provider today.*

SELF-CARE INFORMATION

Plugged ducts in the breast should move and disappear within 48 hours. If not, consult a physician for further evaluation.

Some mothers find manual massage of the area helps the plug to dislodge and move out of the breast. Others prefer warmth, such as a warm, wet towel.

Nursing the baby frequently on the affected breast will help to drain it.

Changing the baby's position can help to move the plug.

Try to understand why the plug happened. Could it be caused by an underwire bra or car seat belt applying pressure on the breast? Then, avoid the cause so that plugs do not reoccur.

IMPORTANT CONDITIONS TO REPORT

Temperature higher than 101°F (38.5°C).

Reddened area on the breast.

NOTES

New mothers are not protected from breast cancer. Prompt evaluation is warranted if a lump does not move in 48 hours.

See also Breast infection; Breast inflammation; Breast lumps; Breast pain; Mastitis

➤ POLYCYSTIC OVARY SYNDROME (PCOS)

DEFINITION   A syndrome caused by hormonal imbalances. Cysts form on the ovaries' surface due to high levels of androgen, and ovulation does not occur. The menstrual cycle may not begin, the uterine lining is not released, and abnormal uterine growths may form.

PCOS is also associated with glucose intolerance and insulin resistance.

Symptoms of PCOS include irregular menstrual periods, elevated male hormone levels in the blood (which can cause excessive facial and body hair), obesity, acne, cystic ovaries, or enlarged ovaries.

SELF-CARE INFORMATION

Some mothers with PCOS struggle to achieve and maintain an adequate milk supply for their babies.[243,244]

IMPORTANT CONDITIONS TO REPORT

Inadequate urination or stooling in breastfeeding infant.

Poor weight gain of breastfeeding infant.

See also Hormones; Obesity; Slow weight gain, baby; Thyroid disease

Footnotes

[243]Vanky, E., Isaksen, H., Moen, M. H., & Carlsen, S. M. (2008). Breastfeeding in polycystic ovary syndrome. *Acta Obstetricia Et Gynecologica Scandinavica, 87*(5), 531–535. doi:10.1080/0001634 0802007676

[244]Marasco, L., Marmet, C., & Shell, E. (2000). Polycystic ovary syndrome: A connection to insufficient milk supply? *Journal of Human Lactation, 16*(2), 143–148.

➤ POOR WEIGHT GAIN IN THE BREASTFED BABY

DEFINITION   Inadequate growth in a nursing infant. Breastfed newborns should lose no more than 7% from their birthweight and have no further weight loss by the 5th day.[245(p.e835)] Once birthweight has been regained, newborns should gain a minimum of 0.5 oz to 1 oz a day on average. New studies indicate that breastfed babies gain even faster than was previously believed, most likely due to the fact that in the past, breastfeeding was done on a schedule (and not as frequently as we now know is ideal).

ASK ABOUT

Age of the baby.
Weight gain pattern.

ASSESSMENT

PROMPT CARE NEEDED?

Are any of the following present?

Meconium bowel movements after 5 days of life.

No yellow stool by day 5.

Fewer than three bowel movements daily in a breastfed newborn after the first 2 days of life.

No urine in 6 hours.

Brick dust urine (uric acid crystals) after 2 days of life.

Dark-colored urine.

Fewer than four urinations daily in the breastfed newborn after day 5 of life.

Noticeably sunken fontanelles (soft spot on the top of the head).

Decreased activity.

Weight loss of more than 7% from birth or further weight loss by day 5.

Cessation of weight gain.

Sleeping at the breast.

IF YES,   *Seek pediatric care now.*

ROUTINE CARE NEEDED?

Are any of the following present?

Baby sleeps at the breast after a few sucks.

Hard to latch on.

No audible swallows.

Pediatric referral for slow weight gain in a breastfed newborn.

IF YES,   *Call lactation care provider now.*

IMPORTANT CONDITIONS TO REPORT

Decrease in number of urinations or stools.

Increased sleepiness, or many hours spent sleeping.

Baby is harder to rouse.

See also Hypotonia; Jaundice

Footnote

[245]AAP Section on Breastfeeding. (2012). Breastfeeding and the use of human milk. *Pediatrics, 129*(3), e827–e841. doi: 10.1542/peds.2011-3552

➤ POSITIONING

DEFINITION   Refers to how the baby is held for feedings. Properly positioning the baby at the breast should allow for the nipple to stretch, the milk to flow, and the mother and the baby to feed in comfort. The mother should feel gentle tugging at the most. She should certainly not feel pain. Pain is a reason to seek help.

SELF-CARE INFORMATION

Proper positioning allows the baby to transfer milk and breathe at the breast without pain for the mother.

If the mother feels pain; the baby has trouble coordinating sucking, swallowing, and breathing; or there is not enough milk transfer, the mother should have a face-to-face evaluation of breastfeeding by a skilled observer.

IMPORTANT CONDITIONS TO REPORT

Breast or nipple pain.

Poor weight gain.

Baby struggling to breathe while nursing (this may not be due to positioning, but may indicate an anatomic issue in the baby).

NOTES

A variety of nursing postures are known. Skilled help and evaluation should be available to the mother.

See also Asymmetric latch; Attachment; Australian posture; Clutch posture; Cradle posture; Reclining posture; Sore nipples; Weight gain, baby–high; Weight gain, baby–low

➤ POSTMATURE BABY

DEFINITION A postmature baby is one who has stayed in utero beyond the capacity of its placenta. Instead of continuing to grow in utero, the baby has begun to lose weight before it is born. Postmature babies often have trouble maintaining their blood sugar and temperature at first. Postmature babies also may need extra encouragement to nurse, so they should nurse as soon as possible after birth and then very frequently.

➤ POSTPARTUM DEPRESSION

DEFINITION A mood disorder occurring in mothers after giving birth. Symptoms of depression are not unusual for women during the early days postpartum. More than 50% of women experience some form of mood disorder during this period. The Edinburgh Postnatal Depression Scale is a proven screening tool for postpartum depression. It can be administered by any provider.

ASK ABOUT

Onset.
Age of the baby.
History of depression.

ASSESSMENT

EMERGENT CARE NEEDED?

Are any of the following present?

Suicidal thoughts.

Thoughts of harming the baby.

| IF YES, | *Seek emergency care now.* |

PROMPT CARE NEEDED?

Are any of the following present?

Persistent sadness.

Inability to function.

Frequent crying.

| IF YES, | *Call healthcare provider or mental health professional now.* |

SELF-CARE INFORMATION

Mood swings are normal in the postpartum period, but may become more severe. Seek support.

Practice skin-to-skin contact in the first hour and frequently thereafter.

Feed the baby at the first sign of hunger cues (signs that say "feed me" include hand-to-face or hand-to-mouth movements, lip smacking, seeking with lips, rooting, and head bobbing).

Feed the baby at least 10 times per 24 hours.

Listen for signs of the baby swallowing.

Allow the baby to end feedings.

Expect at least three infant stools per 24 hours after the first 4 days of life and yellow stools by 5 days.

Good positioning and attachment are crucial to prevent or reduce nipple pain.

If feedings are missed, hand express or pump milk or both to maintain supply.

IMPORTANT CONDITIONS TO REPORT

Exacerbation of symptoms.

Nonresolution of symptoms.

History of depression, mood disorders, premenstrual syndrome, or thyroid disorders.

NOTES

Mood disorders in the postpartum period include symptoms of depression as well as other psychiatric manifestations such as anxiety, obsession and compulsion, etc. It is important to encourage mothers to report any worsening of symptoms.

Women who experienced depression during pregnancy and those with a history of depression, mood disorders, or premenstrual syndrome are at greater risk for postpartum depression.

Hypothyroidism, anemia, and other physical disorders share many symptoms with postpartum depression.

Many breastfeeding women resist reporting depression as they fear that medication may be incompatible with breastfeeding. There are many antidepressant medications that are considered safe for use in breastfeeding women.

See also Anemia; Baby blues; Drugs; Hypothyroidism; Postpartum mood disorders

➤ POSTPARTUM MOOD DISORDERS

DEFINITION   A spectrum of emotional difficulties occurring in the period after birth, including anxiety, baby blues, depression, obsessive-compulsive behavior, panic, posttraumatic stress, and psychosis.

NOTES

Postpartum mood disorders affect most new mothers. Mood disorders cover a broad spectrum from baby blues to postpartum psychosis. While mood disorders are common, they are not to be ignored. Avoid giving false reassurance. Depression can be life threatening for the mother and baby.

Women who experienced depression during pregnancy and those with a history of depression, mood disorders, or premenstrual syndrome are at greater risk for postpartum depression.

Hypothyroidism, anemia, and other physical disorders share many symptoms with postpartum depression.

Consider using the Edinburgh Postnatal Depression scale to evaluate the need for referral for diagnosis and treatment.[246]

A wide range of drugs are used as antidepressants. An up-to-date drug reference should be consulted to determine the safety and possible side effects of individual drugs. Many antidepressants are compatible with breastfeeding.

Newborn and premature babies are at greater risk of side effects due to limited ability to clear drugs from their systems.

See also Baby blues; Drugs; Postpartum depression

Footnote

[246]Cox, J. L., Holden, J. M., & Sagovsky, R. (1987). Detection of postnatal depression. Development of the 10-item Edinburgh Postnatal Depression Scale. *The British Journal of Psychiatry: The Journal of Mental Science, 150,* 782–786.

➤ PREDOMINANT BREASTFEEDING

DEFINITION   A pattern of breastfeeding in which the baby is receiving mother's milk as well as water, water-based drinks, ritual foods (such as teas), and oral rehydration solution, vitamins, minerals, and oral medications.[247(p4)] The predominantly breastfed baby is not receiving any other foods or drinks, including infant formula and other animal milks.

Footnote

[247]World Health Organization. (2008). *Indicators for assessing infant and young child feeding—Part 1. Definitions.* Geneva, Switzerland: WHO.

➤ PREGNANCY, BREASTFEEDING DURING

DEFINITION   Continuing to nurse one child while pregnant with another. If a mother becomes pregnant while she is breastfeeding a baby from a prior pregnancy, she may experience extremely sore nipples and a decrease in her milk supply. It is possible to continue breastfeeding through the pregnancy and then continue nursing the two babies together. This is called "tandem nursing."

SELF-CARE INFORMATION

Deciding to nurse during pregnancy and to practice tandem nursing is an individual choice that the mother makes for herself and her family.

Although there are no reported problems with nursing during pregnancy and no reports of nursing causing premature labor, mothers with a prior history of premature birth or threatened premature labor should consider the risk as they make their decision.

Mothers should seek lactation help for sore nipples and other discomforts of pregnancy.

See also Tandem nursing

➤ PRELACTEAL FEEDS

DEFINITION   Feedings that are given to babies before they go to the breast for the first time.

➤ PREMATURE INFANT

DEFINITION   Any infant born before completion of the 37 weeks after the mother's last menstrual period. Due to increased use of fertility treatment, multiple pregnancies (e.g., twins) account for an increased percentage of all premature births. The problems of prematurity are related to the immaturity of the organ systems.

SELF-CARE INFORMATION

Mothers of premature infants should begin nipple stimulation and milk expression as soon as possible and do so regularly in order to increase the supply for the growing baby. Begin with hand expression and add pumping as the volume warrants.

The hospital nursery will have instructions available for the collection and storage of milk.

For about the first 30 days after she gives birth, the mother of the premature baby will produce milk that is higher in some of the components than the milk of mothers who deliver at term.

Premature babies can learn to breastfeed. Mothers should seek skilled lactation help.

The infant requires specialized care in a nursery until his or her organ systems have developed enough to sustain life without specialized support. Depending on the extent of prematurity, this may take weeks or months.

See also Academy of Breastfeeding Medicine (ABM); Hand expression of breastmilk; NICU, milk storage and handling in; Preterm milk

➤ PRETERM MILK

DEFINITION   For about the first 30 days after she gives birth, the mother of the premature baby will produce milk that is higher in some of the components the baby needs. This breastmilk is called "preterm milk."

The volume and calorie amounts of preterm milk are similar to that of the milk of mothers who have delivered at term. Lactose and fat amounts are comparable.

The components of preterm mothers' milk that are higher than term mothers' milk include protein and nonprotein nitrogen, long-, short- and medium-chain fatty acids, sodium, chloride, and iron.

Preterm babies may require nutrition beyond their mother's milk in order to achieve adequate growth. Because of this, her milk may be fortified or lactoengineered.

See also Bioactive components of breastmilk; Human milk fortification; Lactoengineering; Premature infant

➤ PROCTOCOLITIS

DEFINITION   Inflammation of the colon and rectum, typically caused by allergy or disease process.

Proctocolitis often results in blood in the stool. This finding requires immediate medical evaluation.

This disorder occasionally occurs in breastfed infants.

If the infant is reacting to a protein in its mother's diet, the problem may be improved by an avoidance diet. In this case, the mother may benefit from consultation with a dietitian or nutritionist.

The Academy of Breastfeeding Medicine provides a protocol for managing proctocolitis.

See also Academy of Breastfeeding Medicine (ABM); Allergy in the breastfed infant; Blood in stool

➤ PROGESTIN-ONLY CONTRACEPTIVES

DEFINITION   Fertility suppression methods containing synthetic progesterone. Oral contraceptives have been studied in relation to breastfeeding. The recommendation is that hormonal contraceptives used by nursing mothers should contain only progestin. Methods include oral pills, progestin-laden intrauterine devices, implants, and injections of progestin.

ASK ABOUT

Age of the baby.

Duration of contraceptive use.

Timing of use of contraceptive relative to birth of the baby.

ASSESSMENT

PROMPT CARE NEEDED?

Are any of the following present?

Inadequate weight gain in baby.

Perception of decreased milk supply.

IF YES,   *Call lactation care provider today.*

ROUTINE CARE NEEDED?

Are any of the following present?

> More information desired about contraception and breastfeeding.
>
> More information desired about breastfeeding and family planning or birth control.

IF YES,	*Consult up-to-date drug references, call lactation care provider, and call obstetric care provider.*

SELF-CARE INFORMATION

Consider the **lactational amenorrhea method (LAM)**, other natural family planning methods, and barrier methods of contraception if hormonal contraceptives are not acceptable or if milk supply drops.

IMPORTANT CONDITIONS TO REPORT

Decreased milk supply.

Less stooling or urination in the baby.

See also Birth control; Fertility; Hormonal contraceptive methods; Lactational amenorrhea method (LAM); Medication resources (inside back cover); Oral contraceptives; Natural family planning

➤ PROJECTILE VOMITING

DEFINITION   Projectile vomiting in the infant can be differentiated from vomiting or spitting up by the distance it travels. Projectile vomit clears the chin of the infant. It may travel several feet.

SELF-CARE INFORMATION

Occasional projectile vomiting in an otherwise well infant is not uncommon.

Projectile vomiting even in a baby with no other symptoms can indicate the presence of an underlying problem, such as pyloric stenosis, that requires treatment if persistent.

IMPORTANT CONDITIONS TO REPORT
Persistent projectile vomiting.
Signs that the baby is unwell in combination with projectile vomiting.
Decrease in stools and urinations.
Poor feeding behavior.
Weight loss or failure to gain weight adequately.

See also Pyloric stenosis; Spitting up; Vomiting

➤ PROLACTIN

DEFINITION   Prolactin is the hormone that stimulates the production and secretion of milk. It works to prepare the milk cells to make milk during pregnancy. Male and female humans both have prolactin.

See also Hormones; Milk production

➤ PUMP

DEFINITION   A device designed to remove milk from the lactating breast.

SELF-CARE INFORMATION
A breast pump cannot tell you how much milk you are making.
If you have concerns about milk supply, please call or see a lactation care provider.
Problems with pumps should be reported to the manufacturer and the U.S. Food and Drug Administration (FDA). The FDA's Manufacturer and User Facility Device Experience Database (MAUDE) contains prior complaints filed about pumps. See **DHHS/Food and Drug Administration (FDA)** for more information.

> **NOTES**
>
> A plethora of breast pumps are available. Styles, intended uses, and costs vary widely. There is no one pump that works best for all mothers. It is not appropriate to mix one manufacturer's pump kits with another manufacturer's pump, unless recommended by manufacturer.
>
> Pumps can be rented or purchased from representatives of various companies.
>
> Most pumps (with the exception of rental grade models) are not intended to be shared between women. It is possible for the interior part of these pump motors to be contaminated with microorganisms.
>
> Women will sometimes request a breast pump when they have doubts about their milk supply. Pumps should not be used to quantify or give reassurance about a woman's milk supply. Refer these women to a lactation care provider.

See also **Automatic electric breast pumps; Battery operated breast pump; Breast pump; DHHS/Food and Drug Administration (FDA); Hand expression of breastmilk; Manual pump**

➤ PYLORIC STENOSIS

DEFINITION   Pyloric stenosis happens when the pyloric sphincter (located at the outlet of the stomach) becomes thickened. The food in the stomach is prevented from moving into the small intestine as it should. Vigorous contractions of the stomach begin in an effort to force the stomach contents through the obstruction. As the sphincter tightens, projectile vomiting occurs, usually within 60 minutes after a feeding.

SELF-CARE INFORMATION

Babies can resume nursing after surgery for pyloric stenosis.

During the surgery, the mother should express her milk to keep her breasts comfortable.

Pyloric stenosis happens more frequently in male infants. Only about 1% of babies are diagnosed with pyloric stenosis. The babies are otherwise healthy. Pyloric stenosis is diagnosed less frequently among exclusively breastfed babies. Pyloric stenosis typically presents at 3–6 weeks of age, but may be seen as early as 1 week and as late as 5 months.

Pyloric stenosis is a serious condition that can result in severe dehydration, weakness, and weight loss. Surgery is usually recommended.

See also Projectile vomiting

➤ QUADRUPLETS AND QUINTUPLETS

DEFINITION   Quadruplets (quads) are four babies and quintuplets (quints) are five babies born from the same pregnancy.

ASSESSMENT

ROUTINE CARE NEEDED?

Are any of the following present?

Need for strategies for managing nursing quadruplets or quintuplets.

Need for strategies for managing milk supply for quadruplets or quintuplets.

IF YES,   *Call lactation care provider today.*

SELF-CARE INFORMATION

Hand expression should start as soon as possible after the babies are born with pumping added as volume increases.

Many mothers of multiples have found it helpful to keep a journal of who nursed when, number of wet and dirty diapers, and weight gain for each baby, to ensure that none of the babies is being overlooked.

Mothers of **higher order multiples (HOM)** may have been on bed rest during their pregnancies and can become easily fatigued. Advise them to ask for help.

Suggest easy ways for mothers to snack and drink while caring for multiple babies.

Help mothers to connect to any parent support groups for families with multiples.

Mothers can produce enough milk to support quints and quads, usually with a combination of nursing and milk expression.

See also Higher order multiples (HOM); Medication resources (inside back cover); Multiple infants (twins, triplets, and higher order multiples)

➤ RADIOACTIVE AGENTS

DEFINITION   Chemicals such as iodine, gallium, and technetium that are used in diagnostic tests and therapeutically in treatment of some conditions (e.g., thyroid ablation). Use of these agents in the lactating woman may require a temporary suspension of breastfeeding until the radioactive material has been removed from her milk by expressing and discarding it—usually in a special container.

ASK ABOUT

Age of the baby.
Specific name of radioactive agent being used.

ASSESSMENT

ROUTINE CARE NEEDED?
Are any of the following present?
Use of a radioactive chemical in a lactating woman.

IF YES,   *Consult up-to-date drug references and refer mother back to healthcare provider for consultation.*

SELF-CARE INFORMATION
Express or pump and discard milk during the time of cessation of feeding to maintain breast comfort.
Ask your radiologist for recommendations about how close you can safely be to the baby during the period of temporary suspension of feeding.

NOTES

There is a broad range of radioactive agents in use for diagnostic and therapeutic purposes. Each agent requires a different length of suspension of breastfeeding. It is essential to know the specific agents(s) involved.

X-rays do not have this same effect and may be used safely for the breastfeeding woman. Computed tomography, magnetic resonance, and ultrasound imaging are also compatible with breastfeeding.

See also Hand expression of breastmilk; Medication resources (inside back cover)

➤ RANCID OR SOAPY ODOR OF FROZEN BREASTMILK

See also Soapy odor in human milk

➤ RAPID WEIGHT GAIN

DEFINITION Growth that exceeds expectations. Well-fed breastfed babies gain weight more rapidly in the early months compared to standard growth charts and to formula-fed babies. However, some breastfed babies can be uncomfortable when getting too much milk, and rapid weight gain may be a sign of oversupply.

ASK ABOUT

Age of the baby.
Weight gain pattern of the baby.

ASSESSMENT

ROUTINE CARE NEEDED?

Are any of the following present?

About the mother:

Persistent sore nipples.

Nipples often compressed at the end of nursing.

About the baby:

Weight gain of more than 1 lb per week consistently.

Frequent, explosive, large stools.

Gassy, often unhappy baby, even after feeding.

IF YES,   *Call lactation care provider today.*

SELF-CARE INFORMATION

Oversupply can cause discomfort for mother and baby.

Careful management of the mother's milk supply can increase the baby's comfort.

IMPORTANT CONDITIONS TO REPORT

Symptoms of mastitis, including:

Plugged ducts.

Visible red areas on the breast(s).

Fever higher than 101°F (38.5°C).

Extreme breast discomfort.

Flu-like aching throughout body.

See also Milk flow, too fast

➤ RAYNAUD'S PHENOMENON/SYNDROME

DEFINITION A condition in which blood flow to the extremities is temporarily reduced. Nipple pain may occur because of Raynaud's phenomenon/syndrome.[248] It has also been called "nipple vasospasm." The affected extremity becomes cold and numb and turns white. As the blood flow returns, it may quickly turn blue and then reddish pink. This is the tricolor sign of Raynaud's. There is also a bicolor sign (white and pink). As the color returns, the pain increases. The pain can be brief, lasting for just a few minutes, or it can be prolonged, lasting up to an hour.

The reaction occurs in response to cold, wetness, stress, and certain medications.

Usually the fingers and toes are affected, but the nipples are also extremities and can therefore be affected.

ASK ABOUT

Age of the baby.
History of nipple pain.

ASSESSMENT

ROUTINE CARE NEEDED?

Are any of the following present?

Persistent nipple pain.

Breast pain in reaction to cold, wet, and nursing.

Tricolor sign (white, blue, pink) or bicolor sign (white, pink) of the nipple when cold or wet.

IF YES, *Call obstetric care provider today. Call lactation care provider today.*

SELF-CARE INFORMATION

Nifedipine is a prescription medication (calcium channel blocker) that has been used to treat Raynaud's phenomenon/syndrome in nursing mothers.[249]

Mothers with Raynaud's syndrome are usually advised to avoid caffeine and nicotine.

See also Medication resources (inside back cover); Painful breastfeeding; Sore nipples; Vasospasm of breast and nipple

Footnotes

[248]Lawlor-Smith, L., & Lawlor-Smith, C. (1997). Vasospasm of the nipple—a manifestation of Raynaud's phenomenon: Case reports. *British Medical Journal, 314*(7081), 644–645.

[249]Anderson, J. E., Held, N., & Wright, K. (2004). Raynaud's phenomenon of the nipple: A treatable cause of painful breastfeeding. *Pediatrics, 113*(4), e360–e364.

➤ REACTION TO FOODS IN THE MOTHER'S DIET

DEFINITION   Concern about the impact of foods the mother eats on her milk. Rules about eating or not eating certain foods during lactation are not warranted, may be hard to follow, and may decrease the mother's enjoyment of breastfeeding.

Gassy foods do not make babies gassy. However, there may be individual cases where certain foods affect the baby.

Flavors from foods in the mother's diet do pass into amniotic fluid prenatally and into the milk after birth. This exposure to flavors of the mother's diet may help the child to accept family foods later in childhood.

ASK ABOUT

Age of the baby.
Description and onset of symptoms.

ASSESSMENT

PROMPT CARE NEEDED?
Are any of the following present?
Blood in the stool.

IF YES,   *Call pediatric healthcare provider now.*

ROUTINE CARE NEEDED?
Are any of the following present?
Colic after the mother eats certain foods.
Inconsolable crying after the mother eats certain foods.
Other baby reactions that the mother attributes to foods she eats.

IF YES,   *Call lactation care provider.*

SELF-CARE INFORMATION

The mother's drinking of liquid cow's milk has been associated with colic symptoms in some babies. If this is the case, improvement may be seen after the mother eliminates cow's milk from her diet for at least a week.

If a mother thinks that her baby is reacting to a food in her diet, she should try eliminating it for a period of a week or longer. Keeping a record of foods eaten each day and baby's temperament may help to identify any potential problem foods.

Mothers should seek further information about diet and breastfeeding on an individual basis.

IMPORTANT CONDITIONS TO REPORT

Difficulty breathing.

Difficulty swallowing.

Rapid progression of symptoms.

See also Allergy in the breastfed infant; Cabbage leaves for engorgement; Colic, infantile; Food restrictions postpartum; Maternal diet

➤ **READINESS FOR FAMILY FOODS**

DEFINITION Developmental preparedness of the infant for table foods. The American Academy of Pediatrics (AAP), The United States Breastfeeding Committee (USBC), The United Nations Children's Fund (UNICEF), and The World Health Organization (WHO) recommend exclusive breastfeeding for about the first 6 months of life.

Researchers have shown that flavors from the foods the mother eats in pregnancy and during lactation pass into the milk. When family foods taste familiar, the baby is more accepting of them.

In addition to age, signs of readiness may include:

Increased interest in table foods.

Ability to sit up.

Ability to pick up objects and put them in the mouth.

Decreased tongue thrusting (automatically pushing foods out of the mouth with the tongue).

ASK ABOUT

Age of the baby.

Reason for wanting to start solid foods.

ASSESSMENT

PROMPT CARE NEEDED?

Are any of the following present?

Breastfed baby under 5 months of age with one or more of the following:

A mother who is concerned about her baby's weight gain.

Decreased stooling or urination.

IF YES,   *Call pediatric care provider today and call lactation care provider today.*

ROUTINE CARE NEEDED?

Are any of the following present?

Breastfed baby around 6 months of age, with maternal questions about starting family foods.

IF YES,   *Call lactation care provider.*

SELF-CARE INFORMATION

Babies are not equally interested in starting solid foods. Allow the baby to hold foods—bring them to the mouth to lick and taste.

When babies start solid foods around 6 months, they do not usually have a prolonged time on the semiliquid foods that were popular years ago when starting solids was recommended at younger ages.[250]

Move the baby onto family foods as appropriate.

IMPORTANT CONDITIONS TO REPORT

Difficulty breathing.

Difficulty swallowing.

Rapid progression of symptoms.

See also Allergy in the breastfed infant; Mixed feeds; Solid foods for breastfed babies

Footnote

[250]Rapley, G., & Murkett, T. (2010). *Baby-led weaning: The essential guide to introducing solid foods and helping your baby to grow up a happy and confident eater.* New York, NY: The Experiment.

➤ RECLINING POSTURE

DEFINITION   A posture in which the mother reclines or lies fully on her back with the baby lying on the mother's abdomen. This technique is known as the "laid-back position." The baby has complete head control in this position. This is a restful way for mothers to nurse, and it also allows optimizes the baby's abilities to self-attach and switch position. It can also be beneficial for large-breasted women and situations of oversupply and fast-flowing milk.

See also Australian posture; Milk flow, too fast; Oversupply

➤ REDUCTION SURGERY, BREAST

DEFINITION   A procedure that decreases the size of the breast by removing fat and glandular tissue. Reduction surgery is likely to affect a woman's ability to produce milk.

ASK ABOUT

Date of surgery.
Type of procedure.

ASSESSMENT

PROMPT CARE NEEDED?

Are any of the following present?

Meconium bowel movements after 5 days of life.

No yellow stool by day 5.

Fewer than three bowel movements daily in a breastfed newborn after the first 2 days of life.

No urine in 6 hours.

Brick dust urine (uric acid crystals) after 2 days of life.

Dark-colored urine.

Fewer than four urinations daily in the breastfed newborn after day 5 of life.

IF YES,   *Seek pediatric care now.*

PROMPT CARE NEEDED?

Are any of the following present?

Concerns about milk supply.

Concerns about infant weight gain without symptoms previously listed.

IF YES,   *Call lactation care provider today.*

SELF-CARE INFORMATION

Monitor baby's feeding, stooling, and urination patterns daily.

Practice skin-to-skin contact in the first hour and frequently thereafter.

Feed the baby at the first sign of hunger cues (signs that say "feed me" include hand-to-face or hand-to-mouth movements, lip smacking, seeking with lips, rooting, and head bobbing).

Feed the baby at least 10 times per 24 hours.

Listen for signs of the baby swallowing.

Allow the baby to end feedings.

Expect at least four infant stools per 24 hours after the first 4 days of life.

Good positioning and attachment are crucial to prevent or reduce nipple pain.

If feedings are missed, hand express or pump milk to maintain supply.

IMPORTANT CONDITIONS TO REPORT

Inadequate feeding (fewer than 10 feedings daily in the newborn).

Inadequate stooling pattern (fewer than three stools daily in the newborn after day 4).

Ongoing concerns.

NOTES

It is not possible to predict the degree of lactation success before giving birth. Women who are interested in breastfeeding should be encouraged to do so with ongoing, proactive monitoring of the baby's growth.

Surgical techniques that include complete removal of the nipple are more likely to decrease innervation of the nipple (and thus, effective stimulation and secretion of lactation hormones). Nipple sensation may indicate the extent to which innervation has been altered.

Pedicle techniques, which preserve nipple attachment, may have a lesser impact on potential for milk production.

See also Breast surgery; Insufficient milk supply; Pedicle technique for breast reduction

➤ REFLUX, GASTROESOPHAGEAL (GE)

DEFINITION   Movement of stomach contents up into the esophagus and mouth.

ASK ABOUT

Age of the baby.

History of vomiting/description of vomiting.

History of weight gain or loss.

History of pneumonia or lung problems.

History of choking.

ASSESSMENT

EMERGENT CARE NEEDED?

Are any of the following present?

Difficulty breathing.

Choking.

Difficulty swallowing.

Rapid progression of symptoms.

IF YES,   *Seek emergency care now.*

PROMPT CARE NEEDED?

Are any of the following present?

Decrease in urination.

Decrease in stooling.

Meconium bowel movements after 5 days of life.

No yellow stool by day 5.

Fewer than three bowel movements daily in a breastfed newborn after the first 2 days of life.

No urine in 6 hours.

Brick dust urine (uric acid crystals) after 2 days of life.

Dark-colored urine.

Fewer than four urinations daily in the breastfed newborn after day 5.

Noticeably sunken fontanelles (soft spot on the top of the head).

Decreased activity.

Baby below birthweight at 10–14 days.

Cessation of weight gain.

IF YES,   *Seek pediatric care within 4 hours.*

ROUTINE CARE NEEDED?

Are any of the following present?

Baby spits up regularly after nursing.

Weight gain is adequate.

Urination and stooling pattern is adequate.

IF YES,   *Call lactation care provider today.*

SELF-CARE INFORMATION

Many breastfed babies spit up frequently without any underlying medical cause. A baby who spits up often should be evaluated by his or her healthcare provider.

IMPORTANT CONDITIONS TO REPORT

Difficulty breathing.
Choking.
Difficulty swallowing.
Rapid progression of symptoms.
Decrease in urination.
Decrease in stooling.
Signs of dehydration.

NOTES

Gastroesophageal (GE) reflux in infants is not common in babies who are exclusively breastfed, except in babies who have been previously tube fed.[251] With GE reflux, the stomach contents move up out of the stomach and back into the esophagus.

With GE reflux, babies vomit after eating. The vomiting happens most of the time and is not projectile (does not clear the chin).

See also Gastroesophageal (GE) reflux; Milk flow, too fast

Footnote

[251]Heacock, H. J., Jeffery, H. E., Baker, J. L., & Page, M. (1992). Influence of breast versus formula milk on physiological gastroesophageal reflux in healthy, newborn infants. *Journal of Pediatric Gastroenterology and Nutrition, 14*, 41–46.

➤ REFUSAL OF INFANT TO BREASTFEED

DEFINITION   A situation in which a baby is not willing to nurse. Babies can refuse to breastfeed even from the first nursing, although this is rare. A nursing strike is a sudden refusal of the baby to nurse. This can happen with a baby of any age.

A newborn baby who is refusing to breastfeed is telling us that there is something wrong. Careful evaluation of the baby and the mother's breasts and observation of breastfeeding is important.

ASK ABOUT

Age of the baby.

Nursing history.

History of any recent mother–baby separation.

ASSESSMENT

PROMPT CARE NEEDED?

Are any of the following present?

The baby refuses to nurse.

Onset of inconsolable crying.

The baby refuses other age-appropriate foods.

Change in stooling, urination, or sleep patterns.

Lethargy.

IF YES, *Call pediatric care provider now and call lactation care provider now.*

ROUTINE CARE NEEDED?

Are any of the following present?

The baby refuses to nurse but otherwise seems normal.

IF YES, *Call lactation care provider today and call pediatric care provider today.*

SELF-CARE INFORMATION

Mothers whose babies refuse to nurse should express milk for comfort and to maintain the milk supply. Expressed milk can be fed by cup or spoon.

Many babies who have gone on strike return to the breast once the problem has been resolved.

Do not starve the baby to the breast. Babies need to be fed.

Babies refuse to nurse when something is wrong in their lives. Some of the reasons reported for newborns refusing to nurse include:

Birth injury.

Low milk volume.

Poor positioning technique.

An undiagnosed medical problem in the baby.

Undiagnosed breast cancer in the mother.

Some of the reasons reported for older babies refusing to nurse include:
Teething.
Stuffy nose.
Ear infection.
Baby has bitten the mother, and she yelled; this frightened the baby.
Reaction to being left unattended to cry it out.
Family stress.
Recent separation of mother and baby, such as mother's return to work.

IMPORTANT CONDITIONS TO REPORT
Change in stooling or urination patterns.
Sleepiness, lethargy.
Breathing difficulties.
Vomiting.
Inconsolable crying.

See also **Breast refusal; Goldsmith's sign; Nursing strike; One-sided nursing**

➤ RELACTATION

DEFINITION   Relactation is the bringing back of lactation. A woman who has given birth has been in the state of lactation even if she did not breastfeed. A woman can relactate weeks or months after giving birth.

ASK ABOUT

Lactation history.
Age of the baby.
Duration of time since last breastfeeding (if there was any breastfeeding).
Reason for wanting to relactate (baby's tolerance of other foods).

ROUTINE CARE NEEDED?

Are any of the following present?

Mother desires information about relactation.

Mother desires to relactate.

IF YES, *Call lactation care provider today. Call pediatric care provider today.*

SELF-CARE INFORMATION

The infant's willingness to nurse is an important consideration in whether breast-feeding will be possible.

If the reason the mother did not breastfeed or did not lactate after birth (severe breast reduction for example) is still present, relactation may be very difficult.

Pumping and hand expression or both are excellent ways to collect milk and build up the milk supply in relactating mothers.

NOTES

Mothers may be successful at bringing in a full supply of milk via pumping or hand expression or a combination of both. Transitioning the baby to the breast may take longer.

See also Decrease in milk supply; Increasing milk supply; Milk production; Pump

➤ RETAINED PLACENTAL FRAGMENTS

DEFINITION Small pieces of placenta (fragments) that are retained in the uterus after the placenta is delivered. The fragment continues to be supported but may subsequently break away. When this happens, the area of the uterus continues to bleed. The mother may hemorrhage and lose a considerable amount of blood.

ASK ABOUT

Age of the baby.
Current vaginal bleeding.
Breastfeeding difficulties.

ASSESSMENT

EMERGENT CARE NEEDED?

Are any of the following present?

> Soaking a sanitary napkin with bright red blood at a rate of one napkin or more per hour.
>
> Clots in the bloody discharge.
>
> Foul odor to the discharge (even if occasional).
>
> Dizziness.
>
> Fever.
>
> Abdominal pain.

IF YES,   *Seek emergency care now or call obstetric care provider immediately.*

PROMPT CARE NEEDED?

Are any of the following present?

> Soaking a sanitary napkin with bright red blood at a rate of one napkin every 2–3 hours.
>
> Abdominal tenderness.
>
> Low-grade fever.
>
> Light-headedness.

IF YES,   *Seek obstetric care within 4 hours.*

ROUTINE CARE NEEDED?

Are any of the following present?

> Soaking a sanitary napkin with bright red blood at a rate of one napkin every 3 or more hours.
>
> Abdominal tenderness.

IF YES,   *Seek obstetric care today.*

PROMPT LACTATION CARE NEEDED?

Are any of the following present?

Problems with milk supply in a woman diagnosed with retained placental fragments.

IF YES,   *Call lactation care provider today.*

SELF-CARE INFORMATION

Rapid soaking of a sanitary napkin with bright red blood after the early days post-partum may be associated with retained placental fragments and can be the first sign of hemorrhage.

Retained placental fragments have been associated with the failure to establish an adequate milk supply.

IMPORTANT CONDITIONS TO REPORT

Increase in bright red blood flow.

Bright red blood after 2 weeks postpartum.

NOTES

A sign of retained placental fragments is the continued vaginal flow of red blood after the early days postpartum.

Retained placental fragments are associated in some women with failure to produce sufficient milk due to the influence of the hormone progesterone, which is manufactured by the placenta.

See also Bleeding, postpartum vaginal; Lochia

➤ REVERSE CYCLE BREASTFEEDING

DEFINITION   A nursing style where the working mother nurses when she is with the baby, giving the baby the majority of calories while they are together. Then, when she is away from the baby, the baby needs less expressed milk or other foods.

ASK ABOUT

Age of the baby.

ASSESSMENT

ROUTINE CARE NEEDED?

Are any of the following present?

The mother is going to work and will be separated from her baby.

IF YES, *Call lactation care provider.*

IMPORTANT CONDITIONS TO REPORT

Change in baby's weight gain pattern.

See also Cosleeping; Feeding pattern of breastfed infants; Maternal employment; Night nursings

➤ ROOMING IN

DEFINITION   Rooming in is a hospital arrangement in which the baby stays in the mother's hospital room. The expectation of the UNICEF/WHO Baby-Friendly Hospital Initiative is that in Baby-Friendly hospitals, babies will room in with their mothers most of the 24 hours in a day.

SELF-CARE INFORMATION

Rooming in offers the opportunity for mothers and babies to get to know each other, for observation of feeding cues, for frequent nursing, and for learning together.

According to research studies, mothers who room in with their babies get off to a better start at breastfeeding.

See also Baby-Friendly Hospital Initiative (BFHI); Ten Steps to Successful Breastfeeding

➤ RUSTY-PIPE SYNDROME (RUSTY-PIPE MILK)

DEFINITION Pumped milk with small bloody streaks or small amounts of rust-colored milk. When examined, the milk is positive for the mother's blood. The condition is temporary (lasts only a few days), and babies accept the milk.

ASK ABOUT

Age of the baby.
History of pumping.

ASSESSMENT

ROUTINE CARE NEEDED?
Are any of the following present?
Orange or blood-streaked pumped milk that does not improve over the course of a week.

IF YES, *Call lactation care provider today. Call obstetric care provider today (rusty-pipe milk could also be a sign of intraductal papilloma).*

IMPORTANT CONDITIONS TO REPORT
Recurrence.
Ongoing rusty color in milk.

See also Blood in milk; Papilloma, intraductal; Sore nipples

➤ SALINE OR SILICONE BREAST IMPLANTS

DEFINITION Saline or silicone-filled medical prosthesis surgically inserted into the breast to increase its size.

ASK ABOUT

Date of implant surgery.
Age of the baby.
Location of the surgical incision.

ASSESSMENT

PROMPT CARE NEEDED?

Are any of the following present?

Presence of implants with:

Concerns about milk supply.

Poor weight gain in breastfed baby.

IF YES, *Call lactation care provider now and report to pediatric care provider.*

SELF-CARE INFORMATION

Practice skin-to-skin contact in the first hour and frequently thereafter.
Feed the baby at first sign of hunger cues (signs that say "feed me" include hand-to-face or hand-to-mouth movements, lip smacking, seeking with lips, rooting, and head bobbing).
Feed the baby at least 10 times per 24 hours.
Listen for signs of the baby swallowing.
Allow the baby to end feedings.
Expect at least three infant stools per 24 hours after the first 4 days of life.
Good positioning and attachment are crucial to prevent or reduce nipple pain.
If feedings are missed, hand express or pump milk to reduce fullness or engorgement and maintain supply.

IMPORTANT CONDITIONS TO REPORT

Fewer than four bowel movements daily after day 4 of life.
Ongoing concerns or problems with milk supply.
Ongoing concerns or problems with full breasts or engorgement.

NOTES

Implants can affect milk-making ability to some extent by reducing storage capacity in the breast.

The location and extent of the incision may impact the sensation of the nerves in the nipple area. Loss of or decreased sensation may decrease milk-making potential. Trauma to the nerves may hinder the stimulation of the brain to release prolactin (the milk-making hormone) in response to suckling. Periareolar incisions suggest more potential nerve and duct injury than do incisions underneath the breast.

Babies of women who have had breast augmentation surgery should be followed closely to ensure proper growth.

If the mother reports that she had an implant in one breast only, inquire about the reason for this surgery. If augmentation corrected breast asymmetry, there may be increased concern regarding the mother's ability to make a full milk supply. Marked asymmetry may indicate insufficient glandular tissue in both breasts. The baby and mother should be closely followed.

Concern has been expressed about the possibility of silicon entering the breastmilk, but research has not indicated negative effects.

See also Asymmetric breasts; Augmentation surgery; Breast augmentation; Breast surgery; Engorgement; Weight gain, baby–low

➤ SALTY TASTE OF BREASTMILK

DEFINITION   Reported briny odor or flavor of human milk. Human milk can increase in sodium if the mother has mastitis, if the milk supply is very low, or in some cases during weaning. The sodium in human milk is never as high as it is in formula.

ASK ABOUT

Age of the baby.
Onset of salty taste.
Presence of symptoms.

ASSESSMENT

EMERGENT CARE NEEDED?

Are any of the following present?

Seizures or convulsions.

Lethargy.

Inadequate urine or stool output.

Rapid progression of symptoms.

IF YES, *Seek emergent care now. Call pediatric care provider now.*

PROMPT CARE NEEDED?

Are any of the following present?

About the mother:

Visible red areas on the breast(s).

Fever higher than 101°F (38.5°C).

Extreme breast discomfort.

Flu-like aching throughout the body.

Continued fever after treatment.

Reaction to the antibiotic prescribed.

IF YES, *Seek obstetric care within 4 hours.*

Are any of the following present?

About the baby:

Breastfeeding infant hospitalized for dehydration, jaundice, or hypernatremia associated with poor milk intake.

IF YES, *Call lactation care provider now for feeding assessment.*

ROUTINE CARE NEEDED?

Are any of the following present?

Weaning.

IF YES, *Call lactation care provider.*

SELF-CARE INFORMATION

Breastmilk sodium can increase naturally during gradual weaning, and the milk will taste salty.

NOTES

Breastmilk sodium can increase naturally during gradual weaning. The milk will taste salty at that point. This change can also occur when feeding frequency is limited or little milk is taken from the breast. When a nursing infant is hospitalized with hypernatremia, dehydration, or jaundice, breastfeeding evaluation is always indicated. In addition, infection and neurologic and renal issues will be ruled out.

See also Failure to thrive (FTT); Mastitis; Weaning; Sodium in breastmilk

➤ SCU

See Neonatal Intensive Care Unit (NICU); Special care unit (SCU)

➤ SECRETORY IGA

DEFINITION   A class antibodies produced by the mother and added to her milk by the mammary cells. The *Ig* in *IgA* stands for immunoglobulin. All classes of immunoglobulins (including IgG, IgD, IgM, and IgE) are found in human milk. They are found in higher amounts in colostrum.

SELF-CARE INFORMATION

Nursing in the first hours after birth transfers IgA from the mother to the baby. The IgA coats the baby's intestines, lung surfaces, and other mucous membranes. This begins to protect the baby from bacteria and viruses as soon as possible.

NOTES

Human babies are born without IgA, which coats all of the mucous membranes in adult humans, forming a protective barrier to viruses and bacteria.

See also Bioactive components of breastmilk; Immunoglobulin

➤ SEIZURES

DEFINITION Sudden changes in behavior caused by temporary changes in activity of the brain and nerves. Seizures may be characterized by jerking in the limbs, eyes rolling up, eyelids fluttering, incontinence, twitching, breathing difficulty, and many other symptoms. Seizure is a medical emergency in an infant. Seizure disorder in the breastfeeding mother calls for careful evaluation, including her medications.

ASK ABOUT

Age of the baby.
Onset of seizure.
History of seizures in mother.

ASSESSMENT

EMERGENT CARE NEEDED?

Are any of the following present?

Symptoms of seizure in an infant, including:

Excessive drooling.

Turning blue.

Rolling back eyes.

Uncontrollable shaking in the arms and legs.

IF YES, *Seek emergency care now.*

PROMPT CARE NEEDED?

Are any of the following present?

Questions about breastfeeding in a woman with history of epilepsy or seizure disorder.

Questions about compatibility of seizure control medications with breastfeeding.

IF YES, *Call lactation care provider today and consult up-to-date drug references.*

See also Epilepsy; Medication resources (inside back cover)

➤ SEPARATION OF MOTHER AND BABY

DEFINITION   Occasions where a mother and baby are not in close contact with one another. Ideally, mothers and babies can maintain close contact from the moment of birth throughout the newborn period. Unless there are medical problems for the mother and/or baby, there is no need for mother–baby separation in the early post-partum period.

ASK ABOUT

Age of the baby.
Reason for separation.
Duration of separation.

ASSESSMENT

PROMPT LACTATION CARE NEEDED?

Are any of the following present?

Immediate need to express milk due to hospitalization or surgery.

Drug questions related to maternal hospitalization or surgery.

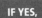 *Call lactation care provider now and consult up-to-date drug references.*

ROUTINE LACTATION CARE NEEDED?

Are any of the following present?

Questions about facilitating milk expression for future separation for reasons of medical procedure, return to work/school, or relief feedings.

IF YES,   *Call lactation care provider.*

SELF-CARE INFORMATION

During long periods of separation, express milk frequently via hand expression or pumping.

Seek to replicate the baby's normal breastfeeding pattern, expressing milk 10–12 times per 24 hours.

See also Expression of mothers' milk; Hand expression of breastmilk; Medication resources (inside back cover); Pump

➤ SEPSIS

DEFINITION   Serious infection in the bloodstream. Sepsis is a life-threatening condition in infants and mothers.

See also Fever; Lethargy; Uncoordinated suckling; Weak suck

➤ SEXUALITY

DESCRIPTION   Sexual activity and intercourse is compatible with breastfeeding, although the low estrogen level of the breastfeeding mother may contribute to vaginal dryness. She may also experience residual discomfort or pain from the birth or episiotomy.

Women may feel differently about sexual relations after the birth of a baby. Many women feel less desire, although some women feel more. No one can predict how a woman will feel.

Breastfeeding is an intimate activity that may make the rest of the family feel left out.

In addition, mothers may feel tired when they have a new baby whether or not they are breastfeeding, and they may not have the energy for sexual activities.

ASK ABOUT

Age of the baby.

ASSESSMENT

ROUTINE MEDICAL CARE NEEDED?
Are any of the following present?
Difficult penetration.
Pain during intercourse.

IF YES,   *Call obstetric care provider.*

ROUTINE LACTATION CARE NEEDED?

Are any of the following present?

Questions about normalcy of feelings.

| IF YES, | *Call lactation care provider.* |

SELF-CARE INFORMATION

Life changes after the birth of a baby, and it is sometimes hard for mothers to know if what they are experiencing is normal. Talking about feelings and physical concerns can help a mother with the adjustment.

IMPORTANT CONDITIONS TO REPORT

Feelings of extreme worry or anxiety.

Difficult or painful penetration.

Pain during intercourse.

See also Fertility; Menstrual cycle

➤ SGA

See Small for gestational age (SGA)

➤ SHEEHAN'S SYNDROME

DEFINITION   Sheehan's syndrome is a condition that may develop when the pituitary gland is deprived of blood and oxygen because of a severe hemorrhage after childbirth. Sheehan's syndrome is a condition that is now uncommon due to modern obstetric care and the availability of blood transfusions.

ASK ABOUT

Age of the baby.
Weight gain pattern of the baby.
History of hemorrhage.

ASSESSMENT

EMERGENT CARE NEEDED?

Are any of the following present?

Soaking a sanitary napkin with bright red blood at a rate of one napkin or
more per hour.

Clots in the bloody discharge.

Foul odor to the discharge (even if occasional).

Dizziness.

Fever.

Abdominal pain.

IF YES,   *Call obstetric care provider now and seek emergency care now.*

PROMPT MEDICAL CARE NEEDED?

Are any of the following present?

Soaking a sanitary napkin with bright red blood at a rate of one napkin every
2–3 hours.

Abdominal tenderness.

Low-grade fever.

Light-headedness.

IF YES,   *Call obstetric care provider now.*

PROMPT LACTATION CARE NEEDED?

Are any of the following present?

Problems with milk supply in a woman with a history of postpartum hemorrhage or heavy bleeding.

IF YES,   *Call lactation care provider today.*

ROUTINE CARE NEEDED?

Are any of the following present?

Soaking a sanitary napkin with bright red blood at a rate of one napkin every 3 or more hours.

Abdominal tenderness.

IF YES, *Call obstetric care provider today.*

IMPORTANT CONDITIONS TO REPORT

Frequent urination and excessive thirst.

Feeling cold frequently.

Feeling dizzy or light-headed.

NOTES

Because of the pituitary damage from the blood loss, the mother may have failure to move into full lactation.

Transient cases of Sheehan's syndrome have been reported.

The amount of damage to the pituitary gland is variable and there may be no other symptoms besides insufficient milk and insufficient milk transfer until later in life. Some women go undiagnosed for many years.

Other symptoms include:

Diabetes insipidus.

Hair loss (especially from the armpit and pubic area).

Hypothyroidism.

Infertility or amenorrhea.

See also Hemorrhage, postpartum; Lochia; Retained placental fragments; Thyroid disease

➤ SIDS

See Sudden infant death syndrome (SIDS)

➤ SKIN-TO-SKIN (STS) CARE

DEFINITION   Skin-to-skin care (STS care or kangaroo care) is a special kind of holding where the baby is skin to skin with the mother. Skin-to-skin care can start right after birth for mothers of term babies and whenever the NICU staff say that a premature baby is ready.

SELF-CARE INFORMATION

Pregnant women should discuss skin-to-skin care with their providers so that the provider knows that it is important to the mother.

Do not just think about skin-to-skin care as something to do for the first few hours after the baby is born. Hold the baby skin to skin often. The baby can hear your heartbeat and feel comforted and warm.

NOTES

Research indicates that premature babies have more optimal outcomes when held skin to skin or in kangaroo care, such as better breastfeeding outcomes, cardiorespiratory stability, decreased crying, and decreased bilirubin levels, when compared with babies in standard NICU care.[252,253,254]

See also Kangaroo care (KC)

Footnotes

[252] Moore, E. R., Anderson, G. C., Bergman, N., & Dowswell, T. (2012). Early skin-to-skin contact for mothers and their healthy newborn infants. *Cochrane Database of Systematic Reviews (Online)*, 5, CD003519. doi:10.1002/14651858.CD003519.pub3

[253] Nyqvist, K. H., Sjödén, P. O., & Ewald, U. (1999). The development of preterm infants' breastfeeding behavior. *Early Human Development*, 55(3), 247–264.

[254]Samra, N. M., El Taweel, A., & Cadwell, K. (2012). The effect of kangaroo mother care on the duration of phototherapy of infants re-admitted for neonatal jaundice. *Journal of Maternal-Fetal and Neonatal Medicine*, 25(8), 1354–1357. doi:10.3109/14767058.2011.634459

➤ SLEEP PATTERNS

DEFINITION   Unique sleep-wake cycles of the infant. Newborn babies have no idea what time it is. They do not have a pattern to their sleep and waking. They do not know if it is night or day, and they are not manipulating their parents.

Night feedings are expected for the first 4 months or so, and then babies might sleep one 5-hour stretch at night. Night waking is normal well into the toddler years.

Many babies continue to nap during the day well into their second year. Preschools and daycare centers structure naps into their day.

ASK ABOUT

Age of the baby.
Weight gain pattern.

ASSESSMENT

PROMPT CARE NEEDED?

Are any of the following present?

Sleep deprivation in the parent.

Anger or other strong reaction to the baby waking at night.

IF YES,   *Call medical care provider today.*

ROUTINE CARE NEEDED?

Are any of the following present?

Concern about:

Night wakening.

Night feedings.

Night crying.

IF YES,   *Call lactation care provider.*

SELF-CARE INFORMATION

Keeping the baby close at night can minimize sleep loss. In addition, babies may transfer more milk.

Try daytime interventions for nighttime wakening problems. Nurse the baby more often during the daytime and avoid long naps in the car seat or home.

IMPORTANT CONDITIONS TO REPORT

Anger at baby waking in the night.

See also Cosleeping; Feeding pattern of breastfed infants; Maternal fatigue; Night nursings; Reverse cycle breastfeeding

➤ SLEEPY BABY

DESCRIPTION A temporary condition in which the baby is difficult to arouse or keep awake during feedings. Some babies are sleepy at first, making it difficult to accomplish 10–12 effective feedings per day after the first day of life. There can be many reasons for sleepiness, such as sepsis (severe infection in the bloodstream), jaundice (which may cause lethargy), drug effects from labor analgesia, difficult labor and birth, and separation from mother.

ASK ABOUT

Age of the baby.
History of sleepiness.
History of weight gain or loss.

ASSESSMENT

EMERGENT CARE NEEDED?

Are any of the following present?

Inability to rouse the baby.

Baby sleeps more than 3 hours between feedings consistently.

Shallow breathing or breathing difficult to observe. (Observe the newborn's breathing for at least 1 minute. Sleeping newborns often exhibit periodic breathing which may include rapid shallow breaths interspersed with brief pauses in breathing.)

Meconium bowel movements after 5 days after birth.

Fewer than three bowel movements daily in the breastfed newborn after the first 2 days of life.

No urine in 6 hours.

Brick dust urine (uric acid crystals) after 2 days of life.

Dark-colored urine.

Fewer than four urinations daily in the breastfed newborn after day 5 after birth.

Low muscle tone or floppiness.

IF YES, *Seek pediatric care now.*

PROMPT CARE NEEDED?

Are any of the following present?

Baby nurses fewer than 10 times in 24 hours.

Baby consistently falls asleep after sucking briefly at the breast.

Baby is not gaining at least 0.5 oz a day.

IF YES, *Call lactation care provider now.*

SELF-CARE INFORMATION

Parents who observe the baby for feeding cues—hand-to-face or hand-to-mouth movements, lip smacking, seeking with lips, rooting, and head bobbing—may find it easier to feed the baby at the baby's best time.

Young babies tend to cluster their feedings. Nurse the baby again when the baby gives the next feeding cue (i.e., watch the baby, not the clock to determine the timing of the next feeding). The baby never completely empties the breast.

Watch for softened body tone and loose hands after feeding to indicate satiety.

IMPORTANT CONDITIONS TO REPORT

Babies that are hard to rouse and sleep longer than 3 hours between nursings should be evaluated.

Babies who fall asleep after a minute or two at the breast should be evaluated.

See also Feeding cues; Hyperbilirubinemia; Hypotonia; Lethargy

➤ SLING/BABY CARRIER

DEFINITION   Cloth device used to hold the baby close to a caregiver's body. Many types exist, from simple pieces of fabric to complex packs. There are many types of slings and baby carriers, from simple cloths to complex packs. Babies and mothers often have a preference based on their comfort and need. Slings that allow breast-feeding may facilitate cue-based breastfeeding for mothers who are simultaneously working or caring for other children.

Some slings and baby carriers allow the mother to have two hands free. Others require the mother to use her arm to support the baby. Some allow the baby to nurse while being carried. Slings that cradle the baby in a flexed position are especially good for babies who are hypertonic or hypotonic.

SELF-CARE INFORMATION

Use the sling or carrier the first few times when the baby is content to help with adjusting to this new experience.

See also Hypertonia; Muscle tone of infant

➤ SLOW WEIGHT GAIN, BABY

DEFINITION   Rate of weight gain that occurs slower than anticipated. Breastfed babies should gain a minimum of 0.5 oz a day on average in the early weeks. New studies indicate that breastfed babies gain even faster than was previously believed, probably because breastfeeding used to be done on a schedule and not as frequently as we now know is ideal. Growth standards using exclusively breastfed babies have been developed by the World Health Organization and are recommended by the Centers for Disease Control and Prevention and the American Academy of Pediatrics. Rates of growth change throughout the first year. Babies are thought to generally double their birthweight by 6 months and triple it by 12 months.

ASK ABOUT

Age of the baby.
Weight gain pattern.

ASSESSMENT

PROMPT CARE NEEDED?

Are any of the following present?

Lethargy.

Hard-to-rouse baby.

Meconium bowel movements after 5 days after birth.

Fewer than three bowel movements daily in breastfed newborn after the first 2 days after birth.

No urine in 6 hours.

Brick dust urine (uric acid crystals) after 2 days after birth.

Dark-colored urine.

Fewer than four urinations daily in the breastfed newborn after day 5 of life.

Noticeably sunken fontanelles (soft spot on the top of the head).

Decreased activity.

Baby below birthweight after 14 days of life.

Cessation of weight gain.

Poor feedings.

Sleeping at the breast.

IF YES,   *Seek pediatric care now.*

ROUTINE CARE NEEDED?

Are any of the following present?

Baby sleeps at the breast after a few sucks.

Difficulty latching on.

No audible swallows.

Pediatric referral for breastfeeding evaluation.

IF YES,   *Call lactation care provider today.*

IMPORTANT CONDITIONS TO REPORT

Decrease in number of urinations or stools.

Increased sleepiness, hours spent sleeping.

Baby is harder to rouse.

See also Growth chart; Hypotonia; Jaundice; Muscle tone of infant

➤ SMALL FOR GESTATIONAL AGE (SGA)

DEFINITION Smaller in weight or length than expected for newborns at their gestational age.

➤ SMOKING

DEFINITION Use of tobacco products. Mothers who smoke may breastfeed. However, all babies should be protected from secondhand smoke.

ASK ABOUT

Age of the baby.
Weight gain pattern of the baby.

ASSESSMENT

ROUTINE CARE NEEDED?

Are any of the following present?

Baby using pacifier.
Frequent feedings.
Smoking in the baby's environment.
Low milk supply.
Poor feeding.
Poor weight gain.
Desire to cut down or stop smoking.

IF YES, *Call lactation care provider today. Report to pediatric care provider today.*

SELF-CARE INFORMATION

Research indicates that mothers who smoke may make and secrete less milk, but if they cut down or stop smoking, their milk supply may rebound.

Babies and children should always be protected from secondhand smoke.

Breastfeeding may mitigate the negative effects of smoking during pregnancy.

Poor weight gain pattern or weight loss.
Poor feeding.
Upper respiratory problems in baby (e.g., coughing or runny nose).

See also Nicotine

➤ SOAPY ODOR IN FROZEN MILK

DEFINITION   Slightly rancid odor or flavor in expressed milk. Human milk contains digestive properties in the form of enzymes. When the baby nurses, these components of milk go right into the baby with the milk. It is one of the reasons breastmilk is so easy for babies to digest. When milk is collected and stored, these active components still function.

NOTES

For some women, the milk takes on a soapy or rancid odor that they notice when the milk is defrosted. The milk is not spoiled. Rather, the odor is the result of the continued activity of digestive enzymes in the milk.

Women who want to stop the digestive activity can gently heat the milk to scalding after collecting it and before freezing. This process usually stops the digestive process.

See also Salty taste of breastmilk

➤ SODIUM IN BREASTMILK

DEFINITION   Salty taste in human milk. Human milk can increase in sodium if the mother has mastitis, if the milk supply is very low, or in some cases during weaning. The sodium in human milk is never as high as it is in formula.

ASK ABOUT

Age of the baby.
Onset of salty taste
Presence of symptoms.

ASSESSMENT

EMERGENT CARE NEEDED?

Are any of the following present?

Seizures or convulsions.

Lethargy.

Inadequate urine or stool output.

Rapid progression of symptoms.

IF YES, *Seek emergency care now. Call pediatric care provider now.*

PROMPT CARE NEEDED?

Are any of the following present?

About the mother:

Visible red areas on the breast(s).

Fever higher than 101°F (38.5°C).

Extreme breast discomfort.

Flu-like aching throughout body.

Continued fever after treatment.

Reaction to antibiotics that are prescribed.

IF YES, *Seek obstetric care within 4 hours.*

Are any of the following present?

About the baby:

Breastfeeding infant hospitalized for dehydration, jaundice, or hypernatremia associated with poor milk intake.

IF YES, *Call lactation care provider now for feeding assessment.*

ROUTINE CARE NEEDED?

Are any of the following present?

Weaning.

IF YES, *Call lactation care provider.*

SELF-CARE INFORMATION

Breastmilk sodium can increase naturally during gradual weaning, and the milk will taste salty.

NOTES

Breast milk sodium can increase naturally during gradual weaning. The milk will taste salty at that point. This change can also occur when feeding frequency is limited or when little milk is taken from the breast. When a nursing infant is hospitalized with hypernatremia, dehydration, or jaundice, breastfeeding evaluation is always indicated. In addition, infection and neurologic and renal issues will be ruled out.

See also Failure to thrive (FTT); Mastitis; Weaning; Salty taste of breastmilk

➤ SOLID FOODS FOR BREASTFED BABIES

DEFINITION   Table foods that are fed to a breastfeeding infant. The American Academy of Pediatrics (AAP), the United States Breastfeeding Committee (USBC), the United Nations Children's Fund (UNICEF) and the World Health Organization (WHO) recommend exclusive breastfeeding for about the first 6 months of life.

Researchers have shown that flavors from the foods the mother eats in pregnancy and during lactation pass into the milk. When foods taste familiar, the baby is more accepting of family foods.

In addition to age, signs of readiness may include:

Increased interest in table foods.

Ability to sit up.

Ability to pick up objects and put them in the mouth.

Decreased tongue thrusting (automatically pushing foods out of the mouth with the tongue).

ASK ABOUT

Age of the baby.

Reason for wanting to start solid foods.

ASSESSMENT

PROMPT CARE NEEDED?

Are any of the following present?

Breastfed baby under 5 months of age.

Mother concerned about the baby's weight gain.

Decreased stooling or urination.

| IF YES, | *Report to pediatric care provider today. Call lactation care provider today.* |

ROUTINE CARE NEEDED?

Are any of the following present?

Breastfed baby around 6 months of age.

Questions about starting family foods.

| IF YES, | *Call lactation care provider or nutritionist.* |

SELF-CARE INFORMATION

Babies are not equally interested in starting solid foods.

Allow the baby to hold foods and bring them to the mouth to lick and taste.

When babies start solid foods around 6 months, they do not usually start with the semi-liquid foods that were popular years ago when starting solids was recommended at younger ages.[255]

Move the baby onto family foods as appropriate.

IMPORTANT CONDITIONS TO REPORT

Difficulty breathing.

Difficulty swallowing.

Rapid progression of symptoms.

See also Allergy in the breastfed infant; Mixed feeds; Readiness for family foods; Solid foods for breastfed babies

Footnote

[255]Rapley, G., & Murkett, T. (2010). *Baby-led weaning: The essential guide to introducing solid foods and helping your baby to grow up a happy and confident eater.* New York, NY: The Experiment.

➤ SORE NIPPLES

DEFINITION   Uncomfortable sensations in the nipples. Pain is not an expected part of breastfeeding and indicates the need for feeding evaluation.

ASK ABOUT

Onset.
Location of pain.
Whether unilateral or bilateral.

ASSESSMENT

PROMPT CARE NEEDED?

Are any of the following present?

> Persistent pain with feeding.
> Persistent pain between feedings.
> Constant pain.
> Pain combined with color change of nipple(s).
> Pain with visible fissure or bleeding of the nipple.

IF YES,   *Call lactation care provider now.*

ROUTINE CARE NEEDED?

Are any of the following present?

> Brief pain at beginning of feeding.
> Mild recurrent pain.

IF YES,   *Report to lactation care provider.*

SELF-CARE INFORMATION

Practice skin-to-skin contact in the first hour and frequently thereafter.
Good positioning and attachment are crucial to prevent or reduce nipple pain.
Feed the baby at first sign of hunger cues (signs that say "feed me" include hand-to-face or hand-to-mouth movements, lip smacking, seeking with lips, rooting, and head bobbing).
Feed the baby at least 10 times per 24 hours.
Listen for signs of the baby swallowing.
Allow the baby to end feedings.
Expect at least three infant stools per 24 hours after the first 4 days of life.

Breastfeeding should not be painful. Advise mothers to seek medical or lactation care for breast pain. When a woman reports that her nipple pain has not resolved after she has improved positioning and latch, consider possibility of other factors such as infection of the nipple area, and/or oral abnormalities such as tongue-tie in the infant.

See also Latch-on; Mastitis; Raynaud's phenomenon/syndrome; Thrush; Tongue-tie

➤ SPECIAL CARE UNIT (SCU)

See Neonatal Intensive Care Unit (NICU)

➤ SPECIAL NEEDS BABY

DEFINITION   Babies with conditions such as inborn errors of metabolism, congenital anomalies, and prematurity. All special needs babies can benefit from breastmilk. The only exception is the baby who has been diagnosed with galactosemia.

ASK ABOUT

Age of the baby.
Special need of the baby.
Weight gain.
Milk transfer.

ASSESSMENT

PROMPT CARE NEEDED?

Are any of the following present?

Baby does not latch onto the breast.
Baby does not stay on the breast.
Baby is not gaining adequately.
Baby does not seem to transfer milk.

IF YES,   *Call lactation care provider now.*

SELF-CARE INFORMATION

As soon after birth as a mother knows that her baby will have special needs, she should begin expressing her milk. When the baby is capable of stimulating the hormones, transferring the milk, and maintaining the milk supply, the mother can reduce the amount of milk expression.

➤ SPITTING UP

DEFINITION   Regurgitation of food from the mouth. Spitting up or vomiting by the infant can be differentiated from projectile vomiting by the distance it travels. Projectile vomiting clears the chin of the infant. It may travel several feet. Spitting up does not clear the chin on its way out.

Spitting up, even after every feeding, may not be an indication that there is anything wrong with the baby. The mother may have a very powerful let-down reflex, for example. Also, a baby's lower esophageal sphincter is normally lower in tone than that of an older child or adult.

SELF-CARE INFORMATION

Occasional spitting up in an otherwise well infant is not uncommon.

Frequent spitting up, even in a baby with no other symptoms, can indicate that there is an underlying problem such as gastroesophageal reflux.

IMPORTANT CONDITIONS TO REPORT

Signs that the baby is unwell in combination with spitting up.

Decrease in stools and urinations.

Poor feeding behavior.

Weight loss, failure to gain adequately.

See also Gastroesophageal (GE) reflux; Let-down reflex; Milk-ejection reflex; Pyloric stenosis

➤ STOOLING PATTERNS

DEFINITION   Routine of production of bowel movements. The frequency and appearance of stools can be an important indication of how well the baby is doing at breastfeeding.

A baby's first stools (meconium) are greenish-black and tarry. The stool is sticky. By the 2nd or 3rd day, the stool becomes less black and more green (transitional stool), and when a large milk volume is available (around day 3) the stool changes to yellow.

After day 3, some babies stool a small stain in the diaper at every nursing. The breastfed newborn (to 6 weeks) should have at least 4 stools daily after day 4 of life. After the early months of life, breastfed babies may stool less frequently, going days between large, soft stools. However, other older breastfed babies may continue to stool frequently.

ASK ABOUT

Age of the baby.
Number of stools per day.
Number of feedings per day.
Weight gain pattern of the baby.

ASSESSMENT

PROMPT CARE NEEDED?

   Are any of the following present?

   No stool in 24 hours in the newborn period.
   Gray or white stool.
   Bloody stool.
   Lethargy (sleepy, difficult to rouse).
   Hard to latch on.
   Subtle feeding cues.
   Weak suck.
   No yellow stool by day 5.
   Weight loss after day 5.

   IF YES,   *Seek pediatric care now and call lactation care provider now.*

ROUTINE CARE NEEDED?

Are any of the following present?

> One or two small stools a day in newborn period.
>
> Fewer than four stools on day 4.
>
> Poor weight gain (less than 0.5 oz a day on average).
>
> Fussy, unsatisfied baby.

IF YES,   *Report to pediatric care provider. Call lactation care provider today.*

SELF-CARE INFORMATION

Improving the number of feedings and the quality of the feedings will increase the number of stools and the stool volume.

Keeping a feeding and diaper diary for a few days can help to describe what is happening to the lactation care provider or healthcare provider.

IMPORTANT CONDITIONS TO REPORT

Decreased stooling.

Increased sleepiness.

See also Bowel movements, infant; Constipation

➤ STORAGE OF BREASTMILK

DEFINITION   Safely preserving expressed milk.

Glass and hard plastic containers with tight lids are recommended for breastmilk storage. All containers should be food grade. Plastic bags designed for milk storage may be used, but prevent spillage and puncture of these bags.

When expressed for the healthy, full-term infant, milk can be safely stored:[256(p230)]

Up to four hours at room temperature (lower than 66°–72°F), but it should be refrigerated immediately if possible (with a frozen gel pack in an insulated lunch bag or cooler if a refrigerator is not available).

For 3–5 days in the refrigerator (32°–50°F).

Up to 3 months in the built-in freezer section (0°–32°F) of a refrigerator.

Up to 6 months in a deep freezer (-20°F or less).

Milk that will not be used fresh within 5 days should be frozen as soon as possible.

When milk is being expressed for the premature or sick infant, it should be handled and stored according to the NICU/SCU guidelines.

See also Collection and storage of breastmilk; Milk storage bags

Footnote

[256]Cadwell, K., & Turner-Maffei, C. (2014). *Pocket guide for lactation management* (2nd ed.). Burlington, MA: Jones & Bartlett Learning.

➤ STS CARE

See Kangaroo care (KC); Skin-to-skin (STS) care

➤ SUDDEN INFANT DEATH SYNDROME (SIDS)

DEFINITION SIDS is the unexpected death of a healthy-appearing baby under the age of 1 year.

SELF-CARE INFORMATION

Learn about safe sleeping practices for babies.

Protect the baby from secondhand smoke.

NOTES

SIDS is rare in the first month of life, and most cases of SIDS occur before 6 months of age.

In the United States there are more SIDS cases in the fall and winter seasons as compared to the spring and summer months.

SIDS is sudden and silent. The baby shows no signs of suffering.

The national "Back to Sleep" campaign encourages parents to put their babies to sleep on their backs. Since the initiation of this campaign, the number of babies to die from SIDS per year has been reduced by 50%.

The CDC reports that of the 4,500 U.S. babies who die each year of no immediate obvious cause, about half are due to SIDS.[257]

The risk of SIDS increases if babies are not put to sleep on their backs, if they are overheated, if they are exposed to secondhand smoke, if they have unsafe bedding, and if they were not exclusively breastfed. The AAP states that SIDS rates are 36% lower among breastfed babies compared with those fed formula.[258]

The American Academy of Pediatrics states:

> Because pacifier use has been associated with a reduction in SIDS incidence, mothers of healthy term infants should be instructed to use pacifiers at infant nap or sleep time after breastfeeding is well established, at approximately 3 to 4 weeks of age.[259(p.e835)]

Babies who are using pacifiers to help regulate their breathing should not be put to bed without their pacifiers until a physician gives the okay.

The AAP provides guidance on other ways to prevent SIDS deaths.[258]

The United Kingdom UNICEF provides guidance on cosleeping.[260]

See also Cosleeping; Crib death; Smoking

Footnotes

[257]CDC. (2012, January 18). Sudden infant death syndrome (SIDS) and sudden, unexpected infant death (SUID). Retrieved from http://www.cdc.gov/sids/

[258]AAP Section on Breastfeeding. (2012). Breastfeeding and the use of human milk. *Pediatrics*, *129*(3), e827–e841. doi:10.1542/peds.2011-3552

[259]AAP Task Force on Sudden Infant Death Syndrome, & Moon, R. Y. (2011). SIDS and other sleep-related infant deaths: Expansion of recommendations for a safe infant sleeping environment. *Pediatrics*, *128*(5), 1030–1039. doi:10.1542/peds.2011-2284

[260]UNICEF UK Baby Friendly Initiative. (2011). Caring for your baby at night: A guide for parents. Retrieved from http://www.unicef.org.uk/Documents/Baby_Friendly/Leaflets/caringatnight_web .pdf

➤ SUPERNUMERARY NIPPLE TISSUE

DEFINITION   Accessory mammary glands and additional (supernumerary) nipples, usually found along the milk line that extends from the underarms to the thighs although they may be found outside of the line as well.

Breast tissue may produce milk, but without a nipple pore, it cannot be released.

During pregnancy and lactation, extra nipple tissue may enlarge and become prominent. A mother may find that what she thought was a mole is actually a supernumerary nipple.

ASK ABOUT

Age of the baby.
Onset of symptoms.

ASSESSMENT

PROMPT CARE NEEDED?

Are any of the following present?

Enlarged, painful areas along the milk line coupled with maternal fever higher than 101°F (38.5°C).

IF YES,   *Call obstetric care provider within 4 hours.*

ROUTINE CARE NEEDED?

Are any of the following present?

Enlarged, painful areas along the milk line.

IF YES,   *Call lactation care provider today.*

SELF-CARE INFORMATION

Comfort measures such as ice packs or moist heat may ease the pain.

The areas will return to normal and become comfortable in a few days.

IMPORTANT CONDITIONS TO REPORT

Fever.

Reddened areas of the body.

Extreme pain in the area of the extra nipple tissue.

See also Accessory breast tissue; Hyperadenia; Hyperthelia

➤ SUPPLEMENTAL FEEDING DEVICES

DEFINITION   Tools used to deliver milk to an infant. These include cups, bottles, spoons, paladai, and at-breast feeders.

See also At-breast supplementation; Bottle feeding; Cup feeding; Paladai

➤ SURGERY

DEFINITION A medical procedure involving cutting into the body. Mothers and babies can have surgery and continue breastfeeding.

Decisions (even in an emergency) must be made about:

How the baby will be fed during the separation.

How the mother's breasts will be kept comfortable during the separation.

If the separation will be prolonged, how the mother's milk supply will be stimulated and maintained.

When and where the mother and baby can be reunited.

Medications or anesthesia used (consult LactMed in order to make evidence-based decisions).

Restrictions after discharge.

SELF-CARE INFORMATION

It is important to ensure that all healthcare providers are informed that the mother and baby are breastfeeding.

See also Breast surgery; Hospitalization; LactMed; Medication resources (inside back cover)

➤ SWADDLING

DEFINITION Wrapping a young baby is called swaddling. Wrapping babies is traditional in some societies. Some babies are happier with the tight feeling of swaddling to remind them of the womb.

NOTES

Babies help to stimulate the mother's lactation hormones with their hands. If swaddling, do not swaddle the hands. Leave the hands free to embrace the breast during the nursing.

Babies nurse best when their hips and knees are flexed. If swaddling, be sure the baby is in a flexed position.

➤ SWITCH NURSING

DEFINITION   Nursing in which the mother moves the baby from one breast to the other and back again during the feeding with the hope that this will stimulate the milk supply.

NOTES

The baby would nurse on the first breast for five minutes. The mother breaks suction and moves the baby to the other breast. She does this several times during the course of one feeding. The feeding should continue until the baby indicates fullness.

See also Cluster feeding; Increasing milk supply

➤ TAIL OF SPENCE

DEFINITION   The tail of Spence is the part of the mammary gland tissue that extends into the underarm (axillary region). Sometimes the tail of Spence is visible and enlarged during lactation.

Because this is part of the mammary gland, lumps, plugs, and other problems can develop here.

SELF-CARE INFORMATION

Examine the tail of Spence for lumps as you would the rest of the breast.

Position the baby to move any milk out of the tail of Spence if milk is not draining efficiently from that area.

IMPORTANT CONDITIONS TO REPORT

Lumps in the armpit that do not move with nursing.

Pain in the armpit.

Reddened areas in the armpit.

Fever and flu-like feelings.

See also Breast structure; Engorgement; Mastitis

➤ TAKING THE BABY OFF THE BREAST

DEFINITION Method of removing the baby's mouth from the breast. Babies make a seal at the breast with their lips and tongue. In addition, the breast is drawn into the mouth and held there firmly during suckling. To take the baby off of the breast, the mother needs to break the seal. She can do this by inserting her clean finger into the corner of the baby's mouth or by pressing down onto her breast to break the seal.

SELF-CARE INFORMATION
Ideally, babies should end the feeding themselves.

IMPORTANT CONDITIONS TO REPORT
Nipple pain.
Baby does not end feeding.
Deep breast pain.

See also Latch-on; Sore nipples; Weaning

➤ TANDEM NURSING

DEFINITION Nursing two babies not from the same pregnancy.

ASK ABOUT

Age of the babies.

ASSESSMENT

ROUTINE CARE NEEDED?
Are any of the following present?
Need for nutrition evaluation.

IF YES, *Seek dietary consultation.*

Are any of the following present?

Mixed feelings about tandem nursing.

Need for practical help or strategies.

Nipple pain in pregnancy.

Help required with weaning.

IF YES,   *Call lactation care provider.*

SELF-CARE INFORMATION

Be open to adjusting expectations to meet reality.

Nurse the younger baby first and frequently.

Find time for nonnursing interactions with the older baby.

NOTES

Usually, the mother has nursed the older baby through the pregnancy, but that is not always the case. Some mothers invite a weaned baby to nurse along with the newborn.

See also Breastfeeding during pregnancy

➤ TASTE OF MILK

DEFINITION   Flavor of human milk. Human milk does not look or taste like cow's milk. At first, during the colostral phase, milk is creamy or yellow in color. Mature milk is more bluish.

Human milk tastes very sweet to the adult palate.

Flavors in the mother's diet do flavor her milk and amniotic fluid. This is probably how babies learn the tastes of their family foods.

In research, babies appear to enjoy volatile flavors such as garlic and carrot in their mothers' milk.[261]

ASSESSMENT

ROUTINE CARE NEEDED?

Are any of the following present?

Fussy baby.

Concerns about the effect of food(s) the mother is eating.

IF YES, *Call lactation care provider.*

SELF-CARE INFORMATION

Eat the foods that your family likes when you are breastfeeding.

Mothers whose babies may be allergic (family history of allergies) should consult their healthcare provider about avoiding foods.

IMPORTANT CONDITIONS TO REPORT

Allergic symptoms in the baby.

See also Allergy in the breastfed infant; Maternal diet

Footnote

[261]Beauchamp, G. K., & Mennella, J. A. (2011). Flavor perception in human infants: Development and functional significance. *Digestion*, *83*(Suppl. 1), 1–6. doi:10.1159/000323397

➤ TB

See Tuberculosis (TB)

➤ TEENAGED MOTHERS

DEFINITION Women under the age of 20 who have children. Adolescent mothers can breastfeed. They have experiences and concerns just as non-teen mothers do.

ASK ABOUT

Age of the baby.
Age of the mother.

ASSESSMENT

ROUTINE CARE NEEDED?

Are any of the following present?

Poor dietary habits.

IF YES,   *Seek dietary consultation.*

Are any of the following present?

Need for support.

Need for practical breastfeeding management strategies.

IF YES,   *Call lactation care provider.*

SELF-CARE INFORMATION

Teenagers who breastfeed have higher bone density later in life, compared to teens who have babies but do not breastfeed.

Teens should be encouraged to eat well to support the needs of their own bodies. Eating well helps provide energy and maintain optimal health. Eating well does not help women make more milk; only more frequent feeding or milk removal can do that.

See also Adolescent breastfeeding; Maternal diet; Milk production

➤ TEETHING

DEFINITION   Eruption of teeth through the gums. Babies do not need to be weaned because they are teething or because they have teeth, although mothers may be told this by friends or family. Because their gums are uncomfortable, teething babies may try chewing at the breast. Mothers may have sore nipples when the baby is teething.

ASK ABOUT

Age of the baby.
Presence of teeth.

ASSESSMENT

ROUTINE CARE NEEDED?

Are any of the following present?

Difficulty nursing during teething period.

Sore nipples during teething period.

Biting at the breast during feeding.

Questions about soothing a breastfeeding, teething baby.

IF YES, *Call lactation care provider.*

Are any of the following present?

Questions about infant tooth care.

IF YES, *Call pediatric care provider or dentist.*

SELF-CARE INFORMATION

Teething is a temporary (but recurring) stage that can be difficult for some babies and families.

IMPORTANT CONDITIONS TO REPORT

Persistent refusal to feed in a teething infant.

See also Biting; Clenching or clamping onto the nipple/areola; Sore nipples

➤ TE FISTULA

See Tracheoesophageal (TE) fistula

➤ TEN STEPS TO SUCCESSFUL BREASTFEEDING

DEFINITION   Optimal steps created by the World Health Organization (WHO) and United Nations Children's Fund (UNICEF) to be practiced in all maternity units worldwide. These steps form the basis of the Baby-Friendly Hospital Initiative.

NOTES

Baby-Friendly USA is the agency responsible for implementing the Baby-Friendly Hospital Initiative in the United States.

The steps for the United States are:

1. Have a written breastfeeding policy that is routinely communicated to all health care staff.
2. Train all health care staff in skills necessary to implement this policy.
3. Inform all pregnant women about the benefits and management of breast-feeding.
4. Help mothers initiate breastfeeding within one hour of birth.
5. Show mothers how to breastfeed and how to maintain lactation even if they should be separated from their infants.
6. Give infants no food or drink other than breastmilk, unless medically indicated.
7. Practice "rooming in"—allow mothers and infants to remain together 24 hours a day.
8. Encourage breastfeeding on demand.
9. Give no pacifiers or artificial nipples to breastfeeding infants.
10. Foster the establishment of breastfeeding support groups and refer mothers to them on discharge from the hospital or clinic.[262](Ten Steps section)

Baby-Friendly USA
Website: www.babyfriendlyusa.org

Footnote

[262]Baby-Friendly Hospital Initiative. (2010). The ten steps to successful breastfeeding. Retrieved from http://www.babyfriendlyusa.org/eng/10steps.html

➤ TEST WEIGHING

DEFINITION   Weighing a baby before and after a breastfeeding to estimate the amount of milk transferred.

Age of the baby.
Reason for test weighing.

ASSESSMENT

PROMPT CARE NEEDED?

Are any of the following present?

Pediatric referral for evaluation of milk supply.

Infrequent feeding (fewer than eight breastfeedings daily).

Insufficient urination or stooling.

Perception of milk supply problem.

IF YES, *Seek lactation care today.*

ROUTINE CARE NEEDED?

Are any of the following present?

Concern about the amount of milk the baby is getting while breastfeeding.

Fear of inadequate milk supply.

IF YES, *Call lactation care provider today.*

SELF-CARE INFORMATION

The test weight reflects only an estimate of the feeding that was test weighed. Babies do not seem to transfer the same amount at each breastfeeding.

IMPORTANT CONDITIONS TO REPORT

The baby is difficult to rouse.

The baby has inadequate urinations or stools.

The baby becomes lethargic.

NOTES

Test weighing with digital scales, accurate to 1 g or 2 g, has been shown in research to be fairly accurate. Test weighing with other types of scales has not been shown to reflect an accurate estimation of intake.

See also Electronic scales; Milk transfer, estimating; Slow weight gain, baby

➤ THAWING AND WARMING FROZEN BREASTMILK

DEFINITION   Techniques used to safely prepare frozen milk for consumption by a baby.

NOTES

Thaw milk in its container.
  Milk can be safely thawed by:
  Placing frozen containers in the refrigerator.
  Holding frozen containers under lukewarm running tap water.
  Placing frozen containers in lukewarm water. Hot water is not recommended due to potential nutrient loss.
Milk should never be boiled or microwaved.
  Milk does not need to be warmed before being fed to the infant.[263(p231)]

See also Collection and storage of breastmilk; Storage of breastmilk

Footnote

[263]Cadwell, K., & Turner-Maffei, C. (2014). *Pocket guide for lactation management* (2nd ed.). Burlington, MA: Jones & Bartlett Learning.

➤ THRUSH

DEFINITION   Overgrowth of *Candida albicans* or other common fungi.

Symptoms of yeast infection of the breast include red, shiny-looking skin on the nipple or areola, flaky skin, and sharp, itching pain that persists between feedings. Infant symptoms of yeast overgrowth or thrush include white patches of growth on the inner buccal surface (cheek) or tongue and occasionally pain on latch. Infants may also have diaper area yeast overgrowth.

ASK ABOUT

Onset.
Medications taken by mother and baby in the past month.

ASSESSMENT

PROMPT CARE NEEDED?

Are any of the following present?

Sharp, itching, persistent nipple pain (not just during feedings).

Flaky, shiny, or itchy skin on the nipple surface.

Presence of white patches in the infant's mouth.

A baby with yeast infection in the diaper area.

IF YES,   *Call the mother's and baby's healthcare providers today.*

ROUTINE CARE NEEDED?

Are any of the following present?

Nipple pain during feeding.

IF YES,   *Call lactation care provider today.*

SELF-CARE INFORMATION

Finish all medications prescribed.

If administering nystatin suspension to the infant, pour a dose into a clean cup or spoon. Half of the dose should be used for each side of the mouth. Suspension may be applied with a cotton swab. A clean swab should be used for each application. Take care not to introduce used swabs into the bottle of suspension.

If the baby uses artificial nipples, pacifiers, etc., these should be boiled at least daily and replaced after completion of yeast treatment.

The mother and baby should be treated simultaneously regardless of which one is symptomatic.

IMPORTANT CONDITIONS TO REPORT

Persistent symptoms after completion of a course of treatment.

Recurrent symptoms.

NOTES

Candida overgrowth may follow or increase after antibiotic treatment.

Recommended treatment for candidiasis is a topical antifungal agent.

If symptoms are not relieved by topical treatment, feeding evaluation should occur to rule out positioning or attachment problems contributing to pain.

The healthcare provider's evaluation should rule out other conditions resulting in redness and pain, including **eczema**, reaction to surface allergens, trauma, **Raynaud's phenomenon**, concomitant bacteria, and infection.

Subsequent treatment with oral antifungal agents may resolve symptoms.

Lactation evaluation should rule out contributing problems with latch or distortion of the nipple in the baby's mouth.

See also Candidiasis; Medication resources (inside back cover); Nipple pain; Yeast infection

➤ THYROID DISEASE

DEFINITION   Disorder in the production of hormones by the thyroid gland. Breast-feeding is not contraindicated for women who have had thyroid disease—either hypothyroidism (low levels of the thyroid hormones) or hyperthyroidism (high levels of the thyroid hormones)—and have normal thyroid levels.

Women with hypothyroidism are prescribed thyroid replacement therapy and can breastfeed. The medications currently used for this condition are compatible with breastfeeding.

A woman whose hyperthyroid problem (thyroiditis) is suspected during pregnancy or lactation presents a special problem in the diagnosis and treatment. The mother should tell all healthcare providers that she is breastfeeding.

Many of the signs and symptoms of thyroid disease can seem normal to a postpartum woman. The symptom that is unique to breastfeeding is difficulty initiating and maintaining an adequate milk supply.

Both high and low levels of thyroid hormones have been shown to affect the milk supply.

Age of the baby.
Weight gain pattern of the baby.

ASSESSMENT

EMERGENT CARE NEEDED?

Are any of the following present?

About the baby:

Extreme lethargy or irritability.

Sudden change in the baby's muscle tone (extremely floppy or stiff) or repetitive jerking movements (e.g., seizure activity).

Baby shows sudden disinterest in feeding.

Inability to wake baby.

Baby does not calm, even with cuddles.

Meconium bowel movements after 5 days of life.

Fewer than three bowel movements daily in breastfed newborn after the first 2 days of life.

No urine in 6 hours.

Brick dust urine (uric acid crystals) after 2 days of life.

Dark-colored urine.

Fewer than four urinations daily in the breastfed newborn after day 5 of life.

Noticeably sunken fontanelles (soft spot on the top of the head).

Decreased activity.

Weight loss of more than 7% from birth.

Weight loss after 5 days of life.

Cessation of weight gain.

Lethargy.

Hard to latch on.

Weak suck.

Sleepy, difficult to rouse.

IF YES, *Seek pediatric care now.*

PROMPT CARE NEEDED?

Are any of the following present?

About the mother:

Signs and symptoms of hypothyroidism, including:

Persistent fatigue.

Weakness.

Weight gain or difficulty losing weight (difficult to ascertain in postpartum).

Coarse, dry hair.

Dry, rough skin.

Hair loss (difficult to notice in pregnant and postpartum women unless it is severe).

Inability to tolerate cold as easily as others in the same environment.

Muscle cramps and aches.

Constipation.

Depression (may be assumed to be baby blues).

Irritability.

Memory loss.

Abnormal menstrual periods (it is normal for breastfeeding women to not menstruate in the first several months postpartum).

Decreased sexual desire (normal in postpartum women).

Signs and symptoms of hyperthyroidism, including:

Palpitations.

Heat intolerance.

Nervousness.

Insomnia.

Breathlessness.

Increased bowel movements.

Light or absent menstrual periods.

Fatigue.

Weight loss.

Fast heart rate.

Trembling hands.

Muscle weakness.

Warm, moist skin.

Hair loss.

IF YES,   *Report to maternal healthcare provider today.*

ROUTINE CARE NEEDED?

Are any of the following present?

Questions about building up milk supply after diagnosis of a thyroid problem.

Questions about drug compatibility.

IF YES,	*Call lactation care provider today and consult up-to-date drug references.*

SELF-CARE INFORMATION

Postpartum thyroid problems can initially present as postpartum depression or just normal tiredness or fatigue. Mothers who struggle with milk supply should have a thorough medical evaluation if the supply does not improve with increased frequency and expression.

IMPORTANT CONDITIONS TO REPORT

Increasing sleepiness in baby.

Increasing fatigue and inability to cope in the mother.

Feelings of hopelessness or depression.

Symptoms of thyroid disease.

See also Hyperthyroidism; Hypothyroidism; Maternal fatigue; Medication resources (inside back cover); Postpartum depression; Slow weight gain, baby

➤ TODDLER AND YOUNG CHILD NURSING

DEFINITION   Continued breastfeeding in a child older than 12 months. Nursing is different as the baby grows through new ages and stages of development. Each stage is a new experience for the mother and child. Breastfeeding is still a valuable experience for toddlers and young children, and breastmilk continues to provide nourishment and immune factors. National and international health authorities recommend that breastfeeding continue as long as mother and baby wish to continue.

ASK ABOUT

Age of the baby.

ASSESSMENT

ROUTINE CARE NEEDED?

Are any of the following present?

Strategies needed for breastfeeding toddlers and young children.

Strategies needed for weaning toddlers and young children.

IF YES, *Call lactation care provider.*

SELF-CARE INFORMATION

Nursing is different at different ages; do not expect the experience to always be the same.

See also Closet nursing; Milk production; Tandem nursing; Weaning

➤ TONGUE EXERCISES

DEFINITION Repeated movements used to train the motion of the tongue. Because the tongue is a muscle, it can be exercised. If a baby is having a problem nursing because of the tongue, occupational therapists, speech and language pathologists, and physical therapists can help babies' tongues become more fit for suckling through specific exercises.

ASK ABOUT

Age of the baby.
Weight gain pattern of the baby.

ASSESSMENT

PROMPT CARE NEEDED?

Are any of the following present?

About the baby:

Lethargy (sleepy, difficult to rouse).

Hard to latch on.

Weak suck.

Extreme irritability.

Sudden change in muscle tone (extremely floppy or stiff) or repetitive jerking movements (e.g., seizure activity).

Sudden disinterest in feeding.

Does not calm, even with cuddles.

Meconium bowel movements after 5 days of life.

Fewer than three bowel movements daily in breastfed newborn after the first 2 days of life.

No urine in 6 hours.

Brick dust urine (uric acid crystals) after 2 days of life.

Dark-colored urine.

Fewer than four urinations daily in the breastfed newborn after day 5 of life.

Weight loss of more than 7% from birth.

Weight loss after 5 days after birth.

Noticeably sunken fontanelles (soft spot on the top of the head).

Decreased activity.

Below birthweight at 10–14 days of life.

Cessation of weight gain.

IF YES, *Seek pediatric care now.*

ROUTINE CARE NEEDED?

Are any of the following present?

Baby appears not to be using tongue correctly during feeding, resulting in difficulty latching onto breast or sustaining feedings.

Nipple pain for the mother.

Clicking sounds heard during feeding.

IF YES, *Call lactation care provider today and refer to occupational therapist, speech and language pathologist, or physical therapist as available and needed.*

SELF-CARE INFORMATION

A baby's tongue can be trained to suckle more effectively by doing specific exercises.

See also Down syndrome (DS); Occupational therapy; Pierre Robin sequence

➤ TONGUE-TIE

DEFINITION   A tight lingual frenulum (the membrane attaching the tongue to the bottom of the mouth). This condition is also referred to as **ankyloglossia**. When the frenulum is tight, it can restrict the movement of the tongue, resulting in breastfeeding problems for some mothers and babies.

ASK ABOUT

Age of the baby.
Appearance of the tongue.

ASSESSMENT

PROMPT CARE NEEDED?

Are any of the following present?

Tight lingual frenulum in the baby.
Persistent nipple or breast pain that is not changed by improving latch.
History of recurrent breast infection.
Milk supply problems.
Poor growth of breastfed infants.

IF YES,   *Call lactation care provider today.*

Are any of the following present?

Presence of tight lingual frenulum in the baby in conjunction with feeding or breast/nipple problems in the breastfeeding mother.

IF YES,   *Report to pediatrician.*

SELF-CARE INFORMATION

Practice skin-to-skin contact in the first hour after birth and frequently thereafter.

Watch for hunger cues (signs that say "feed me" include hand-to-face or hand-to-mouth movements, lip smacking, seeking with lips, rooting, and head bobbing).

Feed the baby at the first sign of hunger cues.

Practice good attachment:

Offer the breast as soon as it is seen.

Wait for the baby to open his or her mouth wide (greater than a 140° angle).

Pull the baby in so that his or her chin touches the breast first, and the nipple enters the open space in the top part of the mouth; this should result in a wide-open mouth on the breast. The baby may need to be in a semiupright position to assist in attaining the widest mouth angle.

The lips should be flanged outward.

The baby's lips should look off center when compared with the areola; the bottom lip should be farther away from the nipple than the top lip.

IMPORTANT CONDITIONS TO REPORT

Unresolved symptoms.

Ongoing concerns.

NOTES

Babies with tongue tie may have difficulty performing the tongue motions required to effectively move milk from a breast or bottle. On visual assessment, the tongue may appear to be heart shaped at the tip. The infant may be unable to extend the tongue beyond the lower gum ridge. The tongue may be held tightly in the posterior part of the mouth as well.

Breastfeeding mothers of babies with tongue-tie may experience sore nipples, mastitis, and milk supply problems.

Babies with tongue-tie should be evaluated for their tongue mobility and possibly for frenotomy or frenectomy.[264,265,266] Mothers should receive lactation assistance to improve positioning and milk removal. Occupational therapists and/or speech language pathologists have specialized skills for assisting babies with ankyloglossia.

See also Ankyloglossia; Nipple pain

Footnotes

[264]Buryk, M., Bloom, D., & Shope, T. (2011). Efficacy of neonatal release of ankyloglossia: A randomized trial. *Pediatrics, 128*(2), 280–288. doi:10.1542/peds.2011-0077

[265]Geddes, D. T., Langton, D. B., Gollow, I., Jacobs, L. A., Hartmann, P. E., & Simmer, K. (2008). Frenulotomy for breastfeeding infants with ankyloglossia: Effect on milk removal and sucking mechanism as imaged by ultrasound. *Pediatrics, 122*(1), e188–194. doi:10.1542/peds.2007-2553

[266]Manfro, A. R. G., Manfro, R., & Bortoluzzi, M. C. (2010). Surgical treatment of ankyloglossia in babies—Case report. *International Journal of Oral and Maxillofacial Surgery, 39*(11), 1130–1132. doi:10.1016/j.ijom.2010.06.007

➤ TORTICOLLIS

DEFINITION Injury and spasms of the muscles of the neck that cause the head to fall to one side, often with the chin pointing to the other side. Womb position and birth injury may contribute to the development of this condition, which develops gradually over the first days of life. Nursing mothers of babies with torticollis may need help finding comfortable positions for nursing.

See also Birth injury

➤ TRACHEOESOPHAGEAL (TE) FISTULA

DEFINITION A small opening between the trachea, which leads from the mouth to the lungs, and the esophagus, which leads from the mouth to the stomach. The two passageways are right next to each other in the throat.

ASK ABOUT

Age of the baby.
Surgical history.

ASSESSMENT

ROUTINE CARE NEEDED?

Are any of the following present?

Problems with milk supply with a baby with TE fistula.

The baby has difficulty breastfeeding after surgery.

| IF YES, | *Call lactation care provider today.* |

SELF-CARE INFORMATION

The mother should begin expressing milk as soon as possible in order to initiate and maintain her milk supply. Her milk may be given to the baby through a feeding tube until the baby is able to go to the breast.

IMPORTANT CONDITIONS TO REPORT

Complications as described by the hospital discharge team.

NOTES

When a baby is born with a TE fistula, there is a chance that food (breastmilk or formula) can easily get into the lungs and cause chemical pneumonia. Therefore, the baby is usually not fed right away.

A TE fistula is considered a surgical emergency.

The mother should begin expressing milk as soon as possible in order to initiate and maintain her milk supply. Her milk may be given to the baby through a feeding tube until the baby is able to go to the breast.

See also Breathing, sucking, swallowing; Hospitalization; Tube feeding

➤ TRANSITIONAL MILK

DEFINITION   Fluid that is a blend of colostrum and mature milk. The stages of human milk are (1) colostrum, (2) transitional milk, and (3) mature milk. Milk content changes gradually from colostrum to mature milk in the first two weeks after the baby is born.

See also Colostrum; Mature milk

➤ TRANSITION TO BREASTFEEDING

DEFINITION   Process of helping a baby learn to feed at the breast after being fed in another manner. Babies may be fed away from the breast for some time and then transition to breastfeeding. For example, a premature baby may be tube fed at first and then need to learn how to suckle at the breast and effectively transfer milk.

ASK ABOUT

Age of the baby.
How the baby is currently being fed (away from the breast).
What the baby is currently being fed.

ASSESSMENT

ROUTINE CARE NEEDED?

Are any of the following present?

Strategies needed to transition baby to breastfeeding.
Desire to feed the baby at the breast.

IF YES,   *Call lactation care provider.*

SELF-CARE INFORMATION

Even after a substantial time being fed away from the breast, babies can be successfully breastfed.

See also At-breast supplementation; Milk production; Premature infant; Relactation; Skin-to-skin (STS) care

➤ TRIPLETS

DEFINITION   Three babies from the same pregnancy. Mothers can make enough milk to support triplets, usually beginning with a combination of expressing and nursing if the babies are premature.

ASSESSMENT

ROUTINE CARE NEEDED?

Are any of the following present?

Strategies needed for managing the nursing of triplets.

Strategies needed for managing milk supply for triplets.

IF YES,   *Call lactation care provider today.*

SELF-CARE INFORMATION

Milk expression should start as soon as possible after the babies are born.

Many mothers of multiples have found it helpful to keep a journal of who nursed when, number of wet and dirty diapers, and weight gain for each baby, to ensure that none of the babies is being overlooked.

Mothers of triplets may have been on bed rest during their pregnancies and can become easily fatigued. Advise them to ask for help.

Suggest easy ways for mothers to snack and drink while caring for triplets.

IMPORTANT CONDITIONS TO REPORT

Lethargy.

Decrease in urine and stools.

Change in breastfeeding behavior.

Problems with feeding.

See also Higher order multiples (HOM); Multiple infants (twins, triplets, and higher order multiples); Premature infant

➤ TUBAL LIGATION

DEFINITION   Tubal ligation is a surgical procedure on women that is commonly referred to as "tying the tubes."

ASSESSMENT

ROUTINE CARE NEEDED?

Are any of the following present?

Nursing after surgery.

| **IF YES,** | *Ask the surgeon about the course of the surgery and recovery and how to decrease the length of time of separation from the baby.* |

ROUTINE CARE NEEDED?

Are any of the following present?

Possibility of drugs and anesthesia passing into the milk.

| **IF YES,** | *Consult up-to-date drug references.* |

SELF-CARE INFORMATION

Always tell your healthcare providers that you intend to breastfeed or that you are breastfeeding.

Ask your healthcare providers if there are choices in drugs and anesthesia that would make the separation from the baby shorter.

When you are reunited with the baby, start with skin-to-skin care.

NOTES

The fallopian tubes transport mature eggs from the ovary to the uterus about one time a month. Sperm travels from the uterus up the fallopian tube. If the sperm encounters a mature egg, fertilization may occur.

Tubal ligation is a form of permanent sterilization. To stop fertilization, the egg is prevented from traveling down the tube and the sperm is prevented from traveling up.

Mothers often make a plan to have a tubal ligation before leaving the hospital after the birth of a baby.

See also Hospitalization; Medication resources (inside back cover); Skin-to-skin (STS) care

➤ TUBE FEEDING

DEFINITION　Delivery of food to a baby through tubing threaded through its nose or mouth and ending in the stomach or small intestine. Sometimes the tube is attached to a pump that feeds the baby continuously. Other times babies are fed a bolus feed through a syringe attached to the tubing.

Premature babies are often tube fed before they can coordinate their suck, swallow, breathe reflex or have the cardiorespiratory stability to feed orally.

Term babies may be tube fed for a variety of medical and surgical reasons.

Colostrum and breastmilk can be fed to the baby through the tube.

Babies who are tube fed are usually given pacifiers to suck on, which helps promote growth through release of beneficial gastric hormones.

ASK ABOUT

Age of the baby.
The baby's feeding history.

ASSESSMENT

ROUTINE CARE NEEDED?

Are any of the following present?

Questions about obtaining a breast pump and learning to hand express breast milk.

Transition to breastfeeding.

Questions about milk supply.

Questions about expressing milk.

Questions about collecting and storing milk.

IF YES,　*Call lactation care provider.*

SELF-CARE INFORMATION

Even though the baby can only be given a small amount of milk, mothers whose babies are being tube fed should maximize their milk production by hand expression and pumping.

Skin-to-skin care offers a way to feel close to the baby even when breastfeeding is not possible.

IMPORTANT CONDITIONS TO REPORT
Decreasing milk supply.

See also At-breast supplementation; Gavage feeding; Premature infant; Skin-to-skin (STS) care; Transition to breastfeeding

➤ TUBERCLES OF MONTGOMERY (MONTGOMERY GLANDS)

See Montgomery glands (Montgomery tubercles)

➤ TUBERCULOSIS (TB)

DEFINITION   A disease that is primarily spread through the air. The disease is spread when a person with active TB coughs, sneezes, speaks, sings, or laughs. Tiny droplets fly through the air.

ASK ABOUT

Age of the baby.
Diagnosis of TB.

ASSESSMENT

PROMPT CARE NEEDED?
Are any of the following present?
Plan for feeding baby during separation needed.

IF YES,   *Call pediatric care provider today. Seek lactation care today.*

ROUTINE CARE NEEDED?

Are any of the following present?

Plan for expressing milk.

TB drug regimen compatibility with breastmilk and breastfeeding.

Transition to breastfeeding.

IF YES,   *Seek lactation care today. Consult up-to-date drug reference.*

SELF-CARE INFORMATION

Treatment for TB can save your life. Take all the medications as prescribed. If you cannot take the drug for some reason, tell your doctor right away.

IMPORTANT CONDITIONS TO REPORT

Declining milk supply.

NOTES

It usually takes lengthy contact with someone who has active TB before another person can become infected.

People who have been treated with appropriate drugs for at least 2 weeks are no longer contagious and do not spread the germ to others.

A mother with newly diagnosed active TB is separated from her baby during the initial 2 weeks of treatment. She can express her milk and it can be fed to her baby. The baby will be tested and may also be treated.

TB can be responsible for mastitis. This is called tuberculosis mastitis. If the mother has this rare form of TB, the organism can be transmitted in her milk.

Except for women with tubercular mastitis, TB has not been found to pass through the milk.

See also Contraindicated conditions; Expression of mothers' milk; Hospitalization; Medication resources (inside back cover); Transition to breastfeeding

➤ TWINS

DEFINITION   Two babies from the same pregnancy. Twins can be identical or fraternal.

ROUTINE CARE NEEDED?

Are any of the following present?

Strategies needed for managing the nursing of twins.

Strategies needed for managing milk supply for twins.

IF YES,   *Call lactation care provider today.*

SELF-CARE INFORMATION

Nurse babies as soon as possible after birth.

If a baby is separated from his or her mother or breastfeeding is not yet effective, hand expression and pumping should start as soon as possible.

Many mothers of multiples have found it helpful to keep a journal of who nursed when, number of wet and dirty diapers, and weight gain for each baby, to ensure that none of the babies is being overlooked.

Mothers of twins may have been on bed rest during their pregnancies and can become easily fatigued. Advise them to ask for help.

Suggest easy ways for mothers to snack and drink while caring for twins.

IMPORTANT CONDITIONS TO REPORT

Lethargy.

Decrease in urine and stools.

Change in breastfeeding behavior.

Problems with feeding.

NOTES

Mothers can make enough milk to support twins. Nursing two babies at the same time boosts milk production.

See also Multiple infants (twins, triplets, and higher order multiples); Premature infant

➤ TYPE 1 DIABETES (IDDM)

DEFINITION   A chronic disease causing high levels of sugar in the blood. Diabetes is caused by too little insulin or resistance to insulin. Also known as insulin dependent diabetes mellitus (IDDM).

ASK ABOUT

Onset.

ASSESSMENT

EMERGENT CARE NEEDED?

Are any of the following present?

Insulin shock (hypoglycemia) in the breastfeeding woman. (Symptoms of insulin shock include rapid pulse, rapid breathing, dizziness or altered consciousness, weakness, blurred vision, headache, sweating, and numbness of hands or feet.)

IF YES,   *Seek emergency care now.*

PROMPT CARE NEEDED?

Are any of the following present?

Difficulty maintaining blood glucose levels during breastfeeding.

IF YES,   *Report to mother's healthcare provider and seek dietary consultation.*

ROUTINE CARE NEEDED?

Are any of the following present?

Breastfeeding questions in the diabetic woman.
Ongoing breastfeeding in the diabetic woman.

IF YES,   *Call lactation care provider today.*

SELF-CARE INFORMATION

Women with diabetes are more prone to infection. Monitor breasts and nipples daily for any red, infected, or painful areas.

If insulin dependent, be aware that less insulin may be required during breastfeeding—watch for signs of low blood sugar.

IMPORTANT CONDITIONS TO REPORT

Any symptoms of infection.

Difficulty regulating blood sugar.

NOTES

Type 1 diabetes is usually diagnosed in childhood. The pancreas makes little or no insulin, requiring daily injections of this hormone in order to regulate sugar metabolism.

Women with this condition can breastfeed their babies and should be encouraged to do so.

Research suggests that women who have experienced gestational diabetes are less likely to develop diabetes if they breastfeed their babies.[267]

See also Autoimmune diseases

Footnote

[267]Kjos, S. L., Henry, O., Lee, R. M., Buchanan, T. A., & Mishell, D. R., Jr. (1993). The effect of lactation on glucose metabolism in women with recent gestational diabetes. *Obstetrics & Gynecology, 82*(3), 451–455.

➤ TYPHOID FEVER

DEFINITION   A life-threatening illness caused by the organism *Salmonella typhi* (*S. typhi*). Although typhoid fever affects about 12.5 million people per year worldwide, there are only about 400 cases per year in the United States.

ASK ABOUT

Age of the baby.

Onset of typhoid fever.

ASSESSMENT

EMERGENT CARE NEEDED?

Are any of the following present?

Mother's inability to care for baby.

Mother's inability to breastfeed or express milk on her own due to her illness.

IF YES, *Seek emergency care now. Seek lactation care soon.*

PROMPT CARE NEEDED?

Are any of the following present?

Compatibility of prescribed drugs with breastfeeding.

IF YES, *Consult up-to-date drug references.*

ROUTINE CARE NEEDED?

Are any of the following present?

Transitioning baby back to breastfeeding.

Lowered milk supply.

IF YES, *Call lactation care provider today.*

SELF-CARE INFORMATION

Take all medications as prescribed, even after you feel better.

Follow all of the self-care instructions (drink extra fluids, rest, etc.).

Practice good hygiene through regular hand washing.

Follow eating and drinking guidelines when traveling to areas of the world with poor sanitation.

IMPORTANT CONDITIONS TO REPORT

Declining milk supply.

The *S. typhi* organism lives only in humans. People with typhoid fever carry the organism in their bloodstream and intestinal tract. They will become ill and shed the organism in their stool. A few people carry the illness but do not become ill. They also shed the organism in their stool.

Typhoid fever can be contracted if food or drink beverages have been handled by a person who is shedding *S. typhi*. Sewage contaminated by *S. typhi* can get into the drinking water and be used for washing food. The food or drink will pass along the organism.

People with typhoid fever usually have a sustained fever as high as 103°F to 104°F (39°C to 40°C). Among other symptoms, they may have stomach pains, feel weak, and lose their appetites.

Vaccines are available. They are advisable for people who are traveling to parts of the world where typhoid fever is common. Travelers should determine whether drinking water in their intended destination is safe.

There is no evidence that *S. typhi* is passed through mothers' milk.

See also Expression of mothers' milk; Hospitalization; Medication resources (inside back cover)

➤ UNCOORDINATED SUCKLING

DEFINITION   Disorder in the pattern of suckling and swallowing at the breast. Efficient milk transfer at the breast depends on a coordinated suck and swallow.

Babies more likely to have an uncoordinated suck at first include:

Babies who are born prematurely.

Babies who have been exposed to certain drugs.

Babies who have neurological impairment.

ASK ABOUT

Age of the baby.

Feeding history.

Weight gain history.

ASSESSMENT

EMERGENT CARE NEEDED?

Are any of the following present?

Difficulty breathing even when not feeding.

Difficulty breathing after feeding.

The baby pulls off of the breast to breathe.

Extreme lethargy or irritability in the baby.

Sudden change in baby's muscle tone (extremely floppy or stiff) or repetitive jerking movements (e.g., seizure activity).

The baby shows sudden disinterest in feeding.

Inability to wake the baby.

The baby does not calm, even with cuddles.

Meconium bowel movements after 5 days of life.

Weight loss of greater than 7% from birth.

Weight loss after 5 days of life.

Fewer than three bowel movements daily in a breastfed newborn after the first 2 days of life.

No urine in 6 hours.

Brick dust urine (uric acid crystals) after 2 days of life.

Dark-colored urine.

Fewer than four urinations daily in the breastfed newborn after day 5 of life.

Noticeably sunken fontanelles (soft spot on the top of the head).

Baby below birthweight at 10–14 days of life.

Cessation of weight gain.

IF YES, *Seek emergent care now and contact pediatric care provider.*

PROMPT CARE NEEDED?

Are any of the following present?

Diagnosis of neuromuscular problem in a breastfeeding baby.

IF YES, *Refer for consultation with occupational, physical, or speech therapist experienced with breastfeeding babies.*

Are any of the following present?

> The baby does not stay on the breast.
>
> The baby is not gaining adequately.
>
> The baby does not seem to transfer milk.

IF YES,   *Call lactation care provider now.*

ROUTINE CARE NEEDED?

Are any of the following present?

> Difficulty maintaining milk supply.

IF YES,   *Call lactation care provider today.*

SELF-CARE INFORMATION

As soon as it is determined that the infant has an uncoordinated suck, the mother should express her milk regularly in order to maintain her supply and to collect milk to feed the baby.

Increased opportunities to practice breastfeeding can be helpful to promote coordinated sucking.

Skin-to-skin holding may improve motor organization of babies.

IMPORTANT CONDITIONS TO REPORT

Inadequate stooling or urinations.

Lethargy.

The baby is difficult to rouse.

Lower milk volume.

See also Alternate breast massage; Botulism, infantile; Breast pump; Lethargy; Sleepy baby; Weak suck; Weight gain, baby–low

➤ UNICEF

See United Nations Children's Fund (UNICEF)

➤ UNILATERAL

DEFINITION   One-sided.

➤ UNITED NATIONS CHILDREN'S FUND (UNICEF)

DESCRIPTION   UNICEF is the driving force that helps build a world where the rights of every child are realized. We have the global authority to influence decision-makers, and the variety of partners at grassroots level to turn the most innovative ideas into reality. That makes us unique among world organizations, and unique among those working with the young.[268](first para)

NOTES

UNICEF International: UNICEF House
Website: www.unicef.org
UNICEF USA
Website: www.unicefusa.org

See also Baby-Friendly Hospital Initiative (BFHI); Baby-Friendly USA, Inc. (BFUSA); Ten Steps to Successful Breastfeeding

Footnote

[268]United Nations Children's Fund. (n.d.). About UNICEF: Who we are. Retrieved from http://www .unicef.org/about/who/index.html

➤ UNITED STATES BREASTFEEDING COMMITTEE (USBC)

DESCRIPTION   The United States Breastfeeding Committee (USBC) is an independent nonprofit coalition of more than 40 nationally influential professional, educational, and governmental organizations, that share a common mission to improve the Nation's [sic] health by working collaboratively to protect, promote, and support breastfeeding.[269]

United States Breastfeeding Committee (USBC)
Email: info@usbreastfeeding.org
Website: www.usbreastfeeding.org
   USBC works to protect, promote, and support breastfeeding through education, advocacy, and communication strategies.

Footnote

[269]United States Breastfeeding Committee. (2008–2011). Home page. Retrieved from http://www
.usbreastfeeding.org

➤ UNITED STATES DEPARTMENT OF AGRICULTURE (USDA), SPECIAL SUPPLEMENTAL FOOD PROGRAM FOR WOMEN, INFANTS, AND CHILDREN (WIC)

DESCRIPTION   WIC's Mission: to safeguard the health of low-income women, infants, and children up to age 5 who are at nutrition risk by providing nutritious foods to supplement diets, information on healthy eating, and referrals to health care . . . Food, nutrition counseling, and access to health services are provided to low-income women, infants, and children under the Special Supplemental Nutrition Program for Women, Infants, and Children, popularly known as WIC.[270](WIC's Mission section)

WIC, Food and Nutrition Service—USDA
Website: www.fns.usda.gov/wic
   WIC provides federal grants to states for supplemental foods, healthcare referrals, and nutrition education for low-income pregnant, breastfeeding, and nonbreastfeeding postpartum women and to infants and children who are found to be at nutritional risk. State and local WIC grantees provide breastfeeding education and often peer counseling and breastfeeding equipment to eligible women.

Footnote

[270]Food & Nutrition Service. (n.d.) About WIC. Retrieved from http://www.fns.usda.gov/wic
/aboutwic/mission.htm

➤ UNITED STATES LACTATION CONSULTANT ASSOCIATION (USLCA)

DESCRIPTION The United States Lactation Consultant Association (USLCA) is the professional association for International Board Certified Lactation Consultants (IBCLCs) and other healthcare professionals who care for breastfeeding families. Mission: To build and sustain a national association that advocates for lactation professionals.[271(p1)]

NOTES

Email: info@uslca.org
Web: www.uslca.org
    USLCA provides education and advocacy for lactation professionals.

See also International Lactation Consultant Association (ILCA)

Footnote

[271]United States Lactation Consultant Association. (2012). Inside USLCA. Retrieved from http ://www.ilca.org/i4a/pages/index.cfm?pageid=3513

➤ UNIVERSAL PRECAUTIONS

DEFINITION Universal precautions are infection control guidelines designed to protect workers from exposure to diseases and certain body fluids. Universal precautions do not apply to breastmilk, except for workers in a milk bank setting.

NOTES

Wearing gloves when handling breastmilk (thawing, heating, and preparing feedings) helps to ensure that the milk will not be contaminated.

➤ URINARY TRACT INFECTION (UTI)

DEFINITION   A urinary tract infection (UTI) is an infection anywhere in the urinary tract. This includes the kidneys, ureter, bladder, and urethra.

ASK ABOUT

Age of the baby.
Onset of UTI.

ASSESSMENT

ROUTINE CARE NEEDED?

Are any of the following present?

Concerns about compatibility with breastfeeding of prescribed medication(s)

IF YES,   *Consult up-to-date drug references.*

SELF-CARE INFORMATION

Follow medical advice and take medication as prescribed.

NOTES

Usually, a UTI is caused by bacteria that can also live in the intestines, in the vagina, or around the urethra, which is at the entrance to the urinary tract. The body typically removes the bacteria.

Signs and symptoms of UTI include:

Burning sensation during urination.

Frequent urge to urinate, even with scanty amount of urine.

Pain in the back or in the lower abdomen.

Cloudy, dark, bloody, or unusual-smelling urine.

Fever or chills.

Breastfeeding is not contraindicated when the mother has a UTI. Breastfeeding confers some protection against urinary tract infections in infants.[272]

See also Acute infection; Medication resources (inside back cover)

Footnote

[272]Pisacane, A., Graziano, L., Mazzarella, G., Scarpellino, B., & Zona, G. (1992). Breast-feeding and urinary tract infection. *Journal of Pediatrics, 120*(1), 87–89.

➤ USBC

See United States Breastfeeding Committee (USBC)

➤ USDA

See United States Department of Agriculture (USDA), Special Supplemental Food Program for Women, Infants, and Children (WIC)

➤ USLCA

See United States Lactation Consultant Association (USLCA)

➤ UTERINE BLEEDING

DEFINITION   Flow of blood from the healing wall of the uterus. Vaginal blood flow is expected after delivery. This blood is also called "lochia." Three types of lochia are recognized, including lochia rubra (red), lochia serosa (pink), and lochia alba (white). Lochia rubra, a red discharge, begins after delivery and continues for 2–3 days. Lochia serosa, a paler, pinkish discharge, continues for the next week or so. Lochia alba, a whitish discharge, starts around the 10th day postpartum and should be resolved within a month.[273]

ASK ABOUT

Onset.
Date of delivery.

ASSESSMENT

EMERGENT CARE NEEDED?

Are any of the following present?

Soaking a sanitary napkin with bright red blood at a rate of one napkin or more per hour.

Clots in the bloody discharge.

Foul odor to the discharge (even if occasional).

Dizziness.

Fever.

Abdominal pain.

IF YES,   *Call obstetric care provider now and seek emergency care now.*

PROMPT MEDICAL CARE NEEDED?

Are any of the following present?

Soaking a sanitary napkin with bright red blood at a rate of one napkin every 2–3 hours.

Abdominal tenderness.

Low-grade fever.

Light-headedness.

IF YES,   *Call obstetric care provider now.*

PROMPT LACTATION CARE NEEDED?

Are any of the following present?

Problems with milk supply in a woman diagnosed with retained placental fragments.

IF YES,   *Call lactation care provider today.*

ROUTINE CARE NEEDED?

Are any of the following present?

Soaking a sanitary napkin with bright red blood at a rate of one napkin every 3 or more hours.

Abdominal tenderness.

IF YES,   *Call obstetric care provider today.*

SELF-CARE INFORMATION

Monitor blood flow.

IMPORTANT CONDITIONS TO REPORT

Continuation of symptoms.
Sudden gushing of blood.
Multiple blood clots passed.
Concerns about milk supply.

NOTES

As time progresses, the volume of lochia should also decrease. Sudden return of bright red blood is of concern and should be evaluated medically. Retained placental fragments can be indicated by ongoing lochia rubra. In this event, mature milk production may not occur until placental fragments are expelled or removed.

See also Hemorrhage, postpartum; Lochia; Retained placental fragments

Footnote

[273]Varney, H., Kriebs, J. M., & Gegor, C. L. (Eds.). (2004). *Varney's midwifery* (4th ed., p. 1043). Sudbury, MA: Jones and Bartlett.

➤ UTI

See Urinary tract infection (UTI)

➤ VACCINATIONS AND IMMUNIZATIONS

DEFINITION   Substances injected or administered to trigger production of antibodies against specific infections. Breastfeeding provides a baby's first immunization (vaccination). After that, breastfed babies should be immunized on the same schedule as babies who are not breastfed.

ROUTINE CARE NEEDED?

Are any of the following present?

Vaccination or immunizations for the mother or baby.

IF YES,   *Consult up-to-date drug references.*

SELF-CARE INFORMATION

Follow medical recommendations for after-immunization care.

Babies are comforted by nursing during and after painful procedures.

IMPORTANT CONDITIONS TO REPORT

The healthcare provider will provide a list of important conditions to report after vaccinations and immunizations.

NOTES

Mothers who are breastfeeding can receive most immunizations except smallpox vaccination. Mothers should not receive the smallpox vaccine even if they are pumping their milk and feeding their babies breastmilk in a bottle.

See also Immunization; Medication resources (inside back cover)

➤ **VARICELLA ZOSTER VIRUS**

DEFINITION   The characteristic lesions, chicken pox, resulting from infection with varicella zoster, a virus of the herpes family. This highly infectious virus is passed via droplet and direct contact with lesions. Exposure can be serious for the newborn. If a mother is judged safe to be with her infant, and she has no lesions on the breast area, breastfeeding is considered safe.

Onset.

Age of the baby.

Infection of any household members.

ASSESSMENT

EMERGENT CARE NEEDED?

Are any of the following present?

Eruption of chicken pox in a newborn infant.

Presence of chicken pox lesions on the breast and nipple area.

IF YES, *Report to healthcare provider immediately.*

NOTES

Mothers who are infected in the early perinatal period may infect their infants by passing droplets and allowing infant contact with lesions. Infection risk may be decreased by administering varicella zoster immunoglobulin (VZIG) to the infant.

If a breastfeeding mother is separated from her baby, she should be encouraged to express or pump her milk eight or more times daily to maintain her milk supply. If she has no lesions on the breast or nipple area, her milk may be given to the baby. Careful hand washing should be practiced to avoid involving the breast or collected milk.

If only siblings are infected, the baby and mother should be isolated and continue breastfeeding.

See Lawrence & Lawrence for an excellent protocol for varicella zoster in the peripartum.[274(p453)]

See also Acute infection

Footnote

[274]Lawrence, R. A., & Lawrence, R. M. (2011). *Breastfeeding: A guide for the medical profession* (7th ed.). St. Louis, MO: Elsevier/Mosby.

➤ VASOSPASM OF BREAST AND NIPPLE

DEFINITION   Sudden constriction of arteries in the breast and/or nipple. Nipple pain may occur because of Raynaud's phenomenon/syndrome.[275] This is a condition in which blood flow to the extremities is temporarily reduced. It has also been called nipple vasospasm. The affected extremity becomes cold and numb and turns white. As the blood flow returns, it may quickly turn blue and then reddish pink. This is the tricolor sign of Raynaud's phenomenon. There is also a bicolor sign (white and pink). As the color returns, the pain increases. The pain can be brief, lasting for just a few minutes, or it can be prolonged, lasting up to an hour.

The reaction occurs in response to cold, wetness, stress, and certain medications.

Usually the fingers and toes are affected, but the nipples are also extremities and can therefore be affected.

ASK ABOUT

Age of the baby.
History of nipple pain.

ASSESSMENT

ROUTINE CARE NEEDED?

Are any of the following present?

Persistent nipple pain.

Breast pain in reaction to cold, wet, and nursing.

Tricolor sign (white, blue, pink) or bicolor sign (white, pink) of the nipple when cold or wet.

IF YES,   *Call obstetric care provider today. Call lactation care provider today.*

SELF-CARE INFORMATION

Nifedipine is a prescription medication (calcium channel blocker) that has been used to treat Raynaud's phenomenon in nursing mothers.[276]

Mothers with Raynaud's phenomenon are usually also advised also to avoid caffeine and nicotine.

See also Painful breastfeeding; Raynaud's phenomenon/syndrome; Medication resources (inside back cover); Sore nipples

Footnotes

[275]Lawlor-Smith, L., & Lawlor-Smith, C. (1997). Vasospasm of the nipple—a manifestation of Raynaud's phenomenon: Case reports. *British Medical Journal, 314*(7081), 644–645.

[276]Anderson, J. E., Held, N., & Wright, K. (2004). Raynaud's phenomenon of the nipple: A treatable cause of painful breastfeeding. *Pediatrics, 113*(4), e360–e364.

➤ VEGETARIANS

DEFINITION   Those who avoid consumption of animal products. Although many vegetarian diets are compatible with breastfeeding, some vegetarian diets (such as macrobiotic and vegan) may not be nutritionally adequate and can put the breastfed infant at risk of malnutrition. The major concerns of vegetarian diets are deficiencies of vitamins B_{12}, B_2, and D, and also the mineral zinc.

ASK ABOUT

Type of diet.
Age of the baby.
Nutritional supplements taken.

ASSESSMENT

EMERGENT CARE NEEDED?

Are any of the following present?

Infant tetany (a condition characterized by painful muscle spasms and tremors).
Infant seizures.

IF YES,   *Seek emergency care now.*

PROMPT CARE NEEDED?

Are any of the following present?

Infant lethargy.

Change in infant feeding behavior.

Infant weight loss after the first 5 days of life.

Slow growth in the breastfed infant of a mother on a macrobiotic diet.

IF YES,   *Seek pediatric care now.*

ROUTINE CARE NEEDED?

Are any of the following present?

Macrobiotic diet of the mother.

Vegan diet of the mother.

Ovo-lacto vegetarian diet of the mother.

IF YES,   *Seek dietary consultation.*

SELF-CARE INFORMATION

Nutritional risks of vegetarian diets are especially associated with protein; vitamins B_{12}, B_2, and D; and zinc deficiencies.

IMPORTANT CONDITIONS TO REPORT

Lethargy and poor feeding behavior.

NOTES

Many people who are vegetarians are knowledgeable about including foods and supplements that balance their diets.

See also Macrobiotic diet of the mother; Maternal diet

➤ VITAMIN SUPPLEMENTS

DEFINITION   Additional nutrients that may be required for infants. The American Academy of Pediatrics recommends that:

> breastfed and partially breastfed infants should be supplemented with 400 IU/day of vitamin D beginning in the first few days of life. Supplementation should be continued unless the infant is weaned to at least 1 L/day or 1 qt/day of vitamin D–fortified formula or whole milk.[277(p1148)]

Vitamin D is ordinarily made in the skin when babies are exposed to sunlight. Today, babies may not be outside enough and when they are, they may be coated in sunscreen, which prevents vitamin D from being formed in the skin. When formula is manufactured, vitamin D is added. Breastfed babies may receive vitamin D separately as a liquid drop.

The need for iron supplementation in preterm and other infants at risk for iron-deficiency anemia should be considered.

Mothers on vegan diets are usually advised to supplement their diets with B vitamins, especially vitamin B_{12}. Vitamin D might also be advised for vegan mothers.

Mothers who are eating a variety of foods may be encouraged to continue taking their prenatal vitamins during lactation.

ASK ABOUT

Age of the baby.

ASSESSMENT

ROUTINE CARE NEEDED?

Are any of the following present?

Questions about vitamin supplements for the baby.

Questions about vitamin supplements for the mother.

IF YES,   *Call medical care provider and seek dietary consultation.*

See also Anemia; Iron; Macrobiotic diet of the mother; Vegetarians

Footnotes

[277]Wagner, C. L., & Greer, F. R. (2008). Prevention of rickets and vitamin D deficiency in infants, children, and adolescents. *Pediatrics, 122*(5), 1142–1152. doi:10.1542/peds.2008-1862

[278]Baker, R. D., Greer, F. R., & The Committee on Nutrition. (2010). Diagnosis and prevention of iron deficiency and iron-deficiency anemia in infants and young children (0–3 years of age). *Pediatrics, 126*(5), 1040–1050. doi:10.1542/peds.2010-2576

[279]AAP Section on Breastfeeding. (2012). Breastfeeding and the use of human milk. *Pediatrics, 129*(3), e827–e841. doi:10.1542/peds.2011-3552

➤ VOMITING

DEFINITION   Regurgitation of food from the mouth. Spitting up or vomiting by the infant can be differentiated from projectile vomiting by the distance it travels. Projectile vomit clears the chin of the infant. It may travel several feet. Spitting up does not clear the chin on its way out.

Spitting up, even after every feeding, may not be an indication that there is anything wrong with the baby. The mother may have a very powerful let-down reflex, for example.

SELF-CARE INFORMATION

Occasional spitting up in an otherwise well infant is not uncommon.

Frequent spitting up, even by a baby with no other symptoms, can indicate that there is an underlying problem, such as gastroesophageal reflux or pyloric stenosis.

IMPORTANT CONDITIONS TO REPORT

Projectile vomiting.

Bilious (green) vomit produced by a newborn (considered a surgical emergency unless proven otherwise).

Signs that the baby is unwell in combination with spitting up.

Decrease in stools and urinations.

Poor feeding behavior.

Weight loss, failure to gain weight adequately.

See also Gastroesophageal (GE) reflux; Let-down reflex; Milk-ejection reflex; Projectile vomiting; Pyloric stenosis

➤ WABA

See World Alliance for Breastfeeding Action (WABA)

➤ WAKING A SLEEPY BABY

DEFINITION   Methods for encouraging feeding in a drowsy baby. Babies cycle between sleep and wakefulness more rapidly than adults. They have twice as many light sleep cycles as adults.

Newborn babies sleep about 18 hours a day on average, but their sleep is more interrupted than that of adults.

When babies cycle into lighter sleep (about every 20 minutes) their eyeballs move under their closed lids. They can nurse well at this stage of sleep, which is called REM (rapid eye movement) sleep.

Some babies seem sleepy at first, making it difficult to get in 10–12 effective nursings a day unless the baby is closely observed for REM sleep, a state during which most babies feed well.

There can be many reasons for sleepiness in the infant, such as jaundice, drug effects from labor analgesia, and a difficult labor and birth.

Babies who are underfed are lethargic and sleepy. The more underfed they are, the more lethargic they become.

Sleepy babies should have a breastfeeding evaluation to determine whether or not they are being adequately fed.

ASK ABOUT

Age of the baby.
Weight gain pattern.
History of sleepiness.

ASSESSMENT

EMERGENT CARE NEEDED?

Are any of the following present?

Inability to rouse the baby.

A baby who sleeps more than 3 hours between feedings consistently.

Shallow breathing or breathing that is difficult to observe. (Observe the newborn's breathing for at least 1 minute. Sleeping newborns often exhibit periodic breathing, which may include rapid shallow breaths interspersed with brief pauses in breathing.)

Meconium bowel movements after 5 days of life.

Fewer than three bowel movements daily in a breastfed newborn after the first 2 days of life.

Weight loss of greater than 7% from birth.

Weight loss after 5 days.

No urine in 6 hours.

Brick dust urine (uric acid crystals) after 2 days of life.

Dark-colored urine.

Fewer than four urinations daily in the breastfed newborn after day 5 of life.

Low muscle tone/floppiness.

IF YES,   *Seek emergent care now. Call pediatric care provider now.*

PROMPT CARE NEEDED?

Are any of the following present?

The baby nurses fewer than 10 times in 24 hours.

The baby consistently falls asleep after sucking briefly at the breast.

The baby is not gaining at least 0.5 oz a day in the newborn period.

The baby does not sustain active suckling or feeding at the breast.

IF YES, *Seek lactation care today.*

SELF-CARE INFORMATION

Babies need to be fed in order to sleep well, but sleepy babies are not necessarily well fed.

Parents who observe the baby for feeding cues—hand-to-face or hand-to-mouth movements, lip smacking, seeking with lips, rooting, and head bobbing—may find it easier to feed the baby at the baby's best time.

Babies tend to cluster their feedings. Nurse the baby again when the baby gives the next feeding cue (i.e., watch the baby, not the clock, to determine the timing of the next feeding). The baby never completely empties the breast.

IMPORTANT CONDITIONS TO REPORT

Babies who are hard to rouse and who sleep longer than 3 hours between nursings should be evaluated.

Babies who fall asleep after a minute or two at the breast should be evaluated.

See also Cosleeping; Feeding cues; Feeding pattern of breastfed infants; Hyperbilirubinemia; Hypotonia; Infant behavior; Lethargy; Milk production

➤ WATER FOR THE NURSING BABY (WATER SUPPLEMENTATION)

DEFINITION Administration of water to a breastfed baby. Water is not needed for the nursing baby, even in hot, dry climates.

Because babies have immature kidneys and a different body composition than adults, they are more vulnerable to water imbalance before 6 months of age.

ASK ABOUT

Age of the baby.

Amount of water being supplemented.

ASSESSMENT

EMERGENT CARE NEEDED?

Are any of the following present in a baby being given extra water?

Seizures or convulsions, particularly facial movements and jerking of a body part.

The baby stops breathing or turns blue.

IF YES,   *Seek emergency care now.*

PROMPT CARE NEEDED?

Are any of the following present?

Giving baby extra water.

More than eight wet diapers a day.

Pale-colored urine.

IF YES,   *Report to pediatric care provider now and seek pediatric care today.*

ROUTINE CARE NEEDED?

Are any of the following present?

Concern about producing enough milk to keep the baby hydrated.

IF YES,   *Call lactation care provider today.*

SELF-CARE INFORMATION

Water is not needed for the nursing baby, even in hot, dry climates.

Because babies have a different body composition than adults, they are more vulnerable to water imbalance.

IMPORTANT CONDITIONS TO REPORT

More than eight wet diapers a day.

Giving baby extra water.

Seizures or convulsions, particularly facial movements and jerking of a body part.

Baby stops breathing or turns blue.

See also Components of breastmilk; Dehydration; Jaundice

➤ WDWN (WELL DEVELOPED, WELL NOURISHED)

DEFINITION An abbreviation used to indicate that an individual appears to be adequately fed.

➤ WEAK SUCK

DEFINITION Poor oral muscle tone or coordination during feeding. Milk production stimulation and milk transfer depend on an effective suck.

Babies more likely to have a weak suck at first include:

Babies who are born prematurely.

Babies who have been exposed to certain drugs.

Babies who have neurological impairment.

ASK ABOUT

Age of the baby.

Feeding history.

Weight gain history.

ASSESSMENT

EMERGENT CARE NEEDED?

Are any of the following present?

Difficulty breathing even when not feeding.

Difficulty breathing after feeding.

The baby pulls off of the breast to breathe.

Extreme lethargy or irritability in the baby.

Sudden change in baby's muscle tone (extremely floppy or stiff) or repetitive jerking movements (e.g., seizure activity).

The baby shows a sudden disinterest in feeding.

Inability to wake the baby.

The baby does not calm, even with cuddles.

Meconium bowel movements after 5 days of life.

Weight loss of greater than 7% from birth.

Weight loss after 5 days.

Fewer than three bowel movements daily in a breastfed newborn after the
first 2 days of life.

No urine in 6 hours.

Brick dust urine (uric acid crystals) after 2 days of life.

Dark-colored urine.

Fewer than four urinations daily in the breastfed newborn after day 5 of life.

Noticeably sunken fontanelles (soft spot on the top of the head).

Baby below birthweight at 10–14 days of life.

Cessation of weight gain.

IF YES,   *Seek emergent care now. Call pediatric provider now.*

PROMPT CARE NEEDED?

Are any of the following present?

Diagnosis of neuromuscular problem in a breastfeeding baby.

IF YES,   *Refer for consultation with occupational, physical, or speech therapist experienced with breastfeeding babies.*

Are any of the following present?

The baby does not stay on the breast.

The baby is not gaining adequately.

The baby does not seem to transfer milk.

IF YES,   *Call lactation care provider now.*

ROUTINE CARE NEEDED?

Are any of the following present?

Difficulty maintaining milk supply.

IF YES,   *Call lactation care provider today.*

SELF-CARE INFORMATION

As soon as it is determined that the infant has an uncoordinated suck, the mother should express her milk regularly in order to maintain her supply and to collect milk to feed the baby.

Increased opportunities to practice breastfeeding can be helpful to promote coordinated sucking.

IMPORTANT CONDITIONS TO REPORT
Inadequate stooling or urinations.
Lethargy.
A difficult-to-rouse baby.
Lower milk volume.

See also Botulism, infantile; Breast pump; Lethargy; Sleepy baby; Uncoordinated suckling; Weight gain, baby–low

➤ WEANING

DEFINITION   Weaning is a process that begins when the breastfed baby is fed other food or drink in addition to mother's milk, and ends when the baby is no longer receiving any mother's milk.

ASK ABOUT

Age of the baby.
Feeding history.

ASSESSMENT

ROUTINE CARE NEEDED?
   Are any of the following present?
      Weaning information required because of prescribed drug.

   IF YES,   *Consult up-to-date drug references.*

ROUTINE CARE NEEDED?
   Are any of the following present?
      Questions about how long breastfeeding should last.
      Need for weaning strategy or management.

   IF YES,   *Call lactation care provider.*

SELF-CARE INFORMATION

Every mother has unique feelings about her breastfeeding experience, including how and when it should end.

Mothers are sometimes instructed to wean for reasons that are not legitimate, such as the onset of the baby's teething.

IMPORTANT CONDITIONS TO REPORT

Breast discomfort.

Fever.

Red streaks on breast.

Concerns about weaning.

See also Abrupt weaning; Closet nursing; Medication resources (inside back cover); Nursing strike

➤ WEIGHT GAIN, BABY—HIGH

DEFINITION   A situation in which a baby is growing faster than anticipated. Well-fed breastfed babies gain more rapidly in the early months based on standard growth charts compared to formula fed babies. It is not thought possible for women to over-feed babies at the breast.

ASK ABOUT

Age of the baby.

Weight gain pattern of the baby.

ASSESSMENT

PROMPT CARE NEEDED?

Are any of the following present?

About the mother:

Reddened areas of the breast.

Fever higher than 101°F (38.5°C).

Extreme breast discomfort.

Flu-like aching throughout body.

Recurrent mastitis.

IF YES,   *Call obstetric care provider now. Seek lactation care today.*

ROUTINE CARE NEEDED?

Are any of the following present?

About the mother:

Persistent sore nipples.

Nipples often compressed at the end of nursing.

About the baby:

Consistent weight gain of more than 1 lb per week.

Frequent, explosive, large stools.

Gassy, often unhappy baby.

IF YES,   *Call lactation care provider.*

SELF-CARE INFORMATION

Oversupply can cause discomfort for the mother and the baby. Careful management of the mother's milk supply can increase the baby's comfort.

IMPORTANT CONDITIONS TO REPORT

Recurrent symptoms.

Unresolved symptoms.

See also Block feeding; Milk flow, too fast; Overactive let-down reflex

➤ WEIGHT GAIN, BABY—LOW

DEFINITION   A situation in which a baby is growing more slowly than anticipated. Breastfed babies should gain a minimum of 0.5 oz to 1 oz a day on average in the early weeks. Breastfed babies gain even faster than was previously believed, probably because in the past, breastfeeding was done on a schedule and not as frequently as we now know is ideal.

ASK ABOUT

Age of the baby.

Weight gain pattern.

ASSESSMENT

PROMPT CARE NEEDED?

Are any of the following present?

Extreme lethargy or irritability in the baby.

Sudden change in the baby's muscle tone (extremely floppy or stiff) or repetitive jerking movements (e.g., seizure activity).

Sudden disinterest in feeding by the baby.

Inability to wake baby.

Baby does not calm, even with cuddles.

Meconium bowel movements after 5 days of life.

Weight loss of greater than 7% from birth.

Weight loss after 5 days.

Fewer than three bowel movements daily in breastfed newborn after the first 2 days of life.

No urine in 6 hours.

Brick dust urine (uric acid crystals) after 2 days of life.

Dark-colored urine.

Fewer than four urinations daily in the breastfed newborn after day 5 of life.

Noticeably sunken fontanelles (soft spot on the top of the head).

Decreased activity.

Baby below birthweight at 10–14 days of life.

Cessation of weight gain.

Sleeping at the breast consistently.

IF YES,   *Seek emergent care now. Call pediatric provider now.*

ROUTINE CARE NEEDED?

Are any of the following present?

The baby sleeps at the breast after a few sucks.

The baby is hard to latch on.

No audible swallows.

Pediatric referral for consultation.

IF YES,   *Seek lactation care today.*

IMPORTANT CONDITIONS TO REPORT
Decrease in number of urinations or stools.
Increased sleepiness or hours spent sleeping.
The baby is harder to rouse.

See also Growth chart; Hypotonia; Jaundice

➤ WEIGHT LOSS, BABY

DEFINITION Decrease in body mass in an infant. Weight loss is not expected after the first 5 days postpartum.

See also Growth chart; Insufficient milk supply; Weight gain, baby–low

➤ WEIGHT LOSS, MOTHER

DEFINITION Decrease in body mass in a nursing woman. Weight loss of up to 5 lb a month in the first months postpartum has not been associated with poorer growth of the nursing baby.

Exclusively breastfeeding mothers are more likely to be closer to their prepregnancy weight at 6 months postpartum when compared to mixed-feeding or formula-feeding mothers.

ASSESSMENT

ROUTINE CARE NEEDED?
Are any of the following present?
Desire to exercise while breastfeeding.
Desire to lose weight while breastfeeding.

IF YES, *Call lactation care provider.*

SELF-CARE INFORMATION

Weight loss of up to 5 lbs a month in the first months postpartum has not been associated with poorer growth of the nursing baby.

Exclusive breastfeeding is the best route to weight loss in the first 6 months postpartum. Continued breastfeeding after 6 months contributes to additional weight loss.

IMPORTANT CONDITIONS TO REPORT

Rapid weight loss of more than 3 lbs per week after the first 6 weeks postpartum.

See also Exclusive breastfeeding; Exercise

➤ WELLSTART INTERNATIONAL

DESCRIPTION   Organization whose mission is "to advance the knowledge, skills, and ability of healthcare providers regarding the promotion, protection, and support of optimal infant and maternal health and nutrition from conception through the completion of weaning."[280](Our Mission section)

NOTES

Wellstart International
Email: info@wellstart.org
Web: www.wellstart.org
   Wellstart offers professional education and support materials, as well as local breastfeeding services.

Footnote

[280]Wellstart International. (2005–2009). Home page. Retrieved from http://www.wellstart.org/

➤ WET DIAPERS

DEFINITION   Evidence of urination in an infant via presence of dampness in the diaper. Wet diapers, in addition to stooling patterns, can be an important indication of breast milk transfer.

ASK ABOUT

Age of the baby.
History of urination.

ASSESSMENT

EMERGENT CARE NEEDED?

Are any of the following present?

No wet diaper or stool in 6–8 hours after the first 2 days of life.

Red dusty urine in diaper after the first 2 days of life.

Urine crystals in diaper after the first 2 days of life.

Lethargy/difficulty rousing the baby.

The baby sleeps at the breast consistently.

IF YES,   *Seek pediatric care now.*

PROMPT CARE NEEDED?

Are any of the following present?

No wet diaper or stool in 4–6 hours after the first 2 days of life.

The baby falls asleep after a few sucks.

Poor latch.

IF YES,   *Seek lactation care now and report to pediatric care provider.*

ROUTINE CARE NEEDED?

Are any of the following present?

Need for reassurance that the baby is getting enough nourishment with no other symptoms.

IF YES,   *Call lactation care provider today.*

SELF-CARE INFORMATION

Wet diapers, in addition to stooling patterns, can be an important indication of breast milk transfer.

IMPORTANT CONDITIONS TO REPORT

No wet diaper or stool in 6 hours after the first 2 days of life.

Red, dusty urine in diaper after the first 2 days of life.

Urine crystals in diaper after the first 2 days of life.

Lethargy.

See also Bowel movements, infant; Stooling patterns; Water for the nursing baby (Water supplementation)

➤ WET NURSING

DEFINITION   Historically, women who nursed babies who were not their own were called wet nurses. Wet nurses usually were not nursing their own babies at the same time and may have been paid for their service.

NOTES

Because of concerns about transmission of HIV, hepatitis, herpes, and other organisms, wet nursing is discouraged in the United States today.

See also Cross nursing; Donor milk

➤ WHO

See Baby-Friendly Hospital Initiative (BFHI); Ten Steps to Successful Breastfeeding; World Health Organization (WHO)

➤ WHO CODE (INTERNATIONAL CODE OF MARKETING OF BREAST-MILK SUBSTITUTES)

DEFINITION   A document adopted by the World Health Assembly in 1981 and amended by several subsequent resolutions as a minimum requirement to protect infant health. The International Code sets forth a series of expectations about the behavior of the infant formula industry, healthcare systems, healthcare providers, governments, and other parties regarding the protection of breastfeeding and ethical marketing of breastmilk substitutes.

➤ WIC PROGRAM

See United States Department of Agriculture (USDA), Special Supplemental Food Program for Women, Infants, and Children (WIC)

➤ WNL (WITHIN NORMAL LIMITS)

DEFINITION   An abbreviation used to indicate that an individual's growth and development is typical.

➤ WORKING MOTHERS

DEFINITION   Mothers who participate in the workforce. Mothers who work for pay may do so away from home or in the home. Employed mothers may be separated from their baby or have the baby nearby. In the United States, more than half of the mothers with babies under the age of 1 year are employed.[281(last para)]

ASK ABOUT

Amount of separation—hours per day, days per week.
Start date of work.
Age of the baby.
The mother's plans to continue breastfeeding.
The mother's plans to express milk.
Accommodations at work for expressing and saving milk.
How the baby will be fed away from the mother.

ASSESSMENT

ROUTINE CARE NEEDED?

Are any of the following present?

Information about managing work and breastfeeding.

IF YES,   *Call lactation care provider.*

SELF-CARE INFORMATION

Stress does not seem to affect milk supply but frequent milk removal is needed to maintain or improve the milk supply.

Milk can be collected and frozen in the early weeks to supplement milk collected after the mother's return to work.

Milk supply is best maintained by hand expression or combining hand expression with pumping using a pump that is intended for that purpose along with breastfeeding.

Select child care facilities carefully.

Expressed milk is a raw food and should be refrigerated immediately if possible. Get information about storage, use, and feeding expressed milk from your lactation care provider.

The timing of return to work and the number of hours spent away from the baby affect the duration of breastfeeding more than the type of work a woman does.

IMPORTANT CONDITIONS TO REPORT

Problems with expressing milk (check that the equipment is working properly).

Breast problems.

Problems with the infant accepting expressed milk.

NOTES

The Patient Protection and Affordable Care Act, passed by Congress in 2010, specifies that:

> Employers are required to provide 'reasonable break time for an employee to express breast milk for her nursing child for 1 year after the child's birth each time such employee has need to express the milk.' Employers are also required to provide 'a place, other than a bathroom, that is shielded from view and free from intrusion from coworkers and the public, which may be used by an employee to express breast milk.'[282](General Requirements section)

Ongoing support and help with problem solving may be needed after returning to work.

See also Breast pump; Collection and storage of breastmilk; Day care; Decrease in milk supply; Storage of breastmilk; Working mothers

Footnotes

[281]U.S. Department of Labor, Bureau of Labor Statistics. (2012, April 26). Employment characteristics of families summary. Retrieved from http://www.bls.gov/news.release/famee.nr0.htm

[282]U.S. Department of Labor. (2010, December). Wage and Hour Division (WHD)—fact sheet. Retrieved from http://www.dol.gov/whd/regs/compliance/whdfs73.htm

➤ WORLD ALLIANCE FOR BREASTFEEDING ACTION (WABA)

DESCRIPTION   The World Alliance for Breastfeeding Action (WABA) is an organization that protects, promotes, and supports breastfeeding worldwide. It is "a global network of individuals and [organizations] concerned with the protection, promotion and support of breastfeeding worldwide. WABA action is based on the Innocenti Declaration, the Ten Links for Nurturing the Future and the Global Strategy for Infant & Young Child Feeding."[283](Main page)

NOTES

WABA coordinates World Breastfeeding Week.
World Alliance for Breastfeeding Action (WABA)
Website: www.waba.org.my

Footnotes

[283]World Alliance for Breastfeeding Action. (n.d.). Untitled. Retrieved from http://www.waba.org.my/

➤ WORLD HEALTH ORGANIZATION (WHO)

DESCRIPTION The World Health Organization (WHO) is a specialized agency of the United Nations that directs and coordinates international health work.

NOTES

WHO's main functions are to give world guidance in the field of health, to set global standards for health to cooperate with governments in strengthening national health programs, and to develop and transfer appropriate health technology, information, and standards.
WHO Headquarters
Website: www.who.int

See also Baby-Friendly Hospital Initiative (BFHI); Ten Steps to Successful Breastfeeding

➤ X-RAY, DIAGNOSTIC

DEFINITION X-ray is a type of high energy radiation. In low doses, X-rays are used to diagnose diseases by making pictures of the inside of the body. Diagnostic X-rays have no effect on lactation.

ASSESSMENT

ROUTINE CARE NEEDED?
Are any of the following present?
Mother requires diagnostic X-ray.

IF YES, *Call lactation care provider now.*

See also Medication resources (inside back cover); Radioactive agents

➤ YEAST INFECTION

DEFINITION Overgrowth of *Candida albicans* or other common fungi.

ASK ABOUT

Onset.
Medications taken in the past month.

ASSESSMENT

PROMPT CARE NEEDED?

Are any of the following present?

Sharp, itching, persistent nipple pain (during as well as between feedings).
Flaky, shiny, or itchy skin on the nipple surface.
Presence of white patches in the infant's mouth.
A baby with yeast infection in the diaper area.

IF YES, *Call the mother's and baby's healthcare providers today.*

ROUTINE CARE NEEDED?

Are any of the following present?

Nipple pain during feeding.

IF YES, *Call lactation care provider today.*

SELF-CARE INFORMATION

Finish all medications prescribed.

If administering nystatin suspension to the infant, pour a dose into a clean cup or spoon. Half of the dose should be used for each side of the mouth. Suspension may be applied with a cotton swab. A clean swab should be used for each application. Take care not to introduce used swabs into the bottle of suspension.

If the baby uses artificial nipples, pacifiers, etc., these should be boiled at least daily and replaced after completion of yeast treatment.

The mother and baby should be treated simultaneously regardless of which one is symptomatic.

IMPORTANT CONDITIONS TO REPORT

Persistent symptoms after completion of a course of treatment.

Recurrent symptoms.

NOTES

Symptoms of yeast infection of the breast include red, shiny-looking skin on the nipple or areola, flaky skin, and sharp, itching pain that persists between feedings. Infant symptoms of yeast overgrowth or thrush include white patches of growth on the inner buccal surface (cheek) or tongue and occasionally pain on latch. Infants may also have diaper area yeast overgrowth.

Candida overgrowth may follow or increase after antibiotic treatment.

Recommended treatment for candidiasis is a topical antifungal agent.

If symptoms are not relieved by topical treatment, feeding evaluation should occur to rule out positioning or attachment problems contributing to pain.

The healthcare provider's evaluation should rule out other conditions resulting in redness and pain, including **eczema**, reaction to surface allergens, trauma, **Raynaud's phenomenon**, concomitant bacteria, and infection.

Subsequent treatment with oral antifungal agents may resolve symptoms.

Lactation evaluation should rule out contributing problems with latch or distortion of the nipple in the baby's mouth.

See also Nipple pain; Candidiasis; Thrush

Appendix A

Sample Triage Documentation Form

SAMPLE INTAKE FORM

DATE ___/___/___   TIME: _____   LC: _____

MOTHER:
Name _____
Telephone _____
Address _____
_____
Referred by _____
Significant Hx _____
OB/CNM _____

INFANT(S):
Name(s) _____
DOB _____ Birthweight _____
Age today _____
Recent weight _____ on _____
Significant Hx _____
_____
Ped/FP _____

Delivered at   _____   Hospital ____ Home
                _____   Birth Center

CALLED CONCERNING:
_____
_____
_____

SUGGESTIONS GIVEN:
_____
_____
_____

DISPOSITION RECOMMENDED:

☐ **Emergent Medical:** Referred to _____

☐ **Prompt Medical:** Referred to ____ Pediatrician   ____ Obstetrician
   ____ Family Practitioner   ____ Other (indicate) _____

☐ **Emergent/Prompt Lactation Care:** ____ Consult Appt Sched for ___ / ___ @ ___
   ☐ Referral to other LC _____

☐ **Routine:** ☐ Mother to call back as needed   ☐ Consult Appt Suggested
   ☐ Referred to _____

Follow-up call planned for ___ / ___ @ ___
   Who will call? ☐ Call Center Staff or ☐ Mother ☐ Information pack sent

Length of call: ____ min.